# Clinical Behavioral Pediatrics
## (PGPS-125)

# Pergamon Titles of Related Interest

**DiMatteo/DiNicola** ACHIEVING PATIENT COMPLIANCE:
The Psychology of the Medical Practitioner's Role
**Karoly/Steffen/O'Grady** CHILD HEALTH PSYCHOLOGY:
Concepts and Issues
**Morris/Kratochwill** PRACTICE OF THERAPY WITH CHILDREN:
A Textbook of Methods
**Morris/Kratochwill** TREATING CHILDREN'S FEARS AND PHOBIAS:
A Behavioral Approach
**Rachman** CONTRIBUTIONS TO MEDICAL PSYCHOLOGY,
Volumes 1 and 2
**Schwartz/Johnson** PSYCHOPATHOLOGY OF CHILDHOOD:
A Clinical-Experimental Approach

# Related Journals*

ANALYSIS AND INTERVENTION IN DEVELOPMENTAL DISABILITIES
APPLIED RESEARCH IN MENTAL RETARDATION
JOURNAL OF CHILD PSYCHOLOGY & PSYCHIATRY
JOURNAL OF PSYCHOSOMATIC RESEARCH
SOCIAL SCIENCE & MEDICINE

**\*Free specimen copies available upon request.**

PERGAMON GENERAL PSYCHOLOGY SERIES
EDITORS
Arnold P. Goldstein, *Syracuse University*
Leonard Krasner, *SUNY at Stony Brook*

# Clinical Behavioral Pediatrics
## An Interdisciplinary
## Biobehavioral Approach

## James W. Varni
*Orthopaedic Hospital and University of
Southern California School of Medicine*

## Pergamon Press

New York   Oxford   Toronto   Sydney   Paris   Frankfurt

Pergamon Press Offices:

**U.S.A.**            Pergamon Press Inc., Maxwell House, Fairview Park,
                     Elmsford, New York 10523, U.S.A.

**U.K.**             Pergamon Press Ltd., Headington Hill Hall,
                     Oxford OX3 0BW, England

**CANADA**           Pergamon Press Canada Ltd., Suite 104, 150 Consumers Road,
                     Willowdale, Ontario M2J 1P9, Canada

**AUSTRALIA**        Pergamon Press (Aust.) Pty. Ltd., P.O. Box 544,
                     Potts Point, NSW 2011, Australia

**FRANCE**           Pergamon Press SARL, 24 rue des Ecoles,
                     75240 Paris, Cedex 05, France

**FEDERAL REPUBLIC**  Pergamon Press GmbH, Hammerweg 6,
**OF GERMANY**        D-6242 Kronberg-Taunus, Federal Republic of Germany

**Copyright © 1983 Pergamon Press Inc.**

**Library of Congress Cataloging in Publication Data**

Varni, James W., 1948-
    Clinical behavioral pediatrics.

    (Pergamon general psychology series)
    Includes indexes.
    1. Pediatrics--Psychological aspects. 2. Sick
children--Psychology. I. Title. II. Series. [DNLM:
1. Child behavior. 2. Child behavior disorders.
3. Pediatrics. 4. Behavioral medicine. WS 100 V321c]
RJ47.5.V37   1983   618.92'0001'9   83-2310
ISBN 0-08-027172-3

*Printed in the United States of America*

*To My Family*

*To The Children*

# Contents

## Part V: BEHAVIORAL AND PSYCHOSOCIAL PROBLEMS

# Preface

During the past several years, the clinical research literature has indicated that the comprehensive care of children with physical handicaps and chronic diseases, as well as the prevention of some chronic diseases, might be significantly influenced by the integration of biobehavioral techniques into ongoing interdisciplinary treatment. This emerging approach, termed *Behavioral Pediatrics*, represents an interdisciplinary and comprehensive field of study which is increasingly receiving clinical attention and application. While the edited text by Russo and Varni, *Behavioral Pediatrics: Research and Practice*, provided the first detailed review of the clinical research literature, the need for a clinical text became apparent.

This clinical text represents the first attempt to provide the clinician and advanced student with an overview of the empirically derived biobehavioral techniques currently utilized in the field of Behavioral Pediatrics. An effort has been made to reference enough of the relevant representative research literature so as to allow the reader to further pursue studies of specific interest. However, at the same time an attempt has been made to provide enough clinical detail to give the reader a working knowledge of the clinical status of the field. Thus, the approach has not been to provide a comprehensive review of the research literature nor a clinical "cookbook," but rather to select published papers with empirical findings which typify the currently generally accepted biobehavioral techniques representing Clinical Behavioral Pediatrics and to describe a number of these studies in sufficient detail so as to give the reader a greater feel for the procedures employed in these studies. Current review papers are often cited so that the interested reader may have access to further studies from the research literature not specifically described in the text.

This clinical text is intended for clinicians and students in pediatric medicine, nursing, behavioral sciences, physical therapy, and other allied health professions, and for clinical researchers who would like an overview of areas not within their area of expertise.

A number of individuals and institutions have made this text possible, both through their financial and colleagual support. Special thanks go to Orthopaedic Hospital, the Crippled Children's Guild, and the Footlighters, Inc., who generously provided the major funding for the preparation of the manuscript through the Behavioral Pediatrics Program at Orthopaedic Hospital. Special thanks go to Ann Squibb Benya, who diligently translated my handwriting into typewritten form, and to Lisa Alexander, who also aided in the manuscript preparation.

Finally, my sincerest appreciation goes to Shelby L. Dietrich, M.D., Co-Director of the Behavioral Pediatrics Program and Assistant Vice President for Medical Affairs at Orthopaedic Hospital, who, as a highly experienced pediatrician and internationally recognized innovator in hemophilia comprehensive team care through her directorship of the Hemophilia Comprehensive Care Center has consistently proven to be a most valued and reliable colleague and trusted friend.

# REFERENCE

Russo, D.C., & Varni, J.W. (Eds.), *Behavioral Pediatrics: Research and Practice*. New York: Plenum Press, 1982.

# Clinical Behavioral Pediatrics
## (PGPS-125)

# Part I

## Basic Orientation and Methodology

# 1
# Behavioral Pediatrics: Historical Perspective and Current Definition

Current trends in research and clinical practice suggest that the role of health-related behaviors in the prevention, development, maintenance, and/or exacerbation of disease is increasingly being recognized in pediatrics. With advances in biomedical science, technology, sanitation, and pharmacology, much of the threat of acute or infectious diseases such as cholera, typhus, and smallpox has been reduced or eliminated. The pediatric clinician's time is no longer consumed with treating rickets, scurvy, poliomyelitis, measles, mumps, and diphtheria. As acute and infectious diseases have become more effectively prevented or treated, a growing emphasis of current pediatric practice has evolved toward the prevention and management of chronic disorders.

Medical treatment of chronic disorders is often aimed at symptom reduction and the arrest of pathology, since the pathogenesis of many chronic conditions is not yet well understood or may not yet be curable given current biomedical knowledge and techniques. As stated by Meenan et al. (1981), "Barring significant basic research breakthroughs, we are probably at a point of diminishing returns in the treatment of most chronic disorders, since we have reached the stage where additional medical or surgical therapy is apt to produce progressively smaller improvements in individual health status [pg. 544]." Consequently, pediatric practice is gradually moving from a focus on acute, infectious diseases where medical treatment is of singular importance to chronic diseases, disorders, and problems in which somatic factors represent only one component of comprehensive care (Varni & Russo, 1980).

With this shift toward disorders where chronic symptomatic management rather than cure represents a primary focus of treatment, issues such as health-related behaviors, coping, life quality, and optimal functional independence become key concerns. Even with the advances in biomedical technology and the costliness of care, little or no improvement in average longevity has been derived in the past decade (Culliton, 1978). However, through changes in health-related behaviors and lifestyle, the average age of initial infirmity may be raised, resulting in a more rectangular morbidity curve and extended vigor farther into a fixed life span (Fries, 1980). Such emerging trends clearly signal the potential contribution of the biobehavioral sciences to medicine (Fabrega & Van Egeren, 1976; Hamburg & Brown, 1978) in prevention, chronic care, and rehabilitation (Cataldo, Russo, Bird, & Varni, 1980; Russo & Varni, 1982).

With this emphasis on the interrelationship between health-related behaviors and disease prevention and management, then the child and his family become increasingly more instrumental in the health care system. Issues concerned with adherence to therapeutic regimens, parent-child interactions, and clinician-parent-child interactions become highly relevant, particularly in complex and long-term interventions. Simply prescribing a medication or exercise regimen is not a sufficient condition to assure the implementation of the regimen; behavioral and psychosocial factors may prevent or impede the therapy process. Attention to the biomedical, psychological, and social dimensions inherent in disease prevention and management requires integrated input from the various disciplines specializing in these areas.

## INTERDISCIPLINARY HEALTH TEAM MODEL

The concept and development of the health team model of care has been proposed as the means by which prevention, diagnosis, treatment, habilitation, and rehabilitation might be provided in a coordinated, comprehensive manner by specialists representing several disciplines (see Halstead, 1976, for review). The comprehensive care of the patient within the health team model requires the consideration of the biomedical, biobehavioral, and psychosocial factors which might influence the patient's health status. Within this model, the pediatric patient and the parents of the child are encouraged to develop greater responsibility for the prevention of illness, the maintenance of health, and the management of chronic problems. Particularly in pediatric chronic disorders where the medical treatment is but one component of comprehensive care, the child's and parent's active involvement in the day-to-day management, habilitation, and rehabilitation of the chronic condition is essential. Whereas in acute disorders a specific medication regimen might cure the illness in a relatively short time period, long-term patient and parent *active* involvement is requisite in pediatric chronic disease and disability management.

The ideal format for the health team model involves an interdisciplinary, integrated approach to patient care (Rothberg, 1981). The difference between an interdisciplinary versus a multidisciplinary approach is an essential concept in optimal health care delivery. Melvin (1980) has clearly defined both approaches. Multidisciplinary refers to activities involving the efforts of professionals from a number of disciplines approaching the patient primarily through an uncoordinated discipline-specific fashion. This approach requires that each professional only know the skills specific to his/her own discipline. In contrast, the interdisciplinary approach requires that physicians, nurses, physical therapists, occupational therapists, medical social workers, psychologists, and other allied health care professionals have a working knowledge of the other team members' skills and specialties. Thus, the interdisciplinary approach is synergistic, integrating the knowledge and skills from the various disciplines into a coordinated plan for patient care.

The interdisciplinary health team model provides the optimal format for the clinical application of behavioral pediatrics. Within this format, the biomedical, biobehavioral, and psychosocial dimensions of the pediatric patient can be considered and subsequently coordinated into a multidimensional and comprehensive health care strategy. This "holistic" approach in many ways challenges the current prevailing biomedical model. The historical development of the biomedical model and "mind-body dualism" provides insight into traditional medical practice, as well as a rationale for the *return* to a holistic view of the patient. The following sections delineate the historical trends which have resulted in the emerging role of clinical behavioral pediatrics in current pediatric comprehensive health care.

## MIND-BODY DUALISM

The current prevailing model of disease is biomedical, with its basis in molecular biology (Engel, 1977). This biomedical model assumes that disease may be completely accounted for by deviations from the norm of somatic parameters, with minimal consideration for biobehavioral and psychosocial variables. This biomedical model is thus characterized by both the reductionistic philosophy that complex phenomena may be explained by a single primary principle and by mind-body dualism which assumes a separation between the mental and somatic processes. As clearly delineated by Engel (1977), this position has previously restricted research advances in the understanding of disease etiology and treatment.

When placed within a historical perspective, the current model of mind-body dualism appears even more tenuous. Both ancient and Renaissance medicine may be characterized as holistic or psychophysiological approaches, consisting of the concept of a spirit or soul with both psychological and physiological properties (McMahon, 1976). Premodern physicians implicated the soul's faculty of imagination in the etiology and cure of disease: images aroused emotions, which set up hormonal imbalances. Digestion and other vital functions were then disturbed, resulting in pathophysiological disorders. This medical tradition ended in the late seventeenth century when the Cartesian dualism of mind and body became the basis of the prevailing medical theory (McMahon & Hastrup, 1980). By redefining the soul or spirit as "immaterial substance" or "mind," Descartes (1596-1659) removed the role of imagination and cognitive functions from the disease process. Imagination and emotional dimensions were redefined as causally ineffective in influencing somatic processes, with reductionistic and mechanistic physiopathology subsequently emerging as the dominant model. Thus, while medicine was holistic in the pre-Cartesian era, the post-Cartesian dualistic era assumed that a holistic psychophysiological model was both a biological and logical impossibility.

The evolution of this reductionistic, dualistic biomedical model in the Western world as defined by Descartes is clearly described by Engel (1977). He cites the concession by the dominant Christian orthodoxy in Europe during the Middle Ages to allow dissection of the human body only by keeping within the church's view that the body was merely a temporary medium for the soul. The church's permission to study the human body depended on a tacit agreement on the dualism of mind (soul) and body. Engel (1977) further states that "this compact may be considered largely responsible for the anatomical and structural base upon which scientific Western medicine eventually was to be built [pg. 131]." Thus, the reductionistic biomedical model, rather than historically derived from scientific data and the empirical approach, originated through religious philosophy and dogma.

In order to accommodate the clinical findings that a reductionistic and mechanistic physiopathological model was in fact an insufficient explanation of disease processes, the diagnostic category known as *psychosomatic* disorders began to emerge (McMahon & Hastrup, 1980). However, to be consistent with the prevailing biomedical model, these psychosomatic disorders were categorized as *nervous* conditions, purely psychological in nature, completely dissociated from physiological processes, and with no physical basis. This accommodation to the biomedical model eventually evolved into the field of psychosomatic medicine.

## PSYCHOSOMATIC MEDICINE

Historically, psychosomatic medicine began to emerge as a recognized discipline in the 1920s. For the first 30 years, the field was characterized by two major schools of thought, the psychodynamic and the psychophysiological perspectives (Lipowski, 1977). The psychodynamic viewpoint was directly influenced by psychoanalytic theory and methods, as exemplified by Alexander's specificity theory, which linked specific unresolved unconscious conflicts causally with specific somatic disorders in the presence of specific, constitutional vulnerability (Alexander, 1950). As theorized by Alexander, these unresolved unconscious conflicts lead to prolonged specific autonomic arousal, representing the somatic concomitant of repressed and suppressed affects.

These specific psychological conflicts were proposed to serve a major and decisive role in the etiology and development of such disorders as rheumatoid arthritis, bronchial asthma, neurodermatitis, peptic ulcer, essential hypertension, and ulcerative colitis. This theoretical framework of psychosomatic diseases subsequently prompted treatment through psychoanalysis or long-term psychotherapy based primarily on recollections, memories, and past associations. This retrospective approach essentially ignored proximal causation and failed to account for such contributory factors as genetic, infectious, immunologic, and traumatic variables in the pathogenesis of disease (Leigh & Reiser, 1977). By the 1950s, the psychodynamic perspective was characterized by widespread disenchantment because of the consistent lack of empirical validation of this approach's tenets (Leigh & Reiser, 1977; Lipowski, 1977).

Concurrently, Wolff and his associates developed the psychophysiological perspective, focusing on conscious psychological processes and their relationship to peripheral physiological changes, emphasizing a theory of psychological stress and symbolic processes as applied to a myriad of somatic diseases (Wolff, 1953). These investigators theorized adaptive, defensive psychophysiological patterns that might result in subsequent tissue damage and disease if prolonged. This perspective continues to have a decisive influence on psychosomatic theory (Lipowski, 1977).

Current psychosomatic theory has been influenced by developments in information and general systems theory, findings on the multicausality of somatic functions and behavior, theories of psychophysiological response specificity and activation, principles of operant conditioning and self-regulation of visceral functions, and concepts of psychosocial stress, cognitive processes, individual susceptibility to disease, and the process of coping (see Lipowski, 1977, for review). Thus, the conceptual model of psychosomatic medicine has moved from a linear, multiple factor causal chain paradigm to a nonlinear, interactional field or systems model (Leigh & Reiser, 1977). In this model, an individual's constitution results from the interplay between genetic factors and early experience, with ongoing development into adulthood influenced by multiple biological and psychosocial variables. Thus, a social and ecological dimension has been added to the previous two-dimensional psychosomatic theory that focused on psychophysiological interactions but disregarded the social milieu. This multidimensional conceptualization has led to a biopsychosocial model of health and disease which transcends psychosomatic theory and provides a general scheme for both adaptive and nonadaptive functioning (Engel, 1977). This broader biopsychosocial model will be discussed in detail in the next section.

A core postulation of current psychosomatic theory proposes that symbolic processes such as conscious and unconscious perceptions, thought, imagery, and memories, subserved by the cerebral structures and functions, influence organismic responding at all levels of functioning, even cellular mechanisms (Lipowski, 1977). These symbolic processes are themselves affected by environmental and biological factors that impinge on cerebral functions. An additional core postulation of current psychosomatic theory points to the role of psychological and physiological tendencies exemplified by specific patterns of cognitive, emotional, behavioral, and physiological responding to specific multidimensional stimuli. Lipowski (1977) has neatly organized these postulations into three major conceptual categories reflecting current psychosomatic theory: psychosocial stress, psychophysiological response specificity, and individual susceptibility to disease.

The concept of psychosocial stress suggests that social situations and psychological states may disturb individual homeostasis, subsequently eliciting physiological changes. It is postulated that the more disturbing a psychosocial stress situation or event, the higher the probability that physiological dysfunction will occur. Any type of life change, including change of residence, divorce of parents, death of a parent, and birth of a sibling, has been postulated to contribute to a psychosocial stress state which may lead to physiological dysfunction (Coddington, 1972a, 1972b; Holmes & Rahe, 1967). As theorized, a clustering of life events or situations, including ongoing family and parent-child dysfunctional interactional patterns (Minuchin, Baker, Rosman, Liebman, Milman, & Todd, 1975), may achieve etiologic significance as a necessary but not sufficient cause of illness, accounting in part for the time of onset of disease (Holmes & Rahe, 1967). This theory has been particularly cited when the medical analysis of onset cause is unclear, such as in juvenile rheumatoid arthritis (Rimon, Belmaker, & Ebstein, 1977) and bronchial asthma (Pinkerton, 1967). However, consistent empirical validation continues to be absent for this particular theoretical framework.

The psychophysiological specificity concept refers to the probability that particular individuals will respond to certain stimulus events and situations with a predictable set of psychological and physiological changes. Finally, the individual susceptibility to disease concept actually encompasses aspects of the prior two concepts, postulating that psychological and social factors contribute to morbidity and the etiology of disease in vulnerable individuals and organ systems. While these three concepts of current psychosomatic theory may have heuristic value, without empirical validation they will remain as interesting theoretical formulations of questionable practical value.

## A BIOPSYCHOSOCIAL MODEL

Engel (1977, 1980) has cogently provided the rationale for a revision and expansion of the existing perspectives of both the biomedical model and psychosomatic medicine. Stating that the term *psychosomatic* perpetuates the concept of Cartesian mind-body dualism, Engel further faults the prevailing biomedical model in general medical practice for its dogmatic adherence to a molecular biology perspective. Engel asserts that the reductionistic biomedical model assumes that biochemical and neurophysiological parameters completely account for any deviations from the norm of measurable biological variables evident in a disease process, essentially excluding the social, psychological, and behavioral dimensions of illness. Engel clearly provides the rationale for a more comprehensive holistic biopsychosocial model, which considers the complex interrelationships between the patient, his social environment, the health care provider, and the overall health care delivery system. For example, psychophysiological responses to social events or situations may interact with existing somatic factors to alter the susceptibility to disease and influence its time of onset, severity, course, and the ultimate communication of symptoms by the patient to the health care system. Further, the clinician's ability to influence and modify the patient's behavior in directions concordant with treatment and health needs requires an understanding of the behavioral and psychosocial dimensions. The tremendous variability observed in patients' responses to disease and subsequent treatment, as well as adherence to therapeutic regimens, cannot be adequately explained through the biochemical dimension alone; the behavioral and psychosocial context intimately determine the process and outcome of disease and treatment (Fabrega & Van Egeren, 1976).

Fabrega and Van Egeren (1976) view the biopsychosocial paradigm from a systems perspective made up of connected and hierarchical subsystems, with changes in any subsystem propagating across the various levels. Thus, psychosocial events may produce or be associated with physiological changes that are transmitted "downwards" through various biochemical and molecular changes; conversely, biochemical and molecular changes may be transmitted "upwards" through physiological subsystems, to cognitive processes, and ultimately to role behaviors in the social ecosystem. Therefore, reciprocal relationships exist among a myriad of subsystems, whereby the health-related behaviors of an individual (e.g., eating, exercising, smoking patterns) may influence the etiology and process of disease, while a disease process may influence what an individual can do, how she feels, how she views herself, and what her functional status is (e.g., sleeping, bathing, grooming, mobility, school or work behaviors).

Finally, a related series of papers have examined the biopsychosocial perspective by considering how health and illness affect the individual's capacity to carry out normal social obligations, as well as the individual's interpretation and reporting of somatic sensations. In this regard, Kasl and Cobb (1966a, 1966b) defined three aspects of health-related behaviors:

1. Health behavior is any activity undertaken by an individual, who perceives himself as healthy, for the purpose of preventing disease or detecting it in an asymptomatic stage;

2. Illness behavior is any activity undertaken by an individual who feels ill to obtain a diagnosis and an appropriate treatment;
3. Sick-role behavior is the activity undertaken by an individual who considers himself ill (not just feels ill) in order to get well.

In this paradigm, health behavior includes appropriate eating, exercise, and stress-reduction behaviors. Sick-role behavior includes not only receiving treatment from appropriate therapists, but a whole range of dependent behaviors that may lead to some degree of neglect of the individual's typical activities of daily living and a reduction in functional status. Illness behavior includes complaining about and reporting of symptoms to relatives, friends, and health care providers. It has been proposed that this reporting and experiencing of symptoms may be in part a learned pattern, involving a focusing on internal feeling states, attending to and interpreting of bodily sensations, and a high level of self-awareness influenced by childhood illness, parental behavior, and life stresses (Campbell, 1978; Mechanic, 1964, 1972, 1979, 1980; Pennebaker & Skelton, 1978; Tessler & Mechanic, 1978). This perspective would suggest an extrasensitivity to and excessive complaining of bodily sensations as a result of situational psychosocial stress or prior learning experiences.

In the next section, it will be evident that these various perspectives on the biopsychosocial model have influenced the formation and definition of the behavioral medicine field. However, the hallmark of behavioral medicine, in contrast to the previously described theoretical models, is its primary emphasis on the *systematic empirical clinical* approach.

## BEHAVIORAL MEDICINE

Behavioral medicine represents a relatively recent and emerging field of inquiry in health care, concerned with the contributory role of biobehavioral factors to health status, the development of treatment strategies in the prevention, treatment, and rehabilitation of disease and disability, and finally, with the enhancement of patient care, hospital services, and health care delivery (Varni & Russo, 1980). While in the past, behavioral approaches have been applied to a myriad of "psychiatric" disorders such as obsessive-compulsive neurosis, depression, and phobias (see Leitenberg, 1976, for review), the field of behavioral medicine represents an independent investigative area. Through the principles derived from these previous research efforts with other clinical populations and problems, the techniques of cognitive-behavior therapy, behavior modification, and biofeedback are now being systematically applied and evaluated as a component in the comprehensive and multidisciplinary management of medical disorders. Work in behavioral medicine is based on the assumption that through the discovery of causal links between disease and health-related behaviors which may contribute to disease development, maintenance, and/or exacerbation, treatments can be developed that modify health-related behaviors, resulting in improved health care and health status.

In 1978, the Academy of Behavioral Medicine Research (Institute of Medicine, National Academy of Sciences) proposed a working definition of behavioral medicine, as a refinement of the 1977 Yale Conference on Behavioral Medicine initial definition (Schwartz & Weiss, 1978), as follows:

> Behavioral medicine is the interdisciplinary field concerned with the development and integration of behavioral and biomedical science knowledge and techniques relevant to the understanding of health and illness and the application of this knowledge and those techniques to prevention, diagnosis, treatment and rehabilitation.

In essence, this working definition proposes a combining of perspectives, strengths, and talents in a truly comprehensive research and clinical effort. Perhaps most salient, behavioral medicine is considered an interdisciplinary empirical endeavor, with its contributions provided within the framework of the existing disciplines of medicine, the allied health professions, and the behavioral sciences. In the long run and following the empirical tradition of previous behavioral applications, behavioral medicine will not be judged on this preliminary definition, but rather on the basis of its practical accomplishments and value to the health care sector.

Current behavioral medicine research and practice may be characterized by three general dimensions (Varni & Russo, 1980):

1. *Focus on Biobehaviors.* This includes health-related behaviors such as eating and exercise patterns, as well as biochemical and neurophysiological functions (e.g., serum medication levels, blood pressure, electromyogram).
2. *Reliance on Measurement.* An emphasis on reliable and valid assessment and measurement instruments is the hallmark of the empirical tradition of behavioral medicine, with the interrelationships between these biobehavioral measures potentially providing clues to the mechanisms of disease.
3. *Relationship between Biobehaviors and Illness.* Understanding the social and physical context of the patient's biobehaviors may help to better empirically elucidate the potential causal relationships between health-related behaviors and the prevention, development, maintenance, and exacerbation of disease such as the potential synergistic effects of inappropriate eating, diet, and exercise patterns and stress on the development and exacerbation of cardiovascular disease.

These three dimensions additionally characterize the field of behavioral pediatrics and will be discussed in detail in Chapter 3.

# BEHAVIORAL PEDIATRICS

In delineating the nature and scope of behavioral pediatrics, it must be recognized that not only is the term not new, but the field has been described in the past by a number of different terms (e.g., developmental, biosocial, or psychosocial pediatrics). Varni and Dietrich (1981) recently traced the origins of this movement in pediatric medicine, indicating that behavioral pediatrics is an emerging and rapidly evolving field of clinical practice and research investigation, currently undergoing a major reconceptualization and redefinition. Within pediatric medicine, the historical focus of behavioral pediatrics has been on the biosocial development and learning difficulties of children and adolescents (Friedman, 1970, 1975; Richmond, 1975), with a primary emphasis on the identification of behavioral and psychosocial adjustment problems and developmental deficits or disabilities as seen by the practicing pediatrician (Brown, 1979; Cullen, 1976; Dworkin, Shonkoff, Leviton, & Levine, 1979; Goldberg, Regier, McInerny, Pless, & Roghmann, 1979; McClelland, Staples, Weisberg, & Berger, 1972; Prazar & Charney, 1980; Starfield, Gross, Wood et al., 1980; Toister & Worley, 1976; Yancy, 1975). However, as a result of recent research and clinical practice, behavioral pediatrics has been reconceptualized and subsequently has emerged as a more comprehensive and multidisciplinary endeavor (Cataldo, 1982; Russo & Varni, 1982; Varni & Dietrich, 1981).

Varni and Dietrich (1981) have proposed an operational definition of behavioral pediatrics reflective of the evolving state of the field, as well as clarified its distinction from related fields. They distinguished it from pediatric psychology by its multidisciplinary approach and from child behavior therapy by its primary focus on medical problems and medical settings. They further distinguished behavioral pediatrics from behavioral medicine given the unique considerations of age, development, and parent-child interactions evident in the child and adolescent populations. These distinctions will most likely become clearer as the field further develops within multidisciplinary medical environments.

In order to establish a comprehensive biobehavioral model for research and clinical practice in behavioral pediatrics, the definition of the field must reflect the specific collaboration of behavioral-medical methods. As specified by Russo and Varni (1982), a definition of behavioral pediatrics should contain the following aspects:

• interdisciplinary in nature
• concerned with the management of acute and chronic disorders, related symptoms, parent training, child self-regulation training, and health staff training
• firmly rooted in the empirical methodologies of its contributing sciences and disciplines

- concerned with long-term care, acute intervention, and prevention
- assessment and treatment that are data-based, concerned with process and outcome measures, and occur with collaborative input and decision-making
- interest in both ambulatory settings and inpatient care environments
- concerned with disease mechanisms and biochemical, physiological and biobehavioral interrelationships

A definition derived from these various parameters would provide the basis for the development of the field of behavioral pediatrics that would best combine the talents of the multiple disciplines involved and produce the most beneficial research and practice. Taking into consideration these various factors, Varni and Dietrich (1981) proposed the following operational definition:

Behavioral pediatrics represents the interdisciplinary integration between biobehavioral science and pediatric medicine, with emphasis on multidimensional and comprehensive diagnosis, prevention, treatment, and rehabilitation of physical disease and disabilities in children and adolescents [pg. 5].

This operational definition of the field provides a comprehensive and multidisciplinary biobehavioral context for research and clinical practice in behavioral pediatrics and should simultaneously serve to focus and integrate the chapters that follow.

## REFERENCES

Alexander, F.G. *Psychosomatic Medicine: Its Principles and Applications.* New York: Norton, 1950.

Brown, G.W. Developmental and behavioral pediatrics: A realistic challenge? *Journal of Developmental and Behavioral Pediatrics,* 1979, **1**, 1–8.

Campbell, J.D. The child in the sick role: Contributions of age, sex, parental status, and parental values. *Journal of Health and Social Behavior,* 1978, **19**, 35–51.

Cataldo, M.F. The scientific basis for a behavioral approach to pediatrics. *Pediatric Clinics of North America,* 1982, **19**, 415–423.

Cataldo, M.F., Russo, D.C., Bird, B.L., & Varni, J.W. Assessment and management of chronic disorders. In J.M. Ferguson & C.B. Taylor (Eds.), *Comprehensive Handbook of Behavioral Medicine.* Vol 3: *Extended Applications and Issues.* New York: Spectrum Publications, 1980.

Coddington, R.D. The significance of life events as etiologic factors in the diseases of children: I. A survey of professional workers. *Journal of Psychosomatic Research,* 1972, **16**, 7–18. (a)

Coddington, R.D. The significance of life events as etiologic factors in the diseases of children: II. A study of a normal population. *Journal of Psychosomatic Research,* 1972, **16**, 205–213. (b)

Cullen, K.J. A six-year controlled trial of prevention of children's behavior disorders. *Journal of Pediatrics,* 1976, **88**, 662–666.

Culliton, B.J. Health care economics: The high cost of getting well. *Science,* 1978, **200**, 883–885.

Dworkin, P.H., Shonkoff, J.P., Leviton, A., & Levine, M.D. Training in developmental pediatrics: How practitioners perceive the gap. *American Journal of Diseases of Children,* 1979, **133**, 709–712.

14     Clinical Behavioral Pediatrics

Engel, G.L. The need for a new medical model: A challenge for biomedicine. *Science*, 1977, **196**, 129–136.
Engel, G.L. The clinical application of the biopsychosocial model. *American Journal of Psychiatry*, 1980, **137**, 535–544.
Fabrega, H., & Van Egeren, L. A behavioral framework for the study of human disease. *Annals of Internal Medicine*, 1976, **84**, 200–208.
Friedman, S.B. The challenge in behavioral pediatrics. *Journal of Pediatrics*, 1970, **77**, 172–173.
Friedman, S.B. Forward to symposium on behavioral pediatrics. *Pediatric Clinics of North America*, 1975, **22**, 515–516.
Fries, J.F. Aging, natural death, and the compression of morbidity. *New England Journal of Medicine*, 1980, **303**, 130–135.
Goldberg, I.D., Regier, D.A., McInerny, T.K., Pless, I.B., & Roghmann, K.J. The role of the pediatrician in the delivery of mental health services to children. *Pediatrics*, 1979, **63**, 898–909.
Halstead, L.S. Team care in chronic illness: A critical review of the literature of the past 25 years. *Archives of Physical Medicine and Rehabilitation*, 1976, **57**, 507–511.
Hamburg, D.A., & Brown, S.S. The science base and social context of health maintenance: An overview. *Science*, 1978, **200**, 847–849.
Holmes, T.H., & Rahe, R.H. The social readjustment rating scale. *Journal of Psychosomatic Research*, 1967, **11**, 213–218.
Kasl, S.V., & Cobb, S. Health behavior, illness behavior, and sick-role behavior: I. Health and illness behavior. *Archives of Environmental Health*, 1966, **12**, 246–266. (a)
Kasl, S.V., & Cobb, S. Health behaviors, illness behavior, and sick-role behavior: II. Sick-role behavior. *Archives of Environmental Health*, 1966, **12**, 531–541. (b)
Leigh, H., & Reiser, M.F. Major trends in psychosomatic medicine: The psychiatrist's evolving role in medicine. *Annals of Internal Medicine*, 1977, **87**, 233–239.
Leitenberg, H. (Ed.). *Handbook of Behavior Modification and Behavior Therapy.* Englewood Cliffs, N.J.: Prentice-Hall, 1976.
Lipowski, Z.J. Psychosomatic medicine in the seventies: An overview. *American Journal of Psychiatry*, 1977, **134**, 233–244.
McClelland, C.Q., Staples, W.I., Weisberg, I., & Bergen, M.E. The practitioner's role in behavioral pediatrics. *Journal of Pediatrics*, 1973, **82**, 325–331.
McMahon, C.E. The role of imagination in the disease process: Pre-Cartesian history. *Psychological Medicine*, 1976, **6**, 179–184.
McMahon, C.E., & Hastrup, J.L. The role of imagination in the disease process: Post-Cartesian history. *Journal of Behavioral Medicine*, 1980, **3**, 205–217.
Mechanic, D. The influence of mothers on their children's health attitudes and behavior. *Pediatrics*, 1964, **33**, 444–453.
Mechanic, D. Social psychologic factors affecting the presentation of bodily complaints. *New England Journal of Medicine*, 1972, **286**, 1132–1139.
Mechanic, D. Development of psychological distress among young adults. *Archives of General Psychiatry*, 1979, **36**, 1233–1239.
Mechanic, D. The experience and reporting of common physical complaints. *Journal of Health and Social Behavior*, 1980, **21**, 146–155.
Meenan, R.F., Yelin, E.H., Nevitt, M., & Epstein, W.V. The impact of chronic disease: A sociomedical profile of rheumatoid arthritis. *Arthritis and Rheumatism*, 1981, **24**, 544–549.
Melvin, J.L. Interdisciplinary and multidisciplinary activities and the ACRM. *Archives of Physical Medicine and Rehabilitation*, 1980, **61**, 379–380.
Minuchin, S., Baker, L., Rosman, B.L., Liebman, R., Milman, L., & Todd, T.C. A conceptual model of psychosomatic illness in children: Family organization and family therapy. *Archives of General Psychiatry*, 1975, **32**, 1031–1038.

Pennebaker, J.W., & Skelton, J.A. Psychological parameters of physical symptoms. *Personality and Social Psychology Bulletin*, 1978, **4**, 524–530.

Pinkerton, P. Correlating physiologic with psychodynamic data in the study and management of childhood asthma. *Journal of Psychosomatic Research*, 1967, **11**, 11–25.

Prazar, G., & Charney, E. Behavioral pediatrics in office practice. *Pediatric Annals*, 1980, **9**, 12–22.

Richmond, J.B. An idea whose time has arrived. *Pediatric Clinics of North America*, 1975, **22**, 517–523.

Rimon, R., Belmaker, R.H., & Ebstein, R. Psychosomatic aspects of juvenile rheumatoid arthritis. *Scandinavian Journal of Rheumatology*, 1977, **6**, 1–10.

Rothberg, J.S. The rehabilitation team: Future direction. *Archives of Physical Medicine and Rehabilitation*, 1981, **62**, 407–410.

Russo, D.C., & Varni, J.W. Behavioral Pediatrics. In D.C. Russo & J.W. Varni (Eds.), *Behavioral Pediatrics: Research and Practice*. New York: Plenum Press, 1982.

Schwartz, G.E., & Weiss, S.M. Yale conference on behavioral medicine: A proposed definition and statement of goals. *Journal of Behavioral Medicine*, 1978, **1**, 3–12.

Starfield, B., Gross, E., Wood, M., Pantell, R., Allen, C., Gordon, B., Moffatt, P., Drachman, R., & Katz, H. Psychosocial and psychosomatic diagnoses in primary care of children. *Pediatrics*, 1980, **66**, 159–167.

Toister, R.P., & Worley, L.M. Behavioral aspects of pediatric practice: A survey of practitioners. *Journal of Medical Education*, 1976, **51**, 1019–1020.

Tessler, R., & Mechanic, D. Psychological distress and perceived health status. *Journal of Health and Social Behavior*, 1978, **19**, 254–262.

Wolff, H.G. *Stress and Disease*. Springfield, Ill.: Charles C. Thomas, 1953.

Varni, J.W., & Dietrich, S.L. Behavioral pediatrics: Toward a reconceptualization. *Behavioral Medicine Update*, 1981, **3**, 5–7.

Varni, J.W., & Russo, D.C. Behavioral medicine approach to health care: Hemophilia as an exemplary model. In M. Jospe, J.E. Nieberding, & B.D. Cohen (Eds.), *Psychological Factors in Health Care*. Lexington, Mass.: Lexington Books, 1980.

Yancy, W.S. Behavioral pediatrics and the practicing pediatrician. *Pediatric Clinics of North America*, 1975, **22**, 685–694.

# 2

# Children's Cognitive Development, Conceptualizations of Illness, and Health Beliefs

It is generally well accepted in pediatric practice that the growing child progresses through a series of logical and systematic stages. An understanding of the relationship between this sequential development and the child's day-to-day functioning is essential in designing and implementing an individualized intervention program for children at different developmental levels. Children's behaviors that may appear random or irrational are actually quite lawful when viewed in the context of the child's particular cognitive developmental level. Environmental events alone are not necessarily what directly affect a child, but rather how she perceives these events, which is in large part a cognitive process. By being aware of cognitive development, certain regularities and patterns emerge in the way children at different ages structure their understanding of the world (Weis, 1975). Further, by comparing the ways that children assimilate their experience of illness to more general cognitive development may result in improved pediatric patient education and treatment programs.

Although physical developmental considerations are particularly important for the infant and very young child, they are a less pervasive aspect of the management of most children after approximately 3 to 4 years of age. However, for developmental disabilities such as cerebral palsy, physical developmental assessment is pertinent irrespective of chronological age. Since physical developmental assessment represents an integral component in the comprehensive management of developmental disabilities, it will be addressed in the chapter on neurology and neuromuscular disorders. Children's cognitive development, on the other hand, is a pervasive concern for all of pediatric practice, whether for the healthy or ill child, particularly as it relates to children's conceptualizations of health and illness.

# COGNITIVE DEVELOPMENT

Cognition refers to symbolic processes, such as mental images and language, which include the diverse areas of learning, thinking, concept formation, perception, memory, ideation, reasoning, and intelligence (Neisser, 1967). Thus, cognition encompasses all the higher mental processes involved in the acquisition, symbolic representation, memory, and use of information. Cognitive style is the term that describes how individuals conceptually organize their experiences with the environment or the way individuals filter and process information so that the environment takes on organized meaning and structure (Goldstein & Blackman, 1978). Cognitive assessment procedures that have been used include interviews, think-aloud protocols, self-report scales, thought listing, thought sampling, spontaneous private speech, and projective techniques (see Meichenbaum & Cameron, 1981, for review). Historically, two major views of cognitive development have received the greatest theoretical attention: structuralism and the mental processes perspective.

Structuralism is concerned with the significance of innate structures and organization, environment, and learning in cognitive development, viewing cognition as the storage of bits of information that become organized through complex associations with each other. On the other hand, rather than emphasizing structure and content, the mental processes perspective is concerned with such mental operations as remembering, judging, feeling, and comparing, that is, the dynamic aspects of cognitive representations rather than solely static content. Modern cognitive development theory actually encompasses both structuralism and the mental processes perspective, as well as new theories derived from linguistics, computer science, and information processing theory (Merluzzi, Rudy, & Glass, 1981). A major influence in the cognitive development of children has been Jean Piaget's "genetic epistemology" approach, an attempt to study the development of the cognitive processes involved in the development of intelligence, thinking, and knowledge in children. In fact, Piaget's influence has been so profound that the vast majority of current studies on cognitive development are within the Piagetian framework. Consequently, the present discussion of children's cognitive development will be stated from the Piagetian perspective given its generally widespread acceptability.

Piaget's cognitive developmental theory is referred to as genetic epistemology, since it is concerned with the ontogenesis of knowledge from infancy to maturity in terms of the dynamic mental processes and functions underlying cognition. This developmental epistemology has been described by Piaget as a naturalistic, biological model involving the interactions between the growing child and his physical and social environment (Piaget, 1970). Piaget considers the four primary factors of child development to be maturation, experience with the physical environment, experience with the social environment, and equilibration or self-regulation, which is necessary for the coordination and integration of the other three factors. Thus, Piagetian theory attributes cognitive development to the maturation of the nervous system, experiences with the physical world, socialization influences, and a general organismic tendency to seek organization and structure (self-regulation).

Piagetian theory may be further characterized as organized around three major unifying principles: (1) The interaction of children with their environment facilitates the process of adaptation; (2) Children progress through cognitive developmental stages, each characterized by qualitatively different cognitive abilities and structures; and (3) Children progress through early developmental stages characterized by illogical thought, with their thinking becoming increasingly capable of dealing with the environment in a logical and rational manner.

Piaget conceptualized cognitive development as a continuous process of organization and reorganization or structures. Piaget referred to operational activities that can be repeated and generalized as a scheme (plural, schemes). For example, the scheme is what is common in the actions of pushing an object with a stick or any other instrument. Schema (plural, schemata) is the term for the figurative aspects of thought, that is, the attempts to represent reality without attempting to transform it (e.g., imagery, perception, and memory). Thus, a schema is a simplified image (e.g., a map), whereas a scheme represents a general concept guiding action.

Schemata and schemes form the framework on which incoming sensory data can fit, but it is a framework that is continuously changing. Each new organization integrates the previous scheme or schema into itself, as well as adding more information to expand it (assimilation) or correcting and changing existing schemes and schemata (accommodation). Piaget uses the term *assimilation* to refer to the integration of external elements into the evolving structures of the child. However, if assimilation alone were involved, there would be no variations in children's structures, and cognitive development would not continue. Rather, cognition development consists of an equilibrium between assimilation and *accommodation,* which Piaget refers to as the modification of schemes or schemata by the elements that are assimilated. When assimilation predominates over accommodation, cognitive development evolves in an egocentric direction. When accommodation predominates over assimilation, rote imitation is the direction of cognitive development. It is the evolving equilibrium between assimilation and accommodation that is fundamental to normal cognitive development. Although this process is considered invariant and continuous, Piaget delineated the process into distinct periods: sensorimotor, preoperational, concrete operational, and formal operational. This is a stage or hierarchical theory of development in which each new period is characterized by new ways of thinking, interacting, and understanding, but within any period there may remain some earlier modes of cognitive development.

Piaget's observations of sequential cognitive development are one of his major contributions to the understanding of children's concept development. Piaget has designated the term *period* to delineate these major developmental milestones, with subdivisions of periods termed *stages*. However, these terms are often used interchangeably by others. A major characteristic of the theory of periods or stages is that they appear in a fixed order of succession since each one of them is necessary for the formation of each following stage. This cognitive developmental theory postulates that there is a general sequence and that the child must move through each lower period/stage before reaching the next one, with the exact timing of this progression varying across individuals and cultural groups. Typically, a given child does not represent a pure stage type. Rather, children will be more or less advanced in certain content areas than in others due to different experiences and the complexity of the particular content area of the stage. Thus, the succession of stages is in a sequential order involving a progressive integration of knowledge and learning experiences between the growing, emerging child and his environment. The major periods/stages are described below.

## Sensorimotor Period

The sensorimotor period spans the time from birth to approximately 2 years of age. During this period the child progresses from instinctual reflexive actions to initial symbolic activities, acquiring the basic knowledge about her physical and social environment that serves as the foundation for subsequent concept development. Through interacting with the environment, seeing, smelling, tasting, hearing, touching, and manipulating objects, the infant learns to attach meaning to sensory information, progressing from responses to the environment that are undifferentiated and nonpurposeful to sensorimotor actions that are organized and purposeful. In order to learn, the infant must be exposed to a variety of experiences with people and objects. Initially, the neonate does not differentiate herself from her mother, but after the first several months of life she views herself as a separate entity, perceiving the world now from a totally egocentric viewpoint. The concept of object permanence develops during the later stages of this period, with the ability to recognize objects and persons as having independent, continued existences. Additionally, the infant begins to develop an initial ability to understand the concepts of causality, imitation, play, and spatiality. At this point, the infant's learning continues on a more conceptual and symbolic level, serving as a basis for general cognitive and intellectual development.

## Preoperational Period

During the early stages of the preoperational period (2 to 7 years of age), the first primitive concepts formed by the child during the latter stages of the sensorimotor period further develop. These "preconcepts" are characterized by action, imagery, and concreteness rather than by cognitive or symbolic representation. While object identity and permanence are present, their stability fluctuates with various environmental changes in which the object appears. According to Piaget (1970), prelogical thinking is typical of children during most of this period, resulting in explanations accounting for cause-effect relationships in terms of the immediate spatial and/or temporal cues that dominate their experience. The view that when two events occur in succession, the first has caused the second is the characteristic cause-effect conceptualization during this period. This lack of logic in thinking is well illustrated by Piaget's classic experiments on conservation. For example, if presented with two identical tall, thin glasses filled with water, a 5-year-old child will acknowledge that they contain the same amounts. If the water from one glass is then poured into a shorter, wide glass and the child is asked if these two glasses still have the same amount to drink, she will likely say that the original glass has more because it is "taller" or that it has less because it is "thinner" than the short, wide glass. Thus, children during this period are misled by centering on a single perceptual aspect of their environment, with their conceptualizations characterized by experiential rather than logical thinking.

As language develops during this period, symbolic activities increase, such as fantasies and symbolic play with toys. The child shows animistic thinking, that is, that inanimate objects have motives and intentions. With further advances in language and memory, symbolic activities with toys, words, pictures, and magical thinking become more involved and complex.

## Concrete Operational Period

Concrete-logical thinking is first manifested by children between 7 and 11 years of age. During this period, reasoning processes and interactions with the environment begin to appear rational and organized. Logical thinking is characterized by integrated, organized mental representations, permitting the understanding of the relationship between simultaneously occurring events. The child begins to grasp the concepts of reversibility, classification, and number. However, reasoning is still limited to the concrete nature of situations in the environment, to observable events. Hypothetical or possible problems of future events are not yet completely within conceptual ability during the initial stages of this period. What is developed is the ability to understand that certain properties of objects such as quantity, number, volume, area, and weight remain invariant (conserved) despite transformations in their physical appearance.

The child is thus able to deal with two elements' properties or relations at the same time. For example, the child can now take into account both the height and width of a glass of colored liquid and recognize that when the liquid is poured into a differently shaped container, the changes in height and width of the container compensate each other so that the total quantity of liquid is conserved. Thus, the development of the concept of conservation enables the child to recognize that although things may change, some defining quality about them remains the same. Further, the development of the ability to classify during this period enables the child to abstract certain qualities of objects that will place them in general categories along such dimensions as color, size, shape, or function. Additionally, this ability to classify enables the child to understand the rules or norms that govern interpersonal and social behavior—that certain actions are classified as socially appropriate, and others are inappropriate.

During this period, children's cognitive processes evolve from primitive egocentric perceptions of events to more abstract and concretely logical reasoning. The child is now able to understand that others are different from him and have different experiences. He can understand that other people have thoughts, feelings, and intentions different from his own. Concrete operations are, therefore, instrumental in overcoming the primitive egocentrism of the preoperational period. Thus, a major developmental shift during this period is an accentuation of the differentiation between self and other, such that the child clearly distinguishes between what is internal and what is external to himself.

## Formal Operational Period

Between 12 to 15 years of age, children develop highly abstract thinking and reasoning abilities termed hypothetico-deductive, considered by Piaget to be the highest, most complex level of cognitive development. The adolescent can now imagine the possibilities inherent in a situation, develop hypotheses concerning what might occur, and make interpretations based on her reasoning, transcending concrete here and now experiences and beginning to think about thoughts and abstractions in and of themselves. After adolescence, cognitive development takes the form of a gradual increase in depth of understanding and a further development of the cognitive abilities first evident during the formal operational period.

# CONCEPTUALIZATIONS OF ILLNESS

Children's understanding and conceptualizations of the causes, prevention, and treatment of illness might be expected to follow a cognitive developmental progression that parallels shifts in cognitive processes in general, emerging from primitive egocentric and magical/fantasy viewpoints to increasingly more abstract thinking and logical reasoning perspectives. Although the development of children's concepts of causality has received considerable research attention in the general child development field, comparatively few studies exist that have investigated children's illness conceptualizations. Studies investigating children's concepts of illness may be most parsimoniously divided into those testing healthy children, and those testing ill and hospitalized children.

## Healthy Children's Concepts of Illness

In one of the earliest studies, Nagy (1951) studied 350 healthy children between 3 to 12 years of age, subsequently identifying four stages of the children's concepts of causality of illness. Children under 6 years of age tended to relate cause and effect to events contiguous in time, in terms of the immediate temporal ordering of the occurrence of each event (Event A causes Event B because Event A is followed immediately by Event B). At 6 to 7 years of age, the children stated that illness was caused by unspecified infection. The 8 to 10 year olds viewed illness as caused by microorganisms. By 11 to 12 years of age, the children recognized that different illnesses were caused by different organisms. Thus, Nagy found a conceptual trend with increasing chronological age from views of illness as caused by a single factor toward an understanding of illness as a complex and multifaceted process. Subsequent investigations have essentially supported the conceptual trends initially reported by Nagy (see Peters, 1978, for review). Two recent studies may be distinguished from these earlier studies by their advances in methodology and improved measurement instruments.

Bibace and Walsh (1980) studied three groups of healthy children, ages 4, 7, and 11, assumed to represent preoperational, concrete operational, and formal operational periods of cognitive development. A "Concept of Illness Protocol" was developed, containing 12 sets of questions examining the child's cognitive processes about a single factor. For example, children's concepts of common illnesses such as a cold, headache, measles, heart attack, and pain were examined, as well as their explanations of personal illnesses or illness of friends and relatives. The protocol was designed to evoke answers that would reveal the children's reasoning processes in contrast to simple yes/no responses.

The aim of the questions was to examine both the children's concepts of causality of illness as well as a definition of the illness. For example, the children were asked, "What is a cold/heart attack?" and "Why do people get sick/measles?" The authors assigned the responses to three general categories designated as prelogical, concrete logical, and formal logical. Within each of these three categories two subcategories were distinguished based on pilot investigations. This resulted in six types of explanations of illness that were developmentally ordered with chronological age. In addition, a category termed *incomprehension* was included to characterize the responses of the very youngest children whose answers appeared irrelevant to the questions asked.

## Prelogical Explanations of Illness

As designated by Piaget, prelogical thinking is typical of children between 2 to 7 years of age, with cause-effect relationships explained in terms of immediate temporal and/or spatial cues. Bibace and Walsh divided the children's prelogical explanations into phenomenism (Category 1) and contagion (Category 2).

*Phenomenism* was categorized as the most developmentally immature explanations of illness. Children during this stage explain the cause of illness as an external concrete phenomenon that may occur simultaneously with illness but is spatially remote. Further, the children do not perceive their actions as related to illness causality. For example, to the question, "How do people get colds?" the child during this stage might answer, "From the wind/trees/sun." To the question, "What makes the measles get better?" the child might answer, "God."

The more mature children in the prelogical period commonly explain illness in terms of a *contagion* that is proximate to, but not touching them. For example, when questioned about the causality of a cold, they might answer, "When someone else gets near you." During this stage, children perceive their contracting an illness as a result of a single activity on their part which is idiosyncratic and unrelated to the illness. Additionally, illness cure is perceived as an external singular event that is independent of the child's actions.

## Concrete Logical Explanations of Illness

During this period, children between approximately 7 to 11 years of age begin to clearly differentiate between themselves and external factors. Bibace and Walsh designated contamination (Category 3) and internalization (Category 4) as the types of explanations during this period.

Early in this period, illness causality is explained in terms of the body's surface coming into contact with a *contaminant* (e.g., germ, dirt) or in terms of the child's engaging in an activity that is morally contaminated or "bad." For example, a cold results when "Someone sneezes into your face, and you get it from the germs." Illness cure is perceived in terms of the child removing his body from contact with the contaminant or by stopping the morally "bad" activity.

The older children in this period explain illness in terms of *internalization;* even though the ultimate cause of the illness may be external, the illness is located inside the body through a process of internalization such as inhaling or swallowing a contaminant or harmful object. Illness cure is seen as the process of an external agent entering and affecting the body in a general and positive way, such as "drinking a medicine."

## Formal Logical Explanations of Illness

After approximately 11 or 12 years of age, children begin to conceptualize cause-effect relationships in a more logical and rational manner. Bibace and Walsh found that both the physiological (Category 5) and psychophysiological (Category 6) explanations of the children were characterized by the greatest amount of differentiation between the external and internal world, such that the source of the illness may be located within the body even though an external cause is identified.

In the *physiologic* stage, children perceive the immediate cause of illness as primarily the nonfunctioning or malfunctioning of an internal body part or body process, explained in a step-by-step sequence of events leading to the illness, with a clear differentiation between immediate and remote causal events. For example, when asked why he was sick, a child responded, "My platelet count was down. In the blood stream they are like white blood cells— they help kill germs. I got sick because there were more germs than platelets. They killed the platelets off." Illness cure is also primarily described as a step-by-step sequence of events involving internal anatomy and physiology.

The more developmentally advanced child views illness within a *psychophysiological* perspective, including psychological factors as well as the previously described physiological processes in illness causality. The child at this stage perceives an effect of thoughts and feelings on physiological functions. For example, a child may describe heart attack causality as, "It can come from being all nerve wracked. You worry too much. The tension can affect your heart." Cure explanation is basically the same as in Category 5, with physiological cures viewed as primarily relevant rather than psychological ones. At this stage, children perceive themselves as having a reasonable amount of control over onset and cure of an illness.

The results of the Bibace and Walsh study are consistent with a cognitive developmental framework. For the 4 year olds, 54 percent gave contagion explanations, and 38 percent gave contamination explanations. For the 7 year olds, 63 percent gave contamination explanations, and 27 percent gave internalization explanations. For the 11 year olds, 54 percent gave internalization explanations, and 34 percent physiologic explanations. Thus, with advancing chronological age the children demonstrated a cognitive developmental progression along the categories designated by Bibace and Walsh, consistent with a Piagetian theoretical framework.

Perrin and Gerrity (1981) tested healthy children entering kindergarten, second, fourth, sixth, and eighth grades. The testing session consisted of eight questions regarding the causes, prevention, and treatment of illness, and 14 questions designed to assess the children's general cognitive development. The questions regarding illness examined the concepts of how children get sick, how they can prevent illness, and how they can get well. The questions regarding general cognitive development examined concepts on the conservation of mass, weight and volume, physical causality, and abstract thinking, all unrelated to illness. A 7-point rating scale was developed for scoring the children's responses, ranging from, "No answer or a response unrelated to the question" to "Organized description of mechanism(s) underlying illness/recovery; abstract principles." Ratings in between scored the responses along such dimensions as global or magical thinking, concrete and rigid answers, and increasingly more realistic understanding of cause-effect relationships. Thus, the rating scale was developed to reflect a hierarchical framework for assessing conceptual development from global to concrete to abstract understanding.

Specifically, a score of 0 was assigned if the child did not answer or responded with a clearly unrelated answer. A score of 1 was assigned to the response "I don't know." A score of 2 designated global, circular, or magical responses that did not indicate an understanding of the causal link between an event and illness. A score of 3 was assigned to answers characterized as concrete, rigid, and stereotypic responses that seemed to be a simple repeating of parental rules without a clear conceptual understanding by the child. The score also reflected a perception of illness causality as one or a few external agents, no internalization process, with no control over illness causality or prevention. A score of 4 reflected the conceptualization of internalization, that some agent (e.g., germ) enters the body in illness causality. A score of 5 indicated a greater delineation of causal agents and illness, as well as beginning an understanding of internal bodily processes. Finally, a score of 6 designated responses describing a coherent underlying mechanism in illness causality and cure.

The results of the study showed a wide range of scores at each age level and to each question. For example, kindergarten children's total mean scores ranged from 1.5 to 3.2, fourth graders scored from 2.7 to 4.4, and eighth grader's responses were scored from 3.4 to 5.4. However, overall mean scores evidenced a developmental trend, gradually increasing with each higher grade level. This was evident for both the set of questions testing illness concepts as well as the set testing general cognitive development. Further, the two sets of questions were highly correlated, with the intercorrelations revealing that illness causality concepts closely paralleled development of concepts of physical causality. However, illness causality concepts were slower to develop than general physical causality concepts. Finally, concepts associated with illness prevention appeared to be more difficult to understand than concepts of illness causation and treatment. In conclusion, the findings were once again supportive of a systematic progression in the understanding of illness-related concepts, with the children's cognitive development in understanding illness paralleling but somewhat behind general cognitive development.

## Ill and Hospitalized Children's Concepts of Illness

It has been suggested by Nagera (1978) that ill and hospitalized children may be expected to function at cognitive developmental stages more appropriate for chronologically younger children. Nagera proposed that the stresses of illness result in regressive behavior and that the most recently acquired skills will be lost most readily. Further, the chance occurrence of an event, unrelated to the illness but contiguous in time or space with illness onset, might also be viewed as a cause-effect relationship. A number of studies have indicated that a common misconception by young ill children is that illness causality, treatment, and hospitalization are punishments for transgressions from parental and societal rules and regulations (see Nagera, 1978, and Weis, 1975, for reviews). This view is apparently not shared by healthy, nonanxious children, but is shared by healthy, anxious children (Brodie, 1974). These misconceptualizations about illness might result in even further stress, resulting in a cycle leading to progressively greater cognitive-behavioral regression. Thus, ill and hospitalized children might be seen as particularly vulnerable to misguided fantasies regarding illness causality and cure. However, recent research investigations have not unequivocally supported these clinical views.

Campbell (1975) studied 264 children, ranging in age from 6 through 12 years; all the children were short-term patients in a pediatric hospital where their median stay was 5 days. They all led normal, active lives until shortly before hospitalization, and all subsequently returned to normal routines shortly after hospitalization. Thus, these children were being treated for acute illnesses. Campbell's findings supported a cognitive developmental framework. Older children gave relatively more attention to specific diseases or diagnoses and to aspects of illness referring to alterations in conventional role behavior. They were also more likely to define illness by statements restricting the illness causality concept, whereas younger children were more apt to mention vague, nonlocalized feelings as a part of their definition. However, there was not a systematic correlation between a measure of the children's overt stress reactions and their cognitive functions, suggesting no relationship between stress and cognitive level. While suggestive, this study's findings are limited by the fact that a control group of healthy children was not included. Only with this matched control group for comparison would the notion of illness-induced cognitive regression be clearly tested for hospitalized children. Additionally, the children were acutely ill; chronically ill children might be more vulnerable for evidencing cognitive developmental delay.

Myers-Vando et al. (1979) tested 12 children chronically ill with congenital heart disease and 12 healthy children, ages 8 to 16 years. Children in the cardiac group were not included if they had experienced surgery or hospitalization in the 6 months prior to testing. To assess general cognitive developmental level, the children were examined using the Piagetian task of physical conservation (clay and water tests) adapted from Bernstein and Cowan (1975). Illness causality was measured by a projective picture task and a semistructured interview. The results showed that eight of the 12 chronically ill and one of the 12 healthy children did not attain an age-appropriate level on the conservation task. However, the illness causality measures did not differentiate between the two groups. Thus, these data failed to support the prediction that the experience of dealing with chronic cardiac illness would result in lower levels of understanding of illness causality (see Introductory Overview to pediatric chronic disorders for a description of a related study by Brewster, 1982). Additionally, a recent study by Feldman and Varni (1983) found that the conceptualizations of health and illness by 27 of 40 children with spina bifida were even higher than their general cognitive development, further questioning the notion that children with chronic disorders evidence lower levels of health/illness understanding.

In addition to acutely ill hospitalized children and chronically ill children, terminally ill children's concepts of illness and death need to be considered. Methodologically, one of the best studies was conducted by Koocher (1973), examining healthy children's views of death. Seventy-five children ranging in age from 6 to 15 years were asked the following four questions: "What makes things die?; How can you make dead things come back to life?; When will you die?; and What will happen then?" The answers were rated along a 3-point continuum ranging from very concrete to rather abstract: (1) Egocentric responses included fantasy reasoning, magical thinking, and/or realistic causes of death characterized primarily by an egocentric viewpoint (e.g., "You die when God reads your name in his book."); (2) Concrete responses included specific means causing death, with or without intention (e.g., "Guns, bows and arrows, rat poison, and getting beat up."); (3) Abstract responses included generalized and abstract clusters of specific causes, that death is a natural process, may involve physical deterioration, or a number of other potential causes such as accidents (e.g., "old age, illness, getting hit by a car or falling off a roof"). The results were again consistent within a cognitive developmental framework, with the children's responses consistent with their general cognitive level as determined by the conservation task in the modalities of mass, number, and volume. It is important to note that general cognitive level was more indicative of the children's responses than chronological age *per se*. For example, concrete-operational children's average age was 10.4 years, but this included a range of 6 to 13 years. Thus, chronological age alone did not appear to be a reliable predictor of the child's level of response. This appears to be a consistent finding across many of the studies on children's concepts of illness and has implications for clinical practice; that is, age alone does not sufficiently predict a child's cognitive level, but in fact the clinician must test both general cognitive development and conceptualizations of illness. In sum, healthy children's conceptualization of death parallels general cognitive development; however, specifically testing terminally ill children's cognitive developmental views of death remains to be empirically investigated (see Ferguson, 1978; Shrier, 1980, for overviews).

Finally, a study by Simeonsson, Buckley, and Monson (1979) tested the illness concepts of hospitalized children (ages 4 to 9 years) representing four broad categories: elective admissions, accidents, chronic conditions, and acute conditions. General cognitive development was assessed through conservation tasks and physical causality questions (e.g., "What makes clouds move?"). Six questions were designed to test illness causality, scored by assignment to one of three stages: (1) Stage I included global, magical, superstitious, or undifferentiated responses as well as "don't know"; (2) Stage II included concrete, specific responses reflecting rule breaking, rule keeping, and/or specific acts and events; and (3) Stage III included abstract verbalizations or expressions of a generalizable principle. Unfortunately, the authors grouped the children's responses so that a differential analysis of the children's concepts from among the four broad categories (i.e., elective admissions, accidents, chronic and acute conditions) was not possible. However, the grouped findings once again supported the cognitive developmental perspective, with the questions dealing with causes for illness, stomachaches, and the conditions for recovery or health maintenance being more sensitive to developmental differences than the questions, "What does medicine do? How do children get bumps and spots?" Nevertheless, it was generally demonstrated that illness causality conceptions were significantly correlated with advances in the concepts of conservation, decentration (i.e., reduction in egocentrism), and physical causality, providing further support for the commonality of cognitive development across a range of phenomena.

In summary, the studies reviewed indicate that healthy, ill, and hospitalized children conceptualize illness in a manner that essentially parallels general cognitive development. However, there are clearly individual differences among children and across the concepts tested by the various questions. The clinical implications of these findings will be discussed later in this chapter.

# HEALTH BELIEFS

Healthy children have been found to gradually develop more complex and complete conceptions of health (Rashkis, 1965) and their perceptions of their internal body parts (Porter, 1974). Natapoff (1978) interviewed 264 first, fourth, and seventh grade children, asking (1) "What does the word health mean?"; (2) "How do you feel when you are healthy?"; (3) "Can you be part healthy and part not healthy at the same time?"; (4) "How can you tell when a family member is healthy?" The children's responses to these questions were more complex, thoughtful, and increasingly longer with age, with the ideas about health showing a clear developmental trend from specific, concrete concerns for health practices to future-oriented interests and abstract thinking. Specifically, the first graders (6 year olds) viewed health as a series of specific health practices (e.g., eating meats and vegetables, getting exercise, and keeping clean). Being healthy enabled them to play with friends, to go outside, and to be with their family. It was not perceived possible to be part healthy and part not healthy at the same time. The fourth graders (9 year olds) were less concerned with specific health practices and more concerned with total body states such as being in good shape and feeling good. They were concerned with the performance of daily activities that required physical fitness. They felt that it was possible to be part healthy and part not healthy. Like the 6 year olds, they used perceptual clues to determine another person's health status, relying on outward, observable behaviors. The 12 year olds also viewed health as feeling good and being able to participate in desired activities while not being sick, but additionally evidenced abstract thinking not found in the younger children. Thirty-two percent of the 12 year olds viewed mental health as a component of overall health. Health was perceived as long-term, involving the mind, body, and the environment, while sickness was viewed as a transient, superimposed state. In sum, all of the children essentially viewed health as a positive state that allowed them to engage in desired activities, rather than as the absence of symptoms or simply the ability to minimally perform activities of daily living (a view of health found to be more common among adults).

The most organized body of empirical work on health beliefs has been conducted within a series of investigations under the rubric of the Health Belief Model. As initially formulated by Rosenstock (see Rosenstock, 1974, for overview), the Health Belief Model (HBM) postulates that the probability of an individual performing a recommended health-related behavior in order to prevent or treat illness depends at least in part on the individual's perceptions of: (1) susceptibility to illness; (2) the seriousness of the consequences of illness on day-to-day functioning; (3) the benefits of health-related behaviors in reducing illness susceptibility and/or seriousness; (4) the potential barriers that may interfere with the performance of the health-related behaviors (e.g., inconvenience, cost, pain). This model has been revised and expanded by Becker and his associates to account for more types of health-related behavior than merely recommended prevention-related health behaviors (Cummings, Becker, & Maile, 1980). Although most of the initial research on the HBM has been restricted to the health beliefs of adults, Becker (Dielman, Leech, Becker, Rosenstock, & Horvath, 1980) has recently studied the health beliefs of 250 children aged 6 to 17 years, identifying six dimensions of children's health beliefs.

These six dimensions were tested by interviewing the children and recording their responses to a 39-item questionnaire. The six dimensions (and a sample item from each) were: (1) General health concerns, e.g., "How much do you worry about getting sick?"; (2) Specific health concerns, e.g., "How worried would you be if you had a fever?"; (3) Perceived general susceptibility to illness, e.g., "How often do you get sick compared to others your age?"; (4) Perceived susceptibility to specific conditions, e.g., "How much of a chance do you think there is (in the next few months) that you might throw up?"; (5) Perceived seriousness of and susceptibility to illness, e.g., "When you're sick, how bad do you usually feel?"; and (6) Perceived parental concern, e.g., "How much does your mother/father seem to worry about you when you get sick?"

For the analysis of the results, the children's ages were grouped into 6-8, 9-11, 12-14, and 15-17 years. Statistically significant age effects were found for five of the six dimensions, suggesting that the level of concern decreases with increasing age. In general, children below age 11 are more likely to express higher levels of specific concerns, perceived susceptibility to specific conditions, perceived general susceptibility, perceived seriousness of and susceptibility to illness, and general health concerns than children between the ages of 12 and 17. With increasing age there was decreased variability in health beliefs, with the younger children differing more among themselves in their beliefs than the older children and a consolidation of health beliefs into a consistent pattern with increasing age. These results are consistent with general cognitive development, indicating a trend from unrelated beliefs that gradually develop into groups of global, undifferentiated belief sets, and finally into differentiated and well-consolidated health beliefs. These findings have implications for health education programs and the teaching of health attitudes and beliefs, suggesting that 6 to 8 year olds are more amenable to modification of health beliefs than older children.

Finally, closely related to aspects of the HBM are the series of studies on health locus of control (HLC). Theoretically, individuals with high levels of perceived internal control (internal locus of control) tend to see themselves as able to determine the outcomes of their encounters with their environment. In contrast, individuals with low levels of internal control (external locus of control) tend to see random, circumstantial events impinging on them and determining their actions; they do not see themselves as able to exert control over their environment. It has been found that children with a high degree of perceived internal control see themselves as better able to prevent or avoid health problems (Gochman, 1971), and perceive themselves as exerting more control over getting well as they grow older (Neuhauser, Amsterdam, Hines, & Steward, 1978).

Parcel and Meyer (1978) developed a Children's Health Locus of Control (CHLC) instrument to systematically assess HLC. Examples of internal/external-oriented questions included: "Good health comes from being lucky. Getting sick just happens. It is my mother's job to keep me from getting sick. I can do many things to fight illness." The results showed that in the tested age range of 7 to 12 years, the CHLC scores tended to become more internal with increases in age, suggesting that locus of control is also consistent within a general cognitive developmental framework.

# IMPLICATIONS AND PRACTICAL APPLICATION

Children increasingly develop progressively more complex ideas to explain (understand) what they perceive and experience, which involves the process of accommodation. Accurate accommodation cannot occur if the information presented requires cognitive skills too far beyond the child's current developmental level. However, if the child perceives new information as containing some previously recognized and assimilated components, then further modification of his cognitive structures is possible so as to accommodate this new information (Weis, 1975). By designing pediatric patient education materials in consideration of children's cognitive development, healthy children may more accurately understand their role in the process of prevention of illness and maintenance of health. For ill and hospitalized children, information provided in accordance with the age, stage, and degree of development of the child may minimize or avoid the additional stresses on the child resulting from misconceptualization of illness causality and treatment (Nagera, 1978). Identifying and understanding the child's conceptual development may be an essential initial step in helping children and their families cope with illness and hospitalization in an optimally adaptive fashion. The family as a unit must be appropriately educated, especially in light of recent findings on the effects of the chronically ill child's condition on siblings' concepts of illness (Carandang, Folkins, Hines, & Steward, 1979). Further, children's understanding of illness causality and treatment may also affect how they perceive of and adhere to treatment regimens, subsequently requiring the individual tailoring of treatment regimen information to each child's cognitive level.

As cogently stated by Peters (1978), "Upon completion of a verbal interchange between child and adult, each may erroneously believe that he has successfully communicated; and each may be erroneously convinced that he has understood [p. 143]." Far too often, adults assume that if they explain something very calmly and rationally, the child will naturally understand the information. We now know, to the contrary, that unless the child is patiently requested to respond to our questions, we will not know how much information has been accurately processed. For instance, Steward and Regalbuto (1975) found that young children viewed the use of a stethoscope as a way to determine life or death, and did not understand, even after they were told, that medicine could be in a syringe. If a child views illness as punishment for transgressions from rules and regulations, the treatment of illness and treatment-related instruments such as stethoscopes and syringes may be seen as a component of the perceived punishment (Brewster, 1982; Peters, 1978). Thus, an overestimation of children's cognitive abilities to understand illness causality and treatment may only further add to their misconceptions and anxiety when ill (Whitt, Dykstra, & Taylor, 1979). On the other hand, appropriately given information may result in greater understanding and a reduction in anxiety.

The following guidelines are intended to facilitate pediatric patient education:

1. Avoid explanatory terminology that may have unintended secondary meanings that children may be cognitively unable to distinguish.
2. The ability to fully understand the abstract conceptualization of an internal process like hemophilia and epilepsy requires attainment of formal operational thought. Explain to the child what she must do using very concrete, behavioral guidelines. Use metaphors appropriate to the child's cognitive level to explain internal processes—for instance, explaining the brain as a telephone and a seizure as a wrong number (see Whitt et al., 1979, for these examples). The use of drawings and play with toys facilitate the use of metaphors.
3. Children use toys and fantasy as activities that help them not only to gain understanding, but also to actively master new situations that would otherwise lead to anxiety. By explaining medical procedures through metaphors and allowing the young child to manipulate some of the instruments in advance of the actual procedure, the young child is given the opportunity to process the new information. For example, the mask used in an anesthetic situation may be handled by the child and compared to those used by pilots or astronauts. Through this play, the child has the opportunity to verbalize his fantasies and concepts of illness and treatment, allowing the clinician to assess any misconceptions that can be altered through further guided play activities by relating the situation to the experiences and fantasies of the young child. For older children, more realistic concepts may be used to explain the procedures, also including the opportunity for mutual discussion of illness and treatment conceptions until appropriate conceptualizations are attained.

The findings from studies on health locus of control also suggest practical guidelines. The child's stage of cognitive development has an effect on the amount of control he feels over the healing process (Neuhauser et al., 1978). As stated by Bibace and Walsh (1980): "At earlier developmental levels, appeals to personal control (for example, a prescription to avoid a certain type of food) are useless, whereas with children at later developmental levels, a sense of personal control should be acknowledged in helping the patient to manage his or her own illness [p. 917]." Thus, younger children, who are more externally oriented, may more easily accept being cared for, whereas older children may respond better to treatment that allows them a measure of control over their own healing process. Young children may initially be provided external sources of reinforcement for health-related behavior with a gradual shift toward reinforcing internal health locus of control as the children become older. This would shift more responsibility for health actions to the children and increase their freedom to make decisions about their health. This requires a skills-oriented approach, gradually teaching the children to self-regulate their health-related behaviors in unison with their health locus of control and cognitive development. The combination of child self-regulation training, parent training, and health staff training incorporates this approach of a gradual shift from external to internal control of health actions and will be evident in the subsequent chapters on treatment programs.

# REFERENCES

Bernstein, A.C., & Cowan, P.A. Children's concepts of how people get babies. *Child Development,* 1975, **46**, 77–91.

Bibace, R., & Walsh, M.E. Development of children's concepts of illness. *Pediatrics,* 1980, **66**, 912–917.

Brewster, A.B. Chronically ill hospitalized children's concepts of their illness. *Pediatrics,* 1982. **69**, 355–362.

Brodie, B. Views of healthy children toward illness. *American Journal of Public Health,* 1974, **64**, 1156–1159.

Campbell, J.D. Illness is a point of view: The development of children's concepts of illness. *Child Development,* 1975, **46**, 92–100.

Carandang, M.L.A., Folkins, C.H., Hines, P.A., & Steward, M.S. The role of cognitive level and sibling illness in children's conceptualizations of illness. *American Journal of Orthopsychiatry,* 1979, **49**, 474–481.

Cummings, K.M., Becker, M.H., & Maile, M.C. Bringing the models together: An empirical approach to combining variables used to explain health actions. *Journal of Behavioral Medicine,* 1980, **3**, 123–145.

Dielman, T.E., Leech, S.L., Becker, M.H., Rosenstock, I.M., & Horvath, W.J. Dimensions of children's health beliefs. *Health Education Quarterly,* 1980, **7**, 219–238.

Feldman, W.S., & Varni, J.W. Conceptualizations of health and illness by children with spina bifida. Manuscript submitted for publication, 1983.

Ferguson, F. Children's cognitive discovery of death. *Journal of the Association for the Care of Children's Health,* 1978, **7**, 8–14.

Gochman, D.S. Some correlates of children's health beliefs and potential health behavior. *Journal of Health and Social Behavior,* 1971, **12**, 148-154.

Goldstein, K.M., & Blackman, S. Assessment of cognitive style. In P. McReynolds (Ed.), *Advances in Psychological Assessment.* San Francisco: Jossey-Bass, 1978.

Koocher, G.P. Childhood, death, and cognitive development. *Developmental Psychology,* 1973, **9**, 369-375.

Meichenbaum, D., & Cameron, R. Issues in cognitive assessment: An overview. In T.V. Merluzzi, C.R. Glass, & M. Genest (Eds.), *Cognitive Assessment.* New York: Guilford Press, 1981.

Merluzzi, T.V., Rudy, T.E., & Glass, C.R. The information-processing paradigm: Implications for clinical science. In T.V. Merluzzi, C.R. Glass, & M. Genest (Eds.), *Cognitive Assessment.* New York: Guilford Press, 1981.

Myers-Vando, R., Steward, M.S., Folkins, C.H., & Hines, P. The effects of congenital heart disease on cognitive development, illness causality concepts, and vulnerability. *American Journal of Orthopsychiatry,* 1979, **49**, 617-625.

Nagera, H. Children's reactions to hospitalization and illness. *Child Psychiatry and Human Development,* 1978, **9**, 3-19.

Nagy, M.H. Children's ideas of the origin of illness. *Health Education Journal,* 1951, **9**, 6-12.

Natapoff, J.N. Children's views of health: A developmental study. *American Journal of Public Health,* 1978, **68**, 995-1000.

Neisser, U. *Cognitive Psychology.* New York: Appleton-Century-Crofts, 1967.

Neuhauser, C., Amsterdam, B., Hines, P., & Steward, M. Children's concepts of healing: Cognitive development and locus of control factors. *American Journal of Orthopsychiatry,* 1978, **48**, 335-341.

Parcel, G.S., & Meyer, M.P. Development of an instrument to measure children's health locus of control. *Health Education Monographs,* 1978, **6**, 149-159.

Perrin, E.C., & Gerrity, P.S. There's a demon in your belly: Children's understanding of illness. *Pediatrics,* 1981, **67**, 841-849.

Peters, B.M. School-aged children's beliefs about causality of illness: A review of the literature. *MCN: American Journal of Maternal Child Nursing,* 1978, **7**, 143-154.

Piaget, J. Piaget's theory. In P.H. Mussen (Ed.), *Carmichael's Manual of Child Psychology.* New York: Wiley, 1970.

Porter, C.S. Grade school children's perceptions of their internal body parts. *Nursing Research,* 1974, **23**, 384-391.

Rashkis, S.R. Child's understanding of health. *Archives of General Psychiatry,* 1965, **12**, 10-17.

Rosenstock, I.M. Historical origins of the Health Belief Model. *Health Education Monographs,* 1974, **2**, 328-335.

Shrier, D.K. The dying child and surviving family members. *Journal of Developmental and Behavioral Pediatrics,* 1980, **1**, 152-157.

Simeonsson, R.J., Buckley, L., & Monson, L. Conceptions of illness causality in hospitalized children. *Journal of Pediatric Psychology,* 1979, **4**, 77-84.

Steward, M., & Regalbuto, G. Do doctors know what children know? *American Journal of Orthopsychiatry,* 1975, **45**, 146-149.

Weis, D.P. Children's cognitive development—Or how children draw "maps." *Child Welfare,* 1975, **LIV**, 567-580.

Whitt, J.K., Dykstra, W., & Taylor, C.A. Children's conceptions of illness and cognitive development. *Clinical Pediatrics,* 1979, **18**, 327-339.

# 3

# Overview of Biobehavioral Principles and Techniques

## BIOBEHAVIORAL ASSESSMENT

Accurate and precise assessment of the relevant behavioral, medical, and physiological parameters provides the essential information required prior to the designing and implementation of a treatment regimen, as well as the necessary process measures required during the treatment and follow-up phases (maintenance).

## Behavioral Parameters

The assessment of health-related behaviors involves a multicomponent process consisting of the identification, measurement, and reliable and valid assessment of the target behavior.

### Identification of Target Behaviors

The selecting or pinpointing of the behaviors targeted for change is initially determined by the patient's self-report information during the history taking interview. The ultimate list of target behaviors may be influenced by further assessments, including patient self-monitoring, direct observation of patient behavior, parental reports, or medical chart review. This process concludes with the precise operational definition of the target behaviors. For example, to state that the patient is noncompliant to a weight control regimen does not provide a specific enough definition of the problem. Rather, it would be more precise to define the various components of the noncompliance pattern targeted for change, such as increasing attendance to clinic appointments, eating fewer high calorie foods, and exercising more frequently. These components can even be more precisely defined, as will be evident in the chapter describing eating, exercise, and diet modification.

*Measurement*

The measurement of behavioral parameters is accomplished through one of the following strategies depending on the characteristics of the target behavior.

*Frequency measures.* This is the recording of the occurrence or rate of the target behaviors on a behavior checklist during a specific time period. Typically used with target behaviors that occur at low or moderate frequency levels and have a clear beginning and end to each ocurrence, such as counting the number of requests per day for analgesic medication during a postoperative inpatient period or the number of repetitions of a particular physical therapy exercise.

*Bipolar measures.* These are frequency measures involving the classification of behaviors into bipolar categories such as occurred/did not occur or correct/incorrect. They are typically used when a list of target behaviors are being observed that have a limited number of possible occurrences, such as recording on a behavior checklist the performance of correct techniques by a parent of a hemophiliac during the preparation and infusion of factor replacement products. The correct techniques would be listed in the required order and simply checked off if they occurred. The percent correct occurrence would then be calculated by dividing the number of correctly performed techniques by the total number of correct techniques necessary for appropriate infusion, multiplied by 100.

*Interval recording measures.* These frequency measures are based on time units rather than overall rate. The target behaviors are observed during a block of time (e.g., 30 minutes), with each block of time further divided into a series of short intervals (e.g., 10 seconds). The target behaviors are then recorded on a behavior checklist as either occurred or did not occur during a 10-second observation interval. Each 10-second observation interval would be followed by a 20-second period for recording the occurrence of the behavior on the checklist. Thus, during a given 60-second period, there would be two 10-second observation intervals and sixty 10-second observation intervals for a 30-minute block of time. The percent occurrence of each target behavior would then be calculated by dividing the number of intervals checked for the occurrence of the behavior by the total number of possible intervals (60 in this example), multiplied by 100. These measures are typically used when the target behaviors occur at moderate to high frequencies and/or without a clear beginning or end (ongoing behaviors), such as recording the number of 10-second intervals that a child cried during a painful medical procedure or the number of intervals that high rate multiple tics occurred during a specific block of time.

*Time-sampling measures.* These are a type of interval recording where the observations are made during brief periods at different times rather than for a specific block of time, similar to taking a photograph or "snapshot" of target behaviors over an extended period of time. For example, such a measurement would be recording whether a patient hospitalized for exfoliative dermatitis treatment is scratching during a 5-second interval taken once an hour. The observer would simply look at the patient, walk out of the room, and then record on a behavior checklist whether scratching had occurred. These "snapshots" taken during the entire day would provide a representative sampling of the patient's total rate of scratching. The percent occurrence of scratching would be calculated by dividing the number of time intervals where scratching occurred by the total number of time-sampling intervals taken for the whole day, multiplied by 100.

*Duration measures.* These are time-based measures of either the total amount of time that the target behaviors are performed, the amount of time before the patient performs the target behavior (latency), or the amount of time between the performance of target behaviors. They are typically used when the target behaviors are continuous or ongoing rather than with a clear beginning or end to each response, such as recording the duration of postoperative hospitalization, the amount of time spent jogging, the latency for a clinic appointment, or the time intervals between the ingestion of prescribed medications on a time-based regimen schedule.

## Reliability

Determining the *reliability* of the assessment measures or *interobserver agreement* requires the simultaneous and independent recording of the target behaviors. Reliability indicates whether the operational definitions of the target behaviors are sufficiently precise and accurate enough for two or more observers to agree on their occurrence or nonoccurrence. Additionally, reliability assessments throughout the various stages of an intervention provide a check on the accuracy of the primary observer(s), since there may be a gradual subjective bias in recording without the feedback from an additional observer(s). Without reliability checks, the possibility exists that the recorded changes in behavior are a function of inaccurate or inconsistent observer recording rather than actual behavior change. An interobserver agreement of at least 80 percent is the conventionally accepted level required in order to have confidence in the reliability of the data collected. This level should be obtained during pilot observations so that subsequent data collected during baseline and treatment phases will be reliable and comparable. Low reliability would typically signal the need for a more precise and specific operational definition of the observed target behaviors before proceeding on to further data collection.

The percentage of interobserver agreement or reliability for frequency and duration measures is calculated by dividing the smaller recorded frequency or duration by one observer by the larger recorded frequency or duration by a second observer, multiplied by 100. The percentage of interobserver agreement or reliability for interval recording measures is calculated by dividing the number of intervals that the observers agreed on the occurrence or nonoccurrence of the target behaviors by the total number of time intervals, multiplied by 100. The percentage of reliability for bipolar and time-sampling measures is calculated by dividing the number of agreements on the occurrence or nonoccurrence of the target behaviors on the behavior checklist by the number of agreements plus disagreements (i.e., total observations) multiplied by 100. Reliability issues are further discussed later in this chapter.

### Validity

The *validity* of the assessment typically refers to the degree of the relationship or correlation between a selected dependent measure and a particular outcome criterion measure; that is, does a change in the dependent measure represent a change in a criterion measure? For example, is the self-report of a change in eating and exercise behaviors an accurate representation of true behavior change in eating and exercise patterns in the patient's home environment? The validity of a self-report measure may be influenced by a number of factors, including wanting to please the therapist, justification for additional medication, and so on. There are no simple formulas for increasing validity except for the strategy of assessing multiple measures, including the various self-report, behavioral, medical, and physiological parameters available. A high correlation between these various parameters consistently across baseline and treatment conditions increases the confidence that the measures accurately reflect a "true" assessment, not just a measurement that is idiosyncratic to a particular assessment technique. Fortunately, in most clinical research and practice, multiple parameters are available for assessment and comparison. Consistency in the direction of change across the various self-report, behavioral, medical, and physiological parameters provides a measure of the validity of each parameter. The various types of validity are discussed in detail later in this chapter.

## Medical Parameters

Examples of medical parameters include the number of analgesics required for pain relief, units of factor replacement products for the treatment of bleeding episodes in hemophilia, articular index score for joint tenderness in arthritic disorders, number of excoriations in exfoliative dermatitis, weight in obesity programs, and prescribed medications for hypertensive patients. The medical parameters may serve as dependent variables that are affected by modifications in the behavioral and physiological parameters. For example, weight loss is typically a function of the modification of eating and exercise behaviors, or the requests for analgesic medication may be decreased subsequent to the training in pain self-regulation and biofeedback techniques.

## Physiological Parameters

The physiological parameters include biochemical, electrodiagnostic, thermography and musculoskeletal measures. Examples of each are described below.

### Biochemical

The assessment of metabolic byproducts of a drug or diet regimen, the identification of a physiological marker placed in a medication, or the direct identification of a therapeutic agent in the blood or urine are typical examples of biochemical measures. Because of individual differences in the absorption, metabolism, and excretion of these agents, biochemical assessment is commonly useful only as a concomitant measure, rather than as a primary dependent variable in a behavioral-medical intervention. An example of a relevant biochemical assessment would be the serum salicylate levels from a patient with rheumatoid arthritis who is on a prophylactic aspirin regimen. The serum salicylate levels may provide a concomitant measure in corroborating the behavioral adherence to the aspirin regimen.

### Electrodiagnostic

Common electrodiagnostic assessments include:

- *Electroencephalography (EEG).* The amplification and recording on an electroencephalograph (electroencephalogram) and analysis of the electrical activity of the brain.
- *Electromyography (EMG).* The amplification and recording on an electromyograph (electromyogram) and analysis of the electrical activity of muscles.
- *Electrocardiography (EKG or ECG).* The amplification and recording on an electrocardiograph (electrocardiogram) and analysis of the electrical activity of the heart.
- *Electrodermal.* The amplification, recording, and analysis of the electrical activity of the skin. Also known as the galvanic skin response (GSR).

### Thermography

Thermography is the recording and analysis of temperature present in specific areas of the body, typically providing relative hot and cold readings on the body surface. Methods include placement of a thermistor on surface skin areas, infrared imaging photography, and the indirect approach of measuring blood flow by plethysmography.

### Musculoskeletal

This involves the recording and analysis of muscle strength/power/endurance parameters as measured by isokinetic and isometric instruments, e.g., the Cybex II dynamometer.

## BIOBEHAVIORAL EVALUATION

The successful development of empirically-based behavioral pediatrics techniques that will have the greatest clinical utility may be most advantageously conducted initially within the context of small groups of patients studied intensely over an extended period of time. While the analysis of large groups of patients may indicate statistically significant changes on pre- to postaveraged measures (outcome), individual differences and therapy process measures are often lost during the statistical analysis. A statistical significance of $p < .01$ (a commonly acceptable level) may not indicate a clinically significant change. Additionally, in clinical practice, the concern is not with an average success rate, but rather with the changes during the treatment course for individual patients. The methodologies for this type of single subject empirical evaluation currently exist (Hersen & Barlow, 1976). Through the intensive study of individual patients and small groups of patients, the most efficacious and potentially utilizable treatment methodologies may be identified. Based upon the empirical outcome of these initial small group studies, these techniques may be subsequently applied to larger numbers of patients with greater confidence. The two methodologies most commonly employed in the empirical evaluation of biobehavioral interventions are the intrasubject reversal design and the multiple-baseline design.

## Reversal Design

In the *reversal design,* a biobehavior is measured during a baseline or pretreatment phase over time until a stable pattern emerges. The treatment variable is then applied while the biobehavior continues to be measured in order to examine whether the intervention produces a clinically significant change in the target biobehavior. This continuous measurement, rather than being simply an averaged pre- and post- (outcome) evaluation, allows for an analysis of the process or course of the hypothesized therapeutic intervention. If a clinically significant change occurs in the biobehavior, the treatment variable is temporarily withdrawn in order to assess whether the change in the biobehavior was a result of the intervention. If so, then the target biobehavior should return to baseline or pretreatment levels (thus a reversal). The intervention variable is then reintroduced and maintained throughout the course of the treatment. The sequential introduction, removal, and reintroduction of the treatment variable is conducted in an attempt to demonstrate a causal relationship and to control for the influence of extraneous variables; that is, to control for the effects of uncontrolled external factors such as passage of time or developmental considerations, a spontaneous remission in the disease, or a relationship change in the home or school setting that motivates the patient to succeed. While any therapeutic change, regardless of the reason, is to be applauded, the treatment variable can be confidently applied to other patients only after a *systematic empirical evaluation.*

## Multiple-Baseline Design

As an alternative to the reversal design, the *multiple-baseline design* is of particular value when a biobehavior appears irreversible or when reversing or returning to baseline levels is clinically undesirable. In the multiple-baseline design, the causal relationship and the control for extraneous variables is demonstrated by the sequential application of the therapeutic intervention at different points in time (therefore, multiple baselines). Multiple baselines may be collected across *biobehaviors, patients,* or *settings.* In the multiple-baseline design across biobehaviors, two or more biobehaviors are identified and measured over time to provide multiple baselines against which the treatment variable can be evaluated. When these baseline measures stabilize, the treatment variable is applied to one biobehavior or a response class (grouping) of related biobehaviors, ideally producing a change, with little or no change in the baseline measures of the other biobehaviors. Rather than reversing the just-produced change by returning to baseline conditions, the treatment is instead maintained and additionally applied to another target biobehavior or group of related biobehaviors (response class). If change now occurs in the second biobehavior contingent on the application of the treatment variable, then evidence is accruing that the intervention effects are valid and not simply a matter of coincidence, passage of time, or some other uncontrolled variable, but that biobehavioral change occurs maximally only when the treatment variable has been applied. Multiple baselines may also be applied across patients and environmental settings or situations in a similar manner.

In the multiple-baseline design across patients, a target biobehavior is identified across two or more patients and measured over time to provide multiple baselines. When these multiple baseline measures on a target biobehavior for different patients stabilize at a relatively constant rate, the treatment is begun with one patient and subsequently for additional patients in the sequential pattern of the design. For the multiple-baseline design across situations or settings, measures are taken on a target biobehavior for a patient or group of patients across different settings (e.g., clinic versus hospital bedroom, hospital versus home versus school setting). Once again, after the biobehavior rate has stabilized in each setting, the treatment variable is sequentially applied in the multiple-baseline design. The selection of the particular multiple-baseline design depends on the characteristics of the target biobehaviors and the treatment regimens.

## Changing-Criterion and Control Patient Designs

Two additional designs may be utilized in evaluating the clinical significance of biobehavioral interventions, but are employed less commonly. The first, the *changing-criterion design,* involves the sequential shaping of a biobehavior toward a target criterion of performance through a gradual series of component criteria. As performance of the biobehavior during treatment successively reaches the criteria levels in the sequence toward the target criterion performance, evidence is accruing that therapeutic change occurs only under the influence of the treatment variable. This design is particularly useful in shaping programs, such as gradually increasing the complexity of a therapeutic regimen.

Finally, the *control patient design* is a variation of the multiple-baseline design across patients and the control group design. This design is less desirable from both an empirical and clinical perspective. Essentially, the design involves matching patient characteristics across two patients or a small number of patients, with half the patients receiving the treatment while the other half continue to be assessed under baseline conditions. The control patient design can be used with as few as one treatment and one control patient, in contrast to the larger sample size traditional control group design, which is subject to a statistical analysis of the averaged pre- and post- (outcome) measures. In the control patient design, the limited number of treatment and control patients allows the continuous recording and evaluation of process measures rather than just pre- and post- (outcome) measures. In the control patient design, both the treatment and control patients are assessed during baseline, with the control patient maintained on baseline while the treatment variable is introduced for the treatment patient. This design may be most useful when adding a new experimental treatment variable to an ongoing regimen for a limited number of patients. If the treatment variable demonstrates a clinically significant change in biobehavioral performance, it may be added to the regimen for the control patient(s). At this point, the design assumes the characteristics of an extended multiple-baseline design across patients. While less desirable, the control patient design does provide some degree of evaluation of treatment techniques in the clinical setting. From a clinical perspective, the larger control group design is not as desirable for initially evaluating a treatment variable, since the control group design focuses on the average performance of a large number of patients. Since the average performance of a group may not accurately reflect individual patient response to a treatment, it is not a specific enough evaluation for the clinical setting. Once again, it is important to emphasize that the *statistically significant* changes in the average pre- and postmeasures of a group of patients does not necessarily indicate a *clinically significant* treatment regimen for individual patients. The value of the afore-mentioned clinical designs (particularly the multiple-baseline design) for evalu-ating treatment regimens for individual patients in clinical settings cannot be too strongly stressed. A number of figures throughout the text will illustrate the applications of these designs across a variety of patients, biobehaviors, and settings.

# ANTECEDENTS OF BIOBEHAVIORS

In addition to identifying and defining the target biobehaviors, a *functional analysis* is essential in specifying the conditions that influence the occurrence or nonoccurrence of the target biobehaviors. These conditions include the events that precede (antecedents) and follow (consequences) the performance of a particular biobehavior, schematically presented as *Antecedents→Biobehav-iors→Consequences. Antecedent events* or *antecedent stimuli* set the occasion for or cue the performance or emission of a biobehavior. Antecedent stimuli may occur at the socioenvironmental, cognitive, and neurophysiological levels. For example, verbal instructions by a therapist may cue the performance of a health-related behavior, the smell of food may set the occasion for eating, seeing someone smoking may be the stimulus for lighting up a cigarette, pain perception may be a stimulus for analgesic intake, or entering a hospital for surgery may be the stimulus for increased heart rate and general overall physiological arousal.

## Stimulus Control

The process whereby specific antecedent stimuli exert control over specific biobehaviors is termed *stimulus control.* In certain situations, antecedent stimuli result in biobehaviors that are reinforced (e.g., satisfaction from eating a favorite food) or are nonreinforced (e.g., no pain relief after ingesting a mild analgesic). The process whereby antecedent stimuli result in reinforcing or nonreinforcing consequences is known as *differential reinforcement.* Through this process of pairing certain antecedent stimuli with reinforcement and certain antecedent stimuli with nonreinforcement, the antecedent stimuli themselves begin to signal the probable consequences of a biobehavior. An antecedent stimulus that signals probable reinforcement is referred to as a *discriminative stimulus.* A discriminative stimulus is distinguished from other antecedent stimuli that have not been paired with reinforcement, i.e., that result in nonreinforcement. The antecedent stimulus that signals nonreinforcement of the biobehavior is termed a *stimulus delta*. The result of differential reinforcement is that a target biobehavior has a higher probability of occurring in the presence of a particular discriminative stimulus than in the presence of a particular stimulus delta that does not lead to reinforcement. For instance, the probability of a child eating and receiving gustatory reinforcement when cookies are on the kitchen table is higher than when celery or carrots are present. To reduce the probability of overeating, the cookies (discriminative stimulus) would be replaced with celery or carrots (stimulus delta). Thus, through differential reinforcement the child makes a discrimination between cookies and carrots, resulting in the stimulus control of eating behaviors—a lower probability of eating behaviors in the presence of carrots and a higher probability of eating behaviors in the presence of cookies.

## Stimulus and Response Generalization

The pairing between antecedent stimuli and reinforcing and nonreinforcing consequences may result in more than a one-to-one relationship. That is, a number of antecedent stimuli may cue the performance of a particular biobehavior, or conversely, one particular antecedent stimulus may cue the performance of a number of biobehaviors. When the effects of the pairing between a particular antecedent stimulus→biobehavior→consequence match extends beyond this one-to-one sequence, the term *generalization* is used.

*Stimulus generalization* refers to the situation whereby a particular biobehavior is cued by a number of similar or related antecedent stimuli. For instance, overeating by a child may be triggered by the presence of a number of sweet antecedent stimuli including cookies, candies, and cake, or a specific physiological response (e.g., anxiety or nausea) in a child may be cued by the presence of a hospital, a person in a white coat, and a hypodermic needle, depending on the child's previous experience with these or similar stimuli.

*Response generalization* refers to the situation whereby a particular antecedent stimulus cues the performance of a number of similar or related biobehaviors (responses). For example, viewing a television commercial on a favorite food may serve to cue eating, drinking, and smoking behaviors (consummatory responses), as well as gastric secretions.

## Prompts

*Prompts* are antecedent stimuli that facilitate the initiation of a biobehavior. Prompts are typically used in treatment programs to increase a particular biobehavior. The prompt serves as a cue or signal for the performance of the biobehavior, and this performance is then typically reinforced. The prompt subsequently becomes a discriminative stimulus for reinforcement. The eventual treatment goal is that the biobehavior is emitted at the desired rate without the need for a prompt. The process of gradually reducing the need for a prompt is termed *fading*. This gradual reduction of the prompt is a necessary condition in the fading process. For instance, in toilet training the young child, a parent would use a number of verbal, physical, and temporal prompts followed by social reinforcement (praise, smiling, hugs). The child might be physically guided to the toilet and helped in undressing every 60 minutes. Eventually, the parent would reduce the physical prompts as the child learned to undress and go to the toilet, simply asking the child every 60 minutes if she has to go to the toilet. These verbal and temporal prompts would then be gradually reduced in frequency by fading out the number of times the parent verbally asked the child about the toileting need. The speed of fading would be dependent on the success of the child in gradually urinating and defecating in the toilet rather than in her pants. By the time the child was 100 percent successful in discriminating the physiological cues leading to urinating and defecating, the frequency of prompts would be essentially zero, even though social reinforcement would continue for successful toileting. In certain situations, prompts may be reduced but not completely faded out. A parent's verbal prompts to a child regarding taking a prescribed medication may be employed on an as-needed basis depending on the child's adherence to the medication regimen. Continuous reinforcement may also be gradually faded out, as described in the next section.

## CONSEQUENCES OF BIOBEHAVIORS

*Consequences* are the events or contingencies that follow the performance of a biobehavior. When temporally contingent on the occurrence of a target biobehavior, these events will either increase or decrease the probability that a target biobehavior will occur again in the future. *Reinforcement* refers to the process whereby the probability of biobehavior performance increases; conversely, *punishment* is the process whereby response probability decreases. As with antecedent stimuli, consequences may occur at the socioenvironmental, cognitive, and neurophysiological levels. For instance, a parent may reinforce a child's physical therapy exercises with praise, hugs, or television time; consuming a potent analgesic may result in significant pain relief; jogging four miles may result in positive self-statements (self-reinforcement) of achievement and self-esteem; or overeating may result in a feeling of guilt and censureship from one's peers.

## Positive Reinforcement

*Positive reinforcement* refers to the *increased* performance of a target biobehavior as a result of the *application* of a consequence contingent on the occurrence of the biobehavior. Typically, positive reinforcers are pleasant events or stimuli such as praise, smiling, hugs, preferred activities (e.g., television time, special trips), or treats (sweets, small toys, comic books, preferred dessert). However, a positive reinforcer is defined after the fact. It is its empirically determined effect on a target biobehavior that operationally defines it as a reinforcer. Thus, parental attention, even when it may be viewed *a priori* as a punishment (e.g., yelling, scolding), may, in fact, increase a misbehavior because any parental attention is reinforcing for the child.

In addition to intuitively apparent reinforcers such as praise and treats, a wide variety of potential reinforcers exist as a result of the *high probability response* premise. Essentially, this premise states that in a given situation where two or more available responses are possible, the one that occurs at a higher or greater frequency (i.e., is preferred and more probable to occur) may serve to reinforce a lower probability or less frequently emitted response. For example, given a choice, a child is more likely or probable to watch television than to engage in physical therapy exercises. By arranging the contingency so that television viewing is dependent on doing a certain number of physical therapy exercises, an increase in exercising may be observed. If television viewing does not function as a reinforcer and increase the exercising, alternative events may be tried as reinforcers such as playing outside with preferred toys. Thus, the reinforcer is defined operationally and empirically by its functional effect on the target response.

It is often more convenient to develop a reinforcement *exchange system* where *tokens* (points, coins, stars, smiling faces) are backed up by preferred events. For instance, thirty repetitions of a physical therapy exercise may be worth three tokens (one token per ten repetitions), which may then be exchanged at a later time for fifteen minutes of either television viewing or playing outside (one token exchanged for each five minutes). Through the use of the high probability premise and the token exchange system, there is a tremendous amount of flexibility and an almost unlimited number of potential reinforcers available in a positive reinforcement program.

### Shaping and Chaining

In attempting to increase a biobehavior through positive reinforcement, it is common to find that the desired response is not occurring, and there are skills deficits as well. In other words, a number of the components of a target biobehavior are not present in the patient's response repertoire. Thus, the target biobehavior never occurs and consequently is never available for positive reinforcement. Through the process of *shaping*, the target biobehavior is gradually achieved by the systematic reinforcement of the early then later components or successive approximations of the target response. For instance, a child would be sequentially reinforced for gradually attaining the composite skills needed for successful bicycle riding, swimming, or the correct performance of a treatment regimen. Typically, prompting is initially employed to cue each desired component response sequentially and then faded out as each component is learned. At the completion of the shaping process, positive reinforcement is contingent only on the total performance of all the components of the target response.

*Chaining* refers to a sequence of responses already in the patient's repertoire that is not yet being emitted in the desired sequential pattern. In contrast to shaping, the last component of the sequence is initially reinforced in chaining and continues to be reinforced with other components gradually added on or chained to this response with an ever increasing criterion for reinforcement. This sometimes is termed backward chaining as opposed to the forward reinforcement process of shaping. Shaping and chaining may be combined when the component skills in a chain are not present, and must first be learned through shaping before they can then be chained together. For example, swimming, bicycle riding, and jogging may be the components in an exercise rehabilitation program, with each component chained into a weekly sequence after initial shaping or training in the component skills of each exercise regimen.

## Negative Reinforcement

*Negative reinforcement* refers to the *increased* performance of a target biobehavior as a result of the *removal* or *avoidance* of a consequence contingent on the occurrence of the biobehavior. Typically, negative reinforcers are unpleasant or aversive events and stimuli such as parental disapproval, pain, and loss of privileges. As with positive reinforcers, a negative reinforcer is operationally defined by an empirical determination of its effect on a target biobehavior.

It is essential to distinguish between negative reinforcement and punishment. As will be described in the next section, *punishment decreases* the probability of biobehavior occurrence. Both positive and *negative reinforcement increase* the probability of performance. In negative reinforcement, the probability of biobehavior occurrence is increased so as to remove, terminate, or escape an aversive stimulus. For example, the probability of adhering to a pain medication regimen is increased when the medication effectively terminates pain perception. Over time and with additional learning trials, a biobehavior may be performed at such an increased rate that there is a complete avoidance of the negative reinforcer. Thus, a patient with arthritis may learn that adhering to a prophylactic aspirin regimen essentially results in a complete avoidance of pain and inflammation.

As with positive reinforcers, the high probability response premise and token exchange system may be used to increase response probability. In this case, physical therapy exercises may be increased so as to remove or completely avoid a usually daily household chore such as throwing out the garbage, or these exercises may be increased to avoid receiving negative points resulting in additional household chores.

## Punishment

*Punishment* refers to the *decreased* performance of a target biobehavior as a result of *either* the *application* of an *aversive* stimulus or the *removal* of a *pleasant* stimulus contingent on the occurrence of a biobehavior. This presentation of unpleasant and aversive events or removal of positive and pleasant events typically includes such consequences as parental disapproval and loss of privileges (e.g., television time). As with positive and negative reinforcement, punishment is operationally defined by an empirical determination of its effect on a target biobehavior, that is, the response probability decreases.

Punishment as the presentation of an aversive event contingent on a response occurs commonly. For example, a child may burn a finger when playing with matches, a parent may scold a child for hitting a sibling, or a child may experience stomach upset and/or parental reprimands after eating too many sweets. Conversely, punishment as the removal of a pleasant event is termed *response cost*. Thus, the response or biobehavior costs a particular preferred pleasant event such as television viewing time, outside playing time, or the loss of tokens.

A variation of response cost involves a certain time interval away from all reinforcement termed *time-out*. During time-out all positive reinforcers are removed for a designated time period contingent on a particular biobehavior. For example, tantrum behavior may be decreased by placing the child on a chair facing a wall for five minutes. During this time period, the child is removed from any parental attention, as well as from all positive reinforcers such as playing with preferred toys. Particularly with younger children, this simple technique can be a powerful punishment procedure for decreasing undesirable biobehaviors, with minimal negative side effects.

## Alternatives to Punishment Procedures

There are three additional methods to *decrease* undesirable biobehaviors which do not require punishment directly. Although they result in a reduction in response occurrence, they do not contain the negative characteristics sometimes implied by the punishment process.

## DRO and DRL

In the method termed *differential reinforcement of other behavior* (DRO), a biobehavior that is incompatible with an undesirable biobehavior is reinforced. For example, adherence to a medical regimen is reinforced rather than punishing noncompliance. In the method termed *differential reinforcement of low rates of responding* (DRL), reinforcement is provided for a gradually decreasing criterion number of undesirable responses or for a gradual increase in the amount of time that a response does not occur; for instance, reinforcement for a sequentially lower number of daily calories consumed, for a lower rate of multiple tic behaviors, or for a longer time period between analgesic medication requests. Even when it is necessary to use punishment procedures, it is always advisable to concurrently systematically reinforce desirable responses that are incompatible with the undesirable responses being punished.

## Extinction

*Extinction* refers to the decreased performance of a target biobehavior as a result of the lack of reinforcement. The distinction between extinction and punishment as procedures (they both result in decreased performance) is important. In punishment, an aversive stimulus is contingently presented on biobehavior performance, or a pleasant stimulus is removed contingent on response occurrence. In extinction, there are no contingencies or consequences; an aversive stimulus is not presented nor is a pleasant stimulus removed contingent on biobehavior performance. Essentially, the occurrence of a previously reinforced response is simply ignored. The target biobehavior typically returns gradually to a prereinforcement level of occurrence. For instance, a parent may attend to a child every time the child complains of a stomachache. After extensive physical examination, it becomes evident that there is no physical cause for the verbal complaints of pain, but they do serve to increase parental attention. By simply ignoring the verbal pain behaviors, the frequency of stomachache complaints will most likely gradually stop occurring. Similarly, if a child has been instructed by a therapist to perform a complex set of physical therapy exercises daily, and the parent eventually stops reinforcing the child either through praise or tokens, then the exercise behaviors are put on extinction and will most likely cease being performed. Thus, nonreinforcement of a biobehavior previously increased or maintained through reinforcement eventually results in the reduction or total elimination of the response to prereinforcement levels.

The extinction or absence of reinforcing consequences for biobehaviors increased and/or maintained through these reinforcers may include both positive and negative reinforcement processes. The extinction of previously positively reinforced biobehaviors is typified by the decrease in exercise behaviors when eventually ignored by the parent. The extinction of previously negatively reinforced biobehaviors is exemplified by the decrease in adherence to an anti-inflammatory drug regimen when joint inflammation and pain are no longer effectively avoided by taking the prescribed drug.

## Contingency Schedules

There are a number of characteristics in the application of consequences that significantly influence the effects of these contingencies on the performance of biobehaviors. A considerable amount of research has indicated that in order to maximize the effect of a consequence on performance there should be: (1) a *close temporal pairing* between the emission of the target biobehavior and its consequence, and (2) a consequence of *sufficient magnitude* to have an effect on performance. Thus, the time delay in applying a consequence should be relatively short or even immediate on the performance of a biobehavior, and the amount of the consequence should be sufficiently great enough so as to be proportional to the desired effect on the response. In addition to these considerations, there are a number of contingency schedules that can further influence the performance and maintenance of biobehavior performance.

### Ratio Schedules

Ratio schedules may be either fixed or variable. A *fixed-ratio schedule* (FR) specifies an unchanging number of biobehavior occurrences prior to the application of a consequence. For example, a FR:5 schedule implies that the response must occur five times before the consequence is applied. A FR:1 schedule implies a continuous or one-to-one schedule. A *variable-ratio schedule* (VR) refers to the application of a consequence on a predetermined varying number of responses. Although the average number of responses is set, the range of responses may be quite variable. For instance, in a VR:10 schedule, an average of every tenth response receives a consequence, but the range may be from the performance of one response to the performance of twenty responses.

### Interval Schedules

Interval schedules may also be either fixed or variable. A *fixed-interval schedule* (FI) specifies that a particular amount of time passes prior to the application of a consequence. As soon as the first response occurs after this time interval, the consequence is applied. For example, a FI:5 schedule refers to the consequence being applied to a target biobehavior only after 5 minutes have passed, irrespective of how many times the response occurred during the 5-minute interval. A *variable-interval schedule* (VI) requires an average time interval before a consequence is applied, with a range of intervals possible. For instance, a VI:5 schedule implies a consequence for biobehavior performance after an average of every 5 minutes, but may range from 1 to 10 minute intervals. Both ratio and interval schedules have important implications for the maintenance of biobehavior performance. Examples of these various schedules will be demonstrated throughout the text.

## Modeling and Observational Learning

*Observational learning* can occur through the observation of modeled biobehaviors by another individual and the resulting consequences for those modeled biobehaviors. Thus, through observing a target response and a positive consequence for that modeled response, a child may begin to emit that response as well. For example, if a sibling receives an increased amount of parental attention for complaining about headaches, a younger sibling may begin to emit this same pattern. Parental health-related behaviors are often learned through observation by their children. This includes not only desirable patterns like appropriate eating and exercise, but also such habits as smoking and alcohol consumption.

As contrasted to the previously discussed explicit shaping and extrinsic reinforcement paradigms, observational learning may occur through the mere observing of modeled responses with the accompanying cognitive activities without the need for explicit shaping and direct reinforcement. In the observational learning paradigm, large chunks of biobehaviors may be learned at one time. A child may learn all about the specific components of a target response (how to behave) in one observation, as well as discriminate the antecedent and consequent conditions that control the occurrence or nonoccurrence of the modeled behavior (when to behave). Modeling and the process of observational learning will be shown in later sections to be a very helpful teaching tool.

## Generalization and Maintenance

*Generalization* refers to the extension of therapeutic gains across situations, settings, and time. Generalization across situations and settings is termed *transfer of learning*. Generalization across time is termed *maintenance*.

A number of strategies have been proposed to improve and enhance generalization. A major recommendation involves programming contingencies in the patient's natural environment that provide ongoing consequences for biobehaviors. Particularly in the pediatric population, parents and teachers may be trained to systematically encourage generalization through programmed contingencies. Additionally, increasing the number of antecedent stimuli available in the natural environment may further cue biobehaviors. Also, contingency schedules that provide consequences on an intermittent or variable schedule rather than on a one-to-one or continuous basis may further enhance generalization after therapeutic levels of responding have been achieved through a one-to-one (response/consequence) contingency. Finally, self-regulation training has been proposed as a set of techniques for enhancing generalization. Examples of these generalization strategies will be provided throughout the text.

## Self-Regulation and Biofeedback

The *self-regulation* of biobehaviors includes the modification of both health-related behaviors and physiological functions. The self-regulation process consists of the following components: (1) *Antecedent stimulus control* involves the systematic identification and use by the patient of specific characteristics of his environment which may cue the performance of a biobehavior; (2) *Self-monitoring* is the systematic observation by the patient of a target biobehavior and involves the recording by the patient of a target biobehavior on an assessment instrument; (3) *Self-instructions* are cognitive strategies and verbal statements that patients are taught to say to themselves as part of a decision-making process to initiate, guide, and maintain biobehaviors; (4) *Self-reinforcement* involves the patient's provision of positive consequences contingent on her performance of a target biobehavior; (5) *Biofeedback* refers to the process whereby physiological functions (e.g., heart rate, skin temperature, EMG) are provided the patient on a moment-to-moment basis via instruments in order to facilitate the self-regulation of these physiological processes. This biological feedback via biofeedback instruments may best be viewed as an initial shaping step toward ultimate instrument-independent self-regulation of these physiological functions in the patient's natural environment.

# MEASUREMENT ISSUES IN BEHAVIORAL PEDIATRICS

## Multidimensional and Comprehensive Assessment

A primary axion in both research and clinical practice in behavioral pediatrics is that data should be obtained through *multidimensional* and *comprehensive* measurement (e.g., medical, physiological, behavioral, self-report). Since the goals, assessment methods, and time basis of medical and behavioral measurement systems have often been dissimilar in the past, the design of behavioral pediatrics measurement systems will require input from all disciplines. As detailed by Varni and Dietrich (1981), the empirical development of these multidimensional and comprehensive biobehavioral measurement instruments should be one of the first tasks of behavioral pediatrics, including such *dimensions* as disease activity, health status, functional status, and psychosocial adjustment.

*Disease activity* refers to the biologic state of the disease; *health status* is a comprehensive assessment of physical, psychological, and social well-being; *functional status* is the patient's level of performance in activities of daily living and is determined by a complex interaction of physiologic variables (e.g., range of joint motion, muscle strength, joint changes), psychosocial parameters (e.g., coping skills, motivation, family support, socioeconomic status), and environmental factors (e.g., transportation, adaptive devices); *psychosocial adjustment* further details and identifies the patient's psychological and social adaption and level of psychosocial functioning. Within these four dimensions may be listed a myriad of *factors,* such as noncompliance to therapeutic regimens, specific physiologic parameters, school attendance, peer relationships, and parent-child interactions, all potential contributory factors to the status of the dimensions identified. Further, these multifactorial variables may be measured through nominal, ordinal, interval, and ratio *scales* (Isaac & Michael, 1981). *Nominal scales* tabulate the frequency or number of unordered occurrences in each factor of a dimension (e.g., gender, job status); *ordinal scales* represent a nonquantitative ordered relationship and indicate only relative position, not how much difference exists between positions on the scale (e.g., joint stiffness ordered as a less severe problem than joint pain); *interval scales* reflect equal distances in the variables being quantitatively ordered where the zero point is arbitrarily determined and does not represent the complete absence of the variable being measured (e.g., a rank ordering in differential severity of school days missed secondary to chronic illness in addition to school days typically missed for acute illnesses); *ratio scales* are the same as interval scales except that there is a true zero point (e.g., zero on a pain intensity scale actually means the absence of pain).

The comprehensive and multidimensional demonstration of the effects of an intervention will not only aid in verifying treatment efficacy, but multifactorial analyses may significantly contribute to knowledge pertinent to the mechanisms of behavioral-medical interrelationships.

## Process and Outcome Measures

There is a special need, particularly in pediatric chronic disorders, to delineate both process and outcome measures given the long-term nature of these conditions and the requirements for ongoing therapy and rehabilitation. Although medicine has been concerned with process and outcome measures, there have been a number of methodological problems with previous work in this area which lends itself to additional research (Brook, Appel, Avery, Orman, & Stevenson, 1971; Greenfield, Nadler, Morgan, & Shine, 1977; Greenfield, Solomon, Brook, & Davies-Avery, 1978; Nobrega, Morrow, Smoldt, & Offord, 1977). Williamson (1971) has identified four measurement categories consisting of: (1) *diagnostic outcomes* representing data that delineate the prognosis and need for treatment; (2) *therapeutic outcomes* representing health status after a long-term intervention; (3) *diagnostic process* which further details the identification of specific needs and therapy; and finally, (4) *therapeutic process* which includes the ongoing progress of the intervention on health status and such potentially contributory factors as noncompliance to therapeutic regimens. The distinction between the process and outcome measurement sets may be a function of different assessment targeted parameters (e.g., joint deterioration versus activities of daily living) or a matter of temporal ordering (e.g., measurements taken during the intervention versus pre- and postassessments).

As pointed out by Fries, Spitz, Kraines, and Holman (1980), disability may be the most important outcome category in chronic disorders. Activities of daily living (ADL) scales are most often used to assess disability associated with chronic disease (Sheikh, Smith, Meade, Goldenberg et al., 1979). In the case of pediatric chronic illness, Pless and Pinkerton (1975) have emphasized the importance of assessing the functional impact of the handicap as well as the extent to which the disease is treated successfully in a purely medical sense, with school attendance suggested as one important ADL outcome measure for children with chronic disease (Parcel, Gilman, Nader, & Bunce, 1979). Thus, for a comprehensive assessment of the relative health-illness status of a patient, measurement must be made in terms of departures from normal role behavioral functioning as well as with reference to health in a physical or medical sense (Reynolds, Rushing, & Miles, 1974). In this regard, the behavioral pediatrics team approach in developing and testing multidimensional and comprehensive process and outcome measurement instruments may ultimately have a profound influence on all aspects of treatment evaluation in pediatric medicine.

## Problem-Oriented Records

The process of organizing and successfully implementing an interdisciplinary behavioral pediatrics team approach requires the utilization of a structure or system set up specifically to effectuate multidisciplinary collaboration. The *Problem-Oriented Record* (POR) system provides an ideal organizing principle for such collaboration (Granger & Greer, 1976; Reinstein, Stass, & Marguette, 1975; Weed, 1968, 1969; Wendland & Crawford, 1976). A major flaw of the traditional chart system has been its inability to indicate adequately complex temporal relationships between clinical, laboratory, and therapeutic parameters (Fries, 1972). The problem-oriented system applies the scientific method of problem solving to comprehensive and multidimensional patient management (Dinsdale, Mossman, Guillickson, & Anderson, 1970; Milhous, 1972; Weed, 1969). The POR system involves four phases:

1. *Data Base.* The first phase in the system is the establishment of an adequate data base consisting of such components as the present illness, chief

complaint, patient profile, past history, psychosocial data, systems review, physical examination, and laboratory findings.

2. *Problem List.* The second phase involves the selection of specific and significant problems identified from the original data base. A list of the patient's medical, psychological, social, and functional problems is thus formulated from the initial data base and organized in numbered sequence at the front of the patient's chart. The numbered list contains every problem in the patient's history, past and present, with new problems added as identified, including potential problem areas in need of prevention. The problem may be listed as a diagnosis (such as arteriosclerotic heart disease), a physiologic finding (such as congestive heart failure), a symptom or physical finding (such as shortness of breath or heart murmur), or an abnormal laboratory result (such as abnormal electrocardiogram). Problems are listed as either active or inactive. As problems are treated and resolved, they are moved from the active to the inactive list, with all problems dated in terms of initial identification, treatment, and resolution.

3. *Specific Plan.* The third phase in the system is the development of a specific management plan for each problem listed, including the identification of problem causes, appropriate treatment, patient education needs, and treatment resolution goals.

4. *Progress Evaluation.* The fourth and final phase of the POR system is the chronologic sequencing of progress notes detailing the process and outcome parameters. Each progress evaluation is divided into four subheadings: subjective data (reported by patient), objective data (observable data, laboratory findings), assessment (has problem changed, by what criteria?), and plan (diagnostic, therapeutic, patient education).

Thus, in essence, the POR is a logistics system and a patient-oriented health care plan for organizing an immense informational data base in such a way as to facilitate a collaborative interdisciplinary health team approach. As such, it provides an ideal model for the implementation of the behavioral pediatrics concept of multidimensional, interdisciplinary, and comprehensive care.

## Reliability and Validity

Only with reliable and valid comprehensive and multidimensional outcome and process measurement instruments will behavioral pediatrics treatment programs be seen as a contribution to the total care of children and adolescents.

### Reliability

Reliability indicates the agreement or consistency between measurements, that is, the extent to which the obtained measures are reproducible (Isaac & Michael, 1981). Reliability coefficients may be determined through: (1) *test-retest reliability* is the correlation between two successive measurements with the same measurement instrument; (2) *alternative forms reliability* is the correlation between the successive measurement by two parallel forms of the same measurement instrument; (3) *split-half reliability* is the correlation between the successive measurement by two equivalent halves of the same measurement instrument; and (4) *interobserver and interrater reliability* is the independent and sometimes simultaneous measurement by two raters or observers using the same forms of a measurement instrument. The type of reliability assessed is determined by the mode of measurement. For example, test-retest reliability would be relevant for a self-administered questionnaire or for the measurement of blood pressure by the same rater (intrarater reliability), simultaneous and independent interobserver reliability would be appropriate for the direct measurement of health-related behaviors in a naturalistic setting, whereas interrater reliability would be utilized in the scoring of a standardized questionnaire.

### Validity

*Internal validity* addresses the issue of whether the treatment intervention was in fact responsible for the observed therapeutic effects, or whether these therapeutic effects were caused by external, extraneous variables not accounted for. These extraneous variables may include the maturation of the patient, patient selection biases, and other uncontrolled events occurring between subsequent measurements for therapeutic changes. *External validity* addresses the issue of whether the observed therapeutic effects are generalizable or relevant to other patient populations and settings and may be influenced by patient selection biases, the setting, and multiple-treatment effects.

Validity also indicates the degree to which a measurement instrument truly measures the factors under investigation. There are three major types of validity coefficients: (1) *content validity* refers to the degree to which the content (items) of the measurement instrument measures what it purports to measure, that is, do the measurement instrument items "look like" they measure the parameters of interest? (an example of *face validity*); (2) *construct validity* refers to the degree to which certain explanatory concepts or constructs (e.g., stress) account for performance on a measurement instrument and is a combination of both logical and empirical examination; and (3) *criterion-related validity* consists of both concurrent validity and predictive validity. *Concurrent validity* is assessed by correlating scores on a measurement instrument with external criteria known or believed to measure the target parameter (when uncertain about external criteria measurement validity, the correlation between a measurement instrument with another measure is termed *convergent validity*). *Predictive validity* refers to the degree to which a measurement correlates with a criterion parameter obtained in the future, that is, whether performance on the measurement instrument predicts a future criterion performance. The above forms of validity are only conceptually independent, and in practice a combination of them are used to increase the degree of validity (Isaac & Michael, 1981). The identification of possible risk factors (e.g., the contribution of type A behavior pattern, smoking, hypercholesterolemia, hypertension, stress, obesity, and physical inactivity to coronary heart disease) represents an example where content, construct, and criterion-related validity have all contributed to the development of a designated symptom complex potentially predictive of a premature myocardial infarction.

Finally, a recent consideration in the validation process has been termed *social validity* (Wolf, 1978). Wolf (1978) delineated three types of social validity: (1) The *social significance* of the goals, that is, are the selected treatment goals important to the patient and society?; (2) The *social appropriateness* of the treatment procedures in terms of the ethics, cost, and practicality of the intervention; and finally, (3) The *social importance* of the treatment effects or *patient satisfaction* with the therapeutic gains. In clinical research and practice, the issue of social validity will increasingly need to be considered an indispensable additional parameter in the evaluation of the effectiveness and relative efficacy of treatment programs (Forehand, Wells, & Griest, 1980; Kazdin, 1977).

# REFERENCES

Brook, R.H., Appel, F.A., Avery, C., Orman, M., & Stevenson, R.L. Effectiveness of inpatient follow-up care. *New England Journal of Medicine,* 1971, **285,** 1509–1514.

Dinsdale, S.M., Mossman, P.L., Gullickson, G., & Anderson, T.P. The problem-oriented medical record in rehabilitation. *Archives of Physical Medicine and Rehabilitation,* 1970, **51,** 488–492.

Forehand, R., Wells, K.C., & Griest, D.L. An examination of the social validity of a parent training program. *Behavior Therapy,* 1980, **11,** 488–502.

Fries, J.F. Time-oriented patient records and a computer databank. *Journal of the American Medical Association,* 1972, **222,** 1536–1542.

Fries, J.F., Spitz, P., Kraines, R.G., & Holman, H.R. Measurement of patient outcome in arthritis. *Arthritis and Rheumatism,* 1980, **23,** 137–145.

Granger, C.V., & Greer, D.S. Functional status measurement and medical rehabilitation outcomes. *Archives of Physical Medicine and Rehabilitation,* 1976, **57,** 103–109.

Greenfield, S., Nadler, M.A., Morgan, M.T., & Shine, K.I. The clinical investigation and management of chest pain in an emergency department: Quality assessment by criteria mapping. *Medical Care,* 1977, **15,** 898–905.

Greenfield, S., Solomon, N.E., Brook, R.H., & Davies-Avery, A. Development of outcome criteria and standards to assess the quality of care for patients with osteoarthrosis. *Journal of Chronic Diseases,* 1978, **31,** 375–388.

Hersen, M., & Barlow, D.H. *Single Case Experimental Designs: Strategies for Studying Behavior Change.* New York: Pergamon Press, 1976.

Isaac, S., & Michael, W.B. *Handbook in Research and Evaluation.* (2nd ed.) San Diego: Edits Publishers, 1981.

Kazdin, A.E. Assessing the clinical or applied importance of behavior change through social validation. *Behavior Modification,* 1977, **1**, 427–452.

Milhous, R.L. The problem-oriented medical records in rehabilitation management and training. *Archives of Physical Medicine and Rehabilitation,* 1972, **53**, 182–185.

Nobrega, F.T., Morrow, G.W., Smoldt, R.K., & Offord, K.P. Quality assessment in hypertension: Analysis of process and outcome methods. *New England Journal of Medicine,* 1977, **296**, 145–148.

Parcel, G.S., Gilman, S.C., Nader, P.R., & Bunce, H. A comparison of absentee rates of elementary school children with asthma and nonasthmatic schoolmates. *Pediatrics,* 1979, **64**, 878–888.

Pless, I.B., & Pinkerton, P. *Chronic Childhood Disorders: Promoting Patterns of Adjustment.* London: Henry Kimpton Publishers, 1975.

Reinstein, L., Stass, W.E., & Marguette, C.H. A rehabilitation evaluation system which complements the problem-oriented medical record. *Archives of Physical Medicine and Rehabilitation,* 1975, **56**, 396–399.

Reynolds, W.J., Rushing, W.A., & Miles, D.L. The validation of a function status index. *Journal of Health and Social Behavior,* 1974, **15**, 271–288.

Sheikh, K., Smith, D.S., Meade, T.W., Goldenberg, E., Brennan, P.J., & Kinsella, G. Repeatability and validity of a modified Activities of Daily Living (ADL) index in studies of chronic disability. *International Journal of Rehabilitation Medicine,* 1979, **1**, 51–58.

Varni, J.W., & Dietrich, S.L. Behavioral pediatrics: Toward a reconceptualization. *Behavioral Medicine Update,* 1981, **3**, 5–7.

Weed, L.L. Medical records that guide and teach. *New England Journal of Medicine,* 1968, **278**, 593–600, 652–657.

Weed, L.L. *Medical Records, Medical Education, and Patient Care: The Problem-Oriented Record as a Basic Tool.* Cleveland: Case Western Reserve University Press, 1969.

Wendland, C.J., & Crawford, C.C. *Team Delivery of Primary Health Care: A Training Manual for Teams in Community Ambulatory Health Centers.* Los Angeles, Department of Health Services, 1976.

Williamson, J.W. Evaluating quality of patient care: A strategy relating outcome and process assessment. *Journal of the American Medical Association,* 1971, **218**, 564–569.

Wolf, M.M. Social validity: The case for subjective measurement. *Journal of Applied Behavior Analysis,* 1978, **11**, 203–214.

# Part II

## Pain, Discomfort, and Stress Associated with Disease, Trauma, and Medical Procedures

# 4

# Acute and Chronic Pain

Pain in children represents a complex developmental process involving cognitive, emotional, motivation, neurochemical, sensory, socioenvironmental, and psychophysiological components that interact to produce differential pain perception and manifestation (see Varni, Katz, & Dash, 1982 for review). The term *pain* is derived from the Latin *poena*, which means punishment. *Pain* is an abstract concept that economically describes a multiplicity of sensations of various etiologies influenced by cultural and social factors (Fabrega & Tyma, 1976). The perception of pain as suffering or as punishment for a moral transgression differentiates it from the neurophysiologic detection of tissue damage (nociception) (Degenaar, 1979). Thus, the meaning of the pain experience adds a further dimension to the child's detection and expression of nociceptive impulses. For the young child in the preabstract stage of cognitive development, the term *pain* may be meaningless. Rather, nociceptive impulses may be perceived as punishment for a real or imagined transgression from societal and parental rules. Consequently, the cognitive developmental stage of the child and stage-related misconceptualizations must be considered when assessing and treating pediatric pain (see Chapter 2).

## BIOBEHAVIORAL ASSESSMENT

Varni et al. (1982) delineated four categories of pediatric pain: (1) pain associated with a disease state (e.g., hemophilia, arthritis, sickle cell anemia); (2) pain associated with an observable physical injury or trauma (e.g., burns, lacerations, fractures); (3) pain not associated with a well-defined or specific disease state or identifiable physical injury (e.g., recurrent abdominal pain syndrome, migraine and tension headaches); and (4) pain associated with medical/dental procedures (e.g., lumbar punctures, bone marrow aspirations, surgery, injections).

The assessment of pediatric pain requires an interdisciplinary, multidimensional, and comprehensive approach, combining self-report, behavioral, cognitive, socioenvironmental, medical, and biological parameters. Given the important modeling role parents and other significant adults play in the observational learning of pain responses by children (Craig, 1982; Varni et al., 1982), then the potential socioenvironmental influences on not only the verbal reports of pain intensity and location, but also such nonverbal expressions as facial grimaces, compensatory posturing, restricted movement, limping, and the absence of developmentally appropriate behaviors must also be considered in the assessment process. Such a comprehensive and multidimensional assessment process is absolutely mandatory prior to the application of any treatment regimen (Katz, Varni, & Jay, in press; Varni et al., 1982; Varni, Kellerman, & Dash, 1983).

## Acute versus Chronic Pain Assessment

There are a number of dimensions that can facilitate a differential assessment of acute versus chronic pain in the pediatric population, subsequently determining an appropriate treatment approach.

### Acute Pain

Acute pain functions as an adaptive biological warning signal, directing attention to an injury or disease, acting as a deterrent against harmful stimuli, and signaling the necessity for immobilization and protection of an injured area. A child's eventual avoidance of hot pavement when barefooted, a hot stove, or boiling water illustrates the adaptive function of acute pain. From a disease perspective, acute pain signals the need for an immediate diagnosis of the underlying pathological process causing the pain, such as acute internal hemorrhaging, which may result from a number of diseases and require immediate and appropriate therapy. However, in some cases of acute pain, the severe intensity of the painful stimulus may be disproportionate to its functional intent as a signaling stimulus. Although neurophysiological mechanisms may differentiate acute and chronic pain (Bonica, 1977; Dennis & Melzack, 1977), it is precisely the severe intensity of acute pain and its associated anxiety that may most parsimoniously distinguish acute and chronic pain (Varni, 1981a; Varni et al., 1982). Thus, the experience of pain contains two components—the original sensation and the emotional reaction to this noxious sensation (nociception). This reactive component in acute pain represents the fearful or anxious response that can modulate the pain sensation, and in acute pain often serves to intensify the reaction to noxious stimulation.

*Anxiety and Acute Pain.* Stress has been defined as a process in which environmental or psychological events, termed stressors, threaten an individual's safety and well-being, with the subsequent stress response accompanied by emotional symptoms such as anxiety, fear and tension, and/or an adaptive coping response (Baum, Grunberg & Singer, 1982). Marks (1981) has attempted to distinguish the terms *anxiety* and *fear* as separate emotions. From a practical standpoint, however, such a distinction may not have any real significance (Johnson & Melamed, 1979).

An attempt has also been made to distinguish the behavioral manifestations of anxiety and acute pain associated with a noxious medical procedure (Shacham & Dant, 1981). As Shacham and Dant (1981) correctly point out, the difficulty in distinguishing between anxiety and pain is the fact that both terms refer to constructs. Katz, Kellerman, and Siegel (1981) suggest that when referring to acute, clinically noxious situations, it may not be feasible to separate anxiety from acute pain, since anxiety is the basic affective state which appears to modulate acute pain perception. Given that both self-report and observational measures of anxiety and emotional reactions in children (e.g., Dearborn & Melamed, 1982; Glennon & Weisz, 1978; Melamed & Siegel, 1975; Spielberger, 1973) seem to overlap with acute pain measures, the suggestion by Katz et al. (1981) that the general term behavioral distress serves to encompass behaviors of negative affect, including anxiety, fear, and pain, appears warranted. However, when correlated with observational measures of behavioral distress, patient self-report data may distinguish between acute pain and anxiety (Katz, Kellerman, & Siegel, 1982). Clearly, this area of investigation requires more assessment research before a clinical distinction can be reliably and validly made.

From a treatment perspective, the behavioral treatment of pediatric anxiety has included *in vivo* and film modeling, *in vitro* and *in vivo* systematic desensitization (gradual hierarchical exposure to anxiety-evoking stimuli, from less to more anxiety eliciting situations, plus relaxation training to elicit a counteranxious response), contingency management, and coping skills training (see Barrios & Shigetomi, 1979, 1980; Graziano, DeGiovanni, & Garcia, 1979; Hatzenbuehler & Schroeder, 1978; Johnson & Melamed, 1979; Thelen, Fry, Fehrenbach, & Frautschi, 1979, for reviews). Studies utilizing *in vivo* systematic desensitization (Ultee, Griffioen, & Schellekens, 1982) and self-instructional training (Fox & Houston, 1981) in the treatment of anxiety-provoking situations suggest the potential compatibility of these anxiety treatment techniques with the overall management of acute pain secondary to noxious medical procedures. Further research on the multidimensionality of the acute pain response may clarify the utilization of anxiety reduction techniques as a component in the comprehensive management of acute pain, particularly acute pain secondary to noxious medical procedures.

*Chronic Pain*

In chronic pain, the fearful or anxious component is absent or greatly diminished as the child demonstrates an adaptive response to the initial acute experience, with the distinguishing reactive features of chronic pain characterized by chronic pain behaviors (e.g., compensatory posturing, restricted movement, limping, the absence of developmentally appropriate behaviors), depressed mood, or inactivity (Fordyce, 1976; Newburger & Sallan, 1981). These chronic pain reactions may become reinforced independently of the original nociceptive impulses and tissue damage and maintained by socioenvironmental influences (Varni, Bessman, Russo, & Cataldo, 1980). The potential for narcotic analgesic dependence becomes greater because of this chronicity, which only further maintains the pain reaction process (Fordyce, 1976; Varni & Gilbert, 1982). Eventually, chronic pain reactions may be emitted completely independent of the original organic pathology and persist even after the pathogenic factor has resolved (Bonica, 1977). This stands in marked contrast to the acute pain reaction, which appears to be more closely associated with the pathogenic factor or noxious stimulus. The distinctions between acute and chronic pain will become more evident when illustrated by the treatment descriptions in the following sections on acute and chronic pain management.

# BIOBEHAVIORAL TREATMENT

The primary biobehavioral treatment techniques utilized in the management of pediatric pain may be categorized into *pain perception regulation* modalities through such self-regulatory processes as guided imagery, meditation, and progressive muscle relaxation, and *pain behavior regulation* which identifies and modifies the socioenvironmental factors that may influence pain expression and rehabilitation (Varni et al., 1982). Self-regulatory processes are the primary treatment modality in the management of pediatric acute pain, whereas self-regulation of pain and pain behavior regulation are utilized in chronic pain syndromes, depending on the particular disorder and the existing socioenvironmental influences. The self-regulation techniques share common features with self-hypnosis, autogenic therapy, meditation, progressive muscle relaxation, and biofeedback training (Varni, 1981a). Laboratory research on experimental pain has indicated the role of distraction, dissociation or refocusing of attention from thoughts concerned with pain, anxiety reduction, suggestions of pain relief, and the imagination of past experiences that were incompatible with pain as potent cognitive variables in the reduction of pain perception (cf. Hilgard, 1975). On the other hand, the pain behavior regulation modality follows the socioenvironmental modification approach initially developed for adult chronic pain patients (cf. Fordyce, 1976). Although similar mechanisms may be operating in both pain perception regulation and pain behavior regulation (e.g., distraction from pain perception as the patient concentrates on emitting developmentally appropriate behaviors or increases in mobility and sleep as pain perception decreases), the focus of treatment has typically identified one or the other treatment modality as the primary management strategy. Following the four pain categories identified by Varni et al. (1982), the next four sections will present the current biobehavioral treatment approaches for pediatric pain.

## Pain Associated with a Disease State

### Chronic Arthritic Pain in Hemophilia

Hemophilia represents a congenital hereditary disorder of blood coagulation, characterized by recurrent, unpredictable internal bleeding episodes affecting any body part, especially the joints and extremities (see Chapter 9). Repeated hemorrhages into the joint areas (hemarthroses) eventually result in a condition similar to osteoarthritis, a chronic disease characterized by destruction of articular cartilage, pathological bone formation, and impaired function (Sokoloff, 1975). Chronic degenerative arthritis represents the most frequent problem confronting the physician who manages the care of adolescent and adult hemophiliacs, with an estimated 75 percent of hemophilic adolescents and adults demonstrating one or more affected joints (Dietrich, 1976). Anti-inflammatory drugs may be employed but are of limited usefulness, with analgesic abuse and dependency of constant concern (Varni & Gilbert, 1982).

Whereas acute pain in the hemophiliac is associated with a specific bleeding episode, chronic arthritic pain represents a substained condition over an extended period of time. Thus, pain perception in the hemophiliac truly represents a complex psychophysiological event, complicated by the existence of both acute bleeding pain and chronic arthritic pain, and requiring differential treatment strategies (Varni, 1981a, 1981b). More specifically, acute pain of hemorrhage provides a functional signal, indicating the necessity of intravenous infusion of factor replacement which temporarily replaces the missing clotting factor, converts the clotting status to normal, and allows a functional blood clot to form. Arthritic pain, on the other hand, represents a potentially debilitating chronic condition which may result in impaired life functioning and analgesic dependence (Varni & Gilbert, 1982). Consequently, the development of an effective alternative to analgesic abuse and dependency in the reduction of perceived chronic arthritic pain that does *not* interfere with the essential functional signal of acute bleeding pain has been the goal of the behavioral medicine approach to hemophilia pain management (Varni, 1981a, 1981b; Varni & Gilbert, 1982).

The treatment techniques were developed after an intensive preintervention survey with a number of hemophilic patients who experienced severe arthritic pain. All reported reduction in perceived arthritic pain associated with increased body warmth, as experienced during warm weather and hot showers. These findings were consistent with data from 30 patients with rheumatoid arthritis or osteoarthritis, with 27 of these patients reporting pain relief and increased range of motion in the involved joint associated with past experiences of warmth or massage (White, 1973). In the same study, application of a counterirritant (10% menthol and 15% methyl salicylate) produced a sensation of heat and active tissue hyperemia resulting in decreased pain perception and increased range of motion. A logical extrapolation of this information and the medical literature on arthritis management (cf. Swezey, 1978) subsequently resulted in the training of increased body temperature specific to the affected arthritic joints, with a thermal biofeedback instrument providing the physiological assessment of skin temperature over the targeted arthritic joint. It was further reasoned that increased body temperature specific to a joint area was a function of vasodilation that would not obfuscate the adaptive value of acute hemorrhage pain. Finally, the most severe and intense site of arthritic pain was targeted for initial intervention, with the rationale that other, less severe sites would covary accordingly within a functional, generalized, biophysiological response class. Data from the first two patients will be reported in detail (Varni, 1981b).

Radiographic examination for both patients revealed severe degenerative arthropathy in a number of joints. During the initial evaluation, each patient was instructed in self-monitoring techniques for the recording of pain episodes. A pain assessment instrument was empirically developed to facilitate self-recording (see Table 9.1). Thermal biofeedback assessment was available only for Patient 2, with his left ankle being the targeted joint for assessment, since he reported the most severe pain with this joint. The thermistor was placed on the site of greatest pain on his left ankle, with readings recorded on a minute-by-minute basis and averaged for each 15-minute trial. During baseline assessment, the patient was requested to close his eyes and imagine a neutral scene of his choice, such as a chair or table.

Following a multiple-baseline design across subjects, treatment was initially begun for Patient 1 after one week of baseline self-recording, and after 3 weeks of baseline self-recording for Patient 2 (see Figure 4.1). Since earlier findings by Wasserman, Oester, Oryshkevich, Montgomery, Poske, and Ruksha (1968) had demonstrated abnormal electromyographic readings in muscles adjacent to arthritic joints, relaxation techniques were included as an additional component in the treatment protocol. Thus, training in the self-regulation of arthritic pain consisted of three sequential phases:

1. A 25-step progressive muscle relaxation sequence involving the alternative tensing and relaxing of major muscle groups (see Table 4.1).

Table 4.1.    Progressive Muscle Relaxation and Meditative Breathing Exercises.

*Progressive Muscle Relaxation Exercises*

1. Take a medium deep breath through your nose and slowly exhale through your mouth.
2. Raise both arms straight out about half way above the couch and breathe normally. Then slowly return arms to the couch.
3. Hold arms out and make a tight fist. Slowly return to couch at count of 10.
4. Raise arms again, and bend fingers away from body. Return to couch at count of 10 and relax.
5. Bend arms at the elbow and tense biceps. Breathe normally, and keep hands loose. Relax hands and arms.
6. Take a medium deep breath and slowly exhale.
7. Wrinkle forehead as much as possible. Hold it, now relax and smooth out your forehead. Study the release of the muscle tension.
8. Squeeze eyes tight and breathe normally. Notice the tension. Relax.
9. Just lie there and relax. Try not to think of anything but the feelings of relaxation and tension release.
10. Open mouth as much as possible. Close mouth gently.
11. Tense lips together. Relax.
12. Bend your head slightly backward. Bring back slowly to natural position. Relax.
13. Bring head down almost to chest. Relax and let head return to natural resting position.
14. Turn head to right and tense neck. Relax and allow head to come back to its natural position.
15. Turn head to left and tense neck. Relax.
16. Arch shoulders back. Hold it. Make certain arms are relaxed. Now relax.
17. Hunch shoulders forward. Make certain to breathe normally and keep arms relaxed.
18. Arch the small of your back and simultaneously tighten your stomach muscles. Hold it. Relax. Take a medium deep breath and slowly exhale completely. Let your body fall onto the couch, completely relaxed.
19. Search upper part of body and actively relax any part that is tense by alternatively tensing and relaxing the muscles involved.
20. Maintaining the upper body relaxation, straighten and raise both legs slightly. Relax.
21. Now raise your legs and bend your feet back so that your toes point toward your face. Notice the tension in your thighs. Relax.
22. Raise your legs and bend your feet the other way, away from your body. Notice tension in calf muscles. Relax.
23. Curl toes downward. Relax.
24. Search your body for any signs of tension and actively relax, contracting and relaxing any tense muscles.
25. Take a medium deep breath, exhale slowly and completely. Now do the meditative breathing exercises.

*Meditative Breathing Exercises*

1. Inhale 10 medium deep breaths through your nose, slowly exhale each breath through your mouth.
2. Say the word *relax* silently to yourself as you exhale.
3. Picture the word *relax* as clearly as possible in your favorite colors.
4. Exhale slowly and completely each time, feeling more and more relaxed with each repetition.

2. Meditative breathing exercises, consisting of medium deep breaths inhaled through the nose and slowly exhaled through the mouth. While exhaling, the patient was instructed to say the word *relax* silently to himself and initially describe aloud and subsequently visualize the word in warm colors, as if written in color chalk on a blackboard.

3. Guided imagery training that was begun after the induction procedures in phases one and two were completed. Initially, the patient was instructed to imagine himself actually in a scene previously experienced as warm and pain free, not simply to observe himself there. The scene was evoked by a detailed multisensory description by the therapist and subsequently described aloud by the patient. Once the scene was clearly visualized by the patient, the therapist's suggestions included imagining the gentle flow of blood from the forehead down all the body parts to the ankle, images of warm colors such as red and orange, and the sensations of warm sand and sun on the involved joint. Further suggestions consisted of statements indicating reduction of pain as the joint progressively felt warmer and more comfortable.

As during baseline, the thermal biofeedback unit served as the physiological assessment device rather than as a training instrument, with the thermistor placed on the left ankle, and the patient instructed to actively attempt to increase the temperature at the joint site using the guided imagery techniques. The patients were also instructed to practice the techniques at home for a minimum of two daily 15-minute sessions and encouraged to individualize and actively explore new cognitive strategies in addition to imagining a warm, pleasant scene of their choice, as long as it involved thermal imagery.

Self-regulation training was clearly effective in significantly reducing the number of days of perceived chronic arthritic pain in both patients, maintained over an eight-month follow-up (Figure 4.1). Thermal control was demonstrated by Patient 2 as indicated by the physiological assessment on his left ankle via an intrasubject reversal design (Figure 4.2). Follow-up probes at six and eight months during guided imagery demonstrated an average increase of 5.6°F over initial baseline conditions, with a range of 84.3°F to 90.6°F, an increase of 6.3°F from lowest initial baseline to highest follow-up measure. Both patients reported that the thermal imagery techniques did *not* reduce their perception of acute bleeding pain.

A subsequent study by Varni (1981a) further supported the findings of this initial study. Varni (1981a) studied three additional hemophiliacs, documenting a decrease in arthritic pain perception and analgesic need without affecting bleeding pain perception and factor replacement requirements (see Chapter 9 for a detailed description of this study). Varni and Gilbert (1982) also applied these self-regulation techniques to a hemophiliac where long-term narcotic analgesic dependence was of primary concern, demonstrating clinically signi-

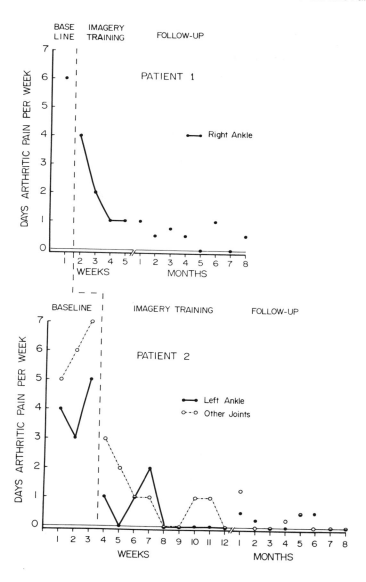

Fig. 4.1.    Days of arthritic pain per week during baseline, guided imagery training, and follow-up for both patients.

Source: Reprinted with permission from J.W. Varni. Behavioral medicine in hemophilia arthritic pain management: Two case studies. *Archives of Physical Medicine and Rehabilitation*, 1981, **62**, 183–187.

ficant changes in both arthritic pain and narcotic analgesic intake (see Figure 4.3 and Table 4.2). In this study, in addition to the pain self-regulation techniques, the patient was also instructed to restrict his analgesic intake to a time interval schedule rather than intake contingent on increasing pain perception or an aversive psychological state (boredom, stress, or depressed mood) and to gradually reduce analgesic intake with increasing success with pain self-regulation. This analgesic regimen of following a time contingent (by-the-clock) schedule and progressively decreasing doses has been previously suggested as the method of choice in deconditioning the relationship between narcotic analgesic dependence and chronic pain (cf. Fordyce, 1976). From a neurochemical perspective, this behavioral strategy may also be most effective in minimizing potential narcotic drug withdrawal side effects.

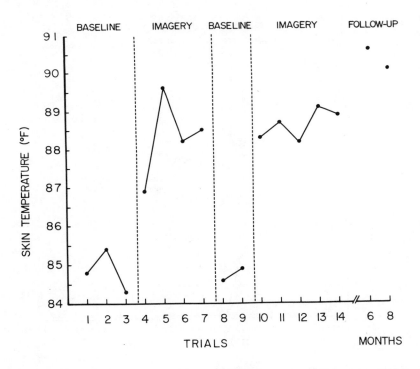

Fig. 4.2.   Skin temperature on patient 2's arthritic left ankle during thermal biofeedback assessment for baseline, guided imagery training, and follow-up conditions.

Source: Reprinted with permission from J.W. Varni. Behavioral medicine in hemophilia arthritic pain management: Two case studies. *Archives of Physical Medicine and Rehabilitation*, 1981, **62**, 183–187.

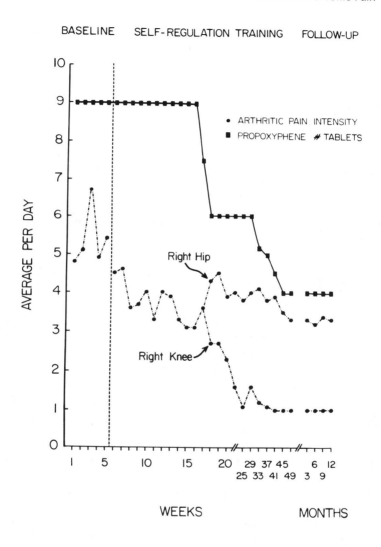

Fig. 4.3.    Daily average of arthritic pain intensity and the number of propoxyphene tablets consumed during baseline, self-regulation training, and follow-up.

Source: Reprinted with permission from J.W. Varni & A. Gilbert. Self-regulation of chronic arthritic pain and long-term analgesic dependence in a hemophiliac. *Rheumatology and Rehabilitation*, 1982, **21**, 171–174.

Table 4.2.    Subjective, Physiological, and Medical Parameters.

| Parameters | Pre | Post | FU |
|---|---|---|---|
| Arthritic pain intensity | | | |
| (1 = mild; 10 = severe) | 5.4 | 2.2 | 2.2 |
| Propoxyphene tablets | | | |
| (self-monitoring data/daily) | 9 (585 mg) | 4 (260 mg) | 4(260 mg) |
| Propoxyphene tablets | | | |
| (pharmacy records/monthly) | 270 (17550 mg) | | 118 (7670 mg) |
| Arthritic joint skin temperature (°F) | 85.0 | 88.5 | 88.2 |
| Stress/tension rating | | | |
| (1 = relaxed; 10 = stressed) | 5.3 | 2.5 | 2.6 |

Source: Reprinted with permission from J.W. Varni & A. Gilbert. Self-regulation of chronic arthritic pain and long-term analgesic dependence in a hemophiliac. *Rheumatology and Rehabilitation*, 1982, **21**, 171–174.

### Pain and Analgesia Management Complicated by Factor VIII Inhibitor in Hemophilia

The treatment of children with hemophilia has evidenced significant advances in recent years as a result of the development of factor replacement products, home infusion programs, and the opportunity for comprehensive care through regional hemophilia centers (Dietrich, 1976). Unfortunately, approximately 10 percent of hemophilic children develop an inhibitor to Factor VIII, presenting a serious problem in the management of bleeding episodes. Although the bleeding frequency is no different, the neutralization of Factor VIII replacement by an inhibitor (antibody) makes the control of bleeding ineffective. A recent advance in the treatment of hemophilic patients with inhibitors has been the use of prothrombin-complex concentrates (PCC), which effect some level of hemostasis through apparent activated by-products present in the reconstituted preparation. However, clinical reports have indicated the lack of complete effectiveness of these products (e.g., Parry & Bloom, 1978). The pain associated with uncontrolled hemorrhage can be extremely severe, with narcotic analgesics traditionally prescribed. Thus, although the acute pain of hemorrhage provides a functional signal indicating the necessity of factor replacement therapy, in the hemophilic child with Factor VIII inhibitor, the intensity of the pain supersedes its functional intent, and analgesic dependence is of constant concern. Consequently, an effective alternative to analgesic dependence in the reduction of perceived pain in the patient with an inhibitor has been greatly needed.

Varni, Gilbert, and Dietrich (1981) reported on a study involving a 9-year-old hemophilic child with Factor VIII inhibitor. At 4 years of age, when the inhibitor developed and subsequent Factor VIII replacement therapy became impossible, the patient began to require narcotics in order to tolerate the pain of each hemorrhage. Progressively, the need for pain medication increased for both bleeding pain and arthritic pain in his left knee secondary to degenerative arthropathy. Since the arthritic pain eventually occurred almost daily, the requests for analgesics further increased so that the acute pain of hemorrhage required ever larger doses for pain relief, even though home PCC therapy and joint immobilization continued for the management of bleeding episodes. As a consequence of bleeding and arthritic pain in the lower extremities, the patient was wheelchair bound nearly 50 percent of the time, hospitalized 16 times in the 4½-year period prior to the study for a total of 80 days after the development of the inhibitor, and analgesic medication was kept at his school for pain control. The final precipitating event in this steadily worsening cycle occurred during an evening visit to the emergency room because of a very painful and severe left knee hemorrhage which had not responded to home PCC therapy; the administration of an adult dose of meperidine and I.V. diazepam provided no pain relief.

Training in the self-regulation of pain perception consisted of techniques developed earlier by Varni (1981a, 1981b), with modification in the guided imagery techniques (pleasant, distracting imagery rather than thermal imagery) required for the bleeding pain intensity. The patient recorded the severity of his pain on a 10-point scale for a 2½-week baseline prior to self-regulation training. The average score for both arthritic and bleeding pain during this period was 7, indicating rather intense pain. At a 1-year follow-up after the initiation of the self-regulation training, the patient reported that both arthritic and bleeding pain were reduced to 2 on the scale when he engaged in the self-regulation techniques. In addition to this measure of pain perception, the patient's evaluation at the 1-year follow-up session on a comparative assessment inventory (see Table 9.2) indicated substantial positive changes in arthritic and bleeding pain, mobility, sleep, and general overall functioning. As seen in Table 4.3, once the patient began using the self-regulation techniques for pain management, there were no further requests for meperidine during the 1-year post-treatment assessment, with substantially decreased amounts of acetaminophen with codeine elixir required. Table 4.3 also shows that significant improvements in other areas of functioning, including improved mobility as evidenced by the physical therapy measures on his arthritic left knee in comparison with his normal right knee on the dimensions of range of motion ($0-150°$ = normal) and quadricep strength (1 = no joint motion, 5 = complete range of motion against gravity with full resistance). Normalization of psychosocial activities are suggested by increased school attendance, decreased hospitalizations, and parental report, which noted a distinct elevation of the child's overall mood, that he was considerably less depressed during pain episodes, since he had the skills to actively reduce his pain perception without depending on pain medication.

Table 4.3.    Parameters Associated with Pain Intensity.

| Parameters | 1-year pre-self-regulation training | 1-year post-self-regulation training |
|---|---|---|
| Pain intensity (1 = mild; 10 = severe) | 7 * | 2 ** |
| Meperidine | 74 tablets (50 mg/ea.) | 0 tablets |
| Acetaminophen/codeine elixir | 438 doses (24 mg codeine/dose) | 78 doses (24 mg codeine/dose) |
| Physical therapy measures | | |
| Range of motion | Normal r. knee 0°—150° Arthritic l. knee 15°—105° | R. knee 0°—150° L. knee 0°—140° |
| Quadricep strength (0—5 scale) | Normal r. knee 4— Arthritic l. knee 3 + | R. knee 4 + L. knee 4 |
| Girth (knee joint circumference) | Not available | R. knee 26 cm L. knee 25.8 cm |
| Ambulation on stairs | 2—3 maximum | No limitation |
| School days missed | 33 | 6 |
| Hospitalizations | | |
| Total days | 11 | 0 |
| Number admissions | 3 | 0 |

* 2.5-week preassessment during pain episodes just prior to self-regulation training.
** 1-year average rating during pain episodes when using self-regulation techniques.

Source: Reprinted with permission from J.W. Varni, A. Gilbert, & S.L. Dietrich. Behavioral medicine in pain and analgesia management for the hemophilic child with factor VIII inhibitor. *Pain*, 1981, **11**, 121–126.

The analysis of the various parameters assessed in this study suggests a significant improvement across a number of areas. As envisioned by the authors, a deteriorating cycle was evident prior to the intervention, schematically represented as: hemorrhage→pain→analgesics/joint immobilization→atrophy of muscles adjacent to the joints/joint deterioration→hemorrhage. Thus, as has been previously suggested (Dietrich, 1976), pain-induced immobilization results in muscle weakness surrounding the joints and sets the occasion for future hemorrhaging. By breaking this deteriorating cycle at the point of pain severity, the patient was offered the opportunity to decrease immobilization and increase therapeutic activities such as swimming, subsequently improving the strength and range of motion in his left knee. With this improved ambulatory status, school attendance and his general activity level were consequently increased. The possibility that this early intervention may have prevented or reduced the likelihood of later drug abuse must also be considered (Varni & Gilbert, 1982). Finally, it is important to reiterate that these procedures were used for a child with an inhibitor. For the hemophiliac without an inhibitor, bleeding pain serves a functional signal and is best managed with factor replacement therapy (see Chapter 9). However, in the present case, no effective medical procedure was available to control severe bleeding pain other than powerful narcotic analgesics, clearly an undesirable therapy modality for recurrent pain.

*Sickle Cell Anemia*

In general, patients with sickle cell anemia manifest a relatively healthy pattern, with periodic sickling crises which may be of sudden onset and occasionally fatal (Lehmann, Huntsman, Casey, Lang, Lorkin, & Comings, 1977). Infarctive or painful crises occur most frequently in the chest, abdomen, and bones. Within the sickle cell pain crisis, the course of events includes sickling, increased blood viscosity resulting in further vascular stasis, more sickling, with vascular obstruction possible, and subsequent infarction leading to tissue anoxia and tissue death, clinically manifested as pain (Lehmann et al., 1977). Thus, the painful crisis, which complicates a chronic hemolytic anemia and is the hallmark of sickle cell anemia, results from the vasoocclusion associated with rigid, tangled, sickled, or crescent-shaped erythrocytes. Environmental pathogenic factors that may induce vasoconstriction associated with sickling include cold climatic conditions, consumption of large quantities of ice water, and swimming. Prophylaxis of infarctive crises and management during crises require keeping the patient warm, administering oxygen, and, at times, transfusions of blood. The recurrent nature of the acute, painful vasoocclusive crises may result in analgesic dependence (Lehmann et al., 1977).

Since vasoconstriction represents a major component of the sickling crisis, therapy aimed at specifically producing vasodilation and associated warmth may have a therapeutic impact on the painful nature of the crisis. Such was the rationale for a study by Zeltzer, Dash, and Holland (1979), teaching self-hypnosis techniques. Specifically, the investigators employed eye fixation and progressive relaxation as the induction, leading to guided imagery techniques centering around a pleasant, pain-free scene, with suggestions of increased body warmth and vasodilation. A thermal biofeedback unit was used periodically to monitor peripheral temperature (the thermistor was placed on an index finger). Each patient was instructed to practice the techniques at the perceived onset of a sickling crisis. Zeltzer et al. (1979) anecdotally reported significant reductions over an 8-month follow-up on the frequency and intensity of pain crises as well as analgesic intake, with increased peripheral skin temperature observed during the utilization of guided imagery as measured by the thermal biofeedback unit. Of particular significance, a comparison of the hospital records 12 months preintervention and 8 months postintervention demonstrated marked reductions in pain-related outpatient visits and in the number and total days of hospitalizations.

*Reflex Sympathetic Dystrophy*

Reflex sympathetic dystrophy is a syndrome characterized by pain in an extremity and associated evidence of dysfunction of the autonomic nervous system; the signs and symptoms observed in the involved extremity include burning or aching pain, discoloration (cyanosis, plethora, or erythema), swelling and joint stiffness, hyperhydrosis, and altered sensation (hyperesthesia, hypesthesia, or paresthesia) (Bernstein, Singsen, Kent, Kornreich, King, Hicks, & Hanson, 1978; Fermaglich, 1977; Wettrell, Hallbook, & Hultquist, 1979). Treatment typically has involved a vigorous course of physical therapy (Bernstein et al., 1978).

Carron and associates (Richlin, Carron, Rowlingson, Sussman, Baugher, & Goldner, 1978; Stilz, Carron, & Sanders, 1977) have utilized transcutaneous nerve stimulation (TNS) (see Melzack, 1975, for review) in the management of pain in two young children diagnosed as evidencing reflex sympathetic dystrophy. Although pain was successfully reduced in both children subsequent to TNS, further empirical evaluation is needed.

## Pain Associated with Physical Injury

*Burns: Acute Pain Phase*

Severe pain complicates the treatment of acute severe burn injury, particularly during procedures such as wound debridement, dressing, and physical therapy (Klein & Charlton, 1980). Even with the appropriate utilization of such narcotic analgesics as morphine, meperidine, and codeine, and psychotropic drugs such as diazepam (Valium), most patients' pain is rated at least in the moderate range during debridement (Perry & Heidrich, 1982).

Muscle relaxation, deep breathing, and attention diversion have recently been successfully utilized to facilitate pain management in adult burn patients (Wernick, Jaremko, & Taylor, 1981). Wakeman and Kaplan (1978) worked with child, adolescent, and adult burn patients using progressive deep muscle relaxation suggestions, dissociations, pleasant scene imagery, and suggestions for pain control. Children and adolescents, aged 7 to 18 years old, required significantly less pain medication subsequent to self-hypnosis training when compared to both a medication-only control group and to adult burn patients receiving self-hypnosis training.

*Burns: Chronic Pain Phase*

An important consideration of the pediatric burn patient study to be described was the rationale developed for the treatment program which was essential in presenting the behavioral program to the medical and professional staff managing the child and enlisting their cooperation in implementing the program. The treatment rationale entailed the proposition that attending to pain complaints in attempts to comfort the child may not always be in the child's long-term best interest, but that demonstrations of affection, concern, and comfort may be rearranged to maximize rehabilitation and improve the child's psychological status by increasing the probability of "well" behaviors. Thus, the study was designed to test empirically the observation that pediatric chronic pain behaviors may be influenced by the child's social environment. The objectives of the investigation were to: (1) identify the influences of adult attention and demand situations on the emission of chronic pain behaviors, (2) devise a treatment strategy useful in decreasing chronic pain behaviors and increasing the child's rehabilitative or "well" behaviors, and (3) assess the practical efficacy of the procedures by training the nursing staff and the physical therapist to carry on the behavioral treatment.

The patient was a 3-year-old child who had been hospitalized for 10 months for the treatment of second and third degree burns to her buttocks, legs, and perineum as the result of immersion in hot water, with the circumstances surrounding the burn incident indicating the possibility of child abuse (Varni, Bessman, Russo, & Cataldo, 1980). The patient's development had been normal previous to the injury; afterward, however, skills were lost and further development was slightly delayed. Secondary complications to the burn condition included heart murmur, sepsis, and ulcerative lesions which required extensive intravenous therapy. Scar contractures and subsequent decreased range of motion in both knees made it necessary for the patient to wear Jobst stockings and knee extension splints to prevent contractures while undergoing a series of operations for plastic surgery. At the time of the initiation of the behavioral program, the patient was exhibiting an array of chronic pain behaviors which interfered significantly with her rehabilitation and constructive patient-caregiver interactions. Furthermore, these pain responses appeared to increase in both intensity and frequency in attention seeking and demand avoidance situations. Data were obtained in three different settings: (1) clinic room where the patient wore the knee extension splints in a contrived setting; (2) bedroom where the patient wore the splints in the natural hospital environment; and (3) physical therapy situation during which the physical therapist focused on improved range of motion and independent ambulation.

Three categories of chronic pain behaviors were recorded: (1) crying, which ranged in intensity from sobbing to screaming; (2) verbal pain behaviors, which consisted of such statements as "My leg/ankle/foot/stomach hurts," "Ouch," or "I can't stand up"; and (3) nonverbal pain behaviors consisting of any gestural response expressing pain or discomfort such as facial grimaces, rubbing her legs or buttocks, or not standing. In addition, a rehabilitative activity measure, number of steps descended, was measured in physical therapy, since it was essential for improving the child's range of motion and independent ambulation.

During the baseline assessment, it became evident that the child's pain behaviors were a function of adult attention and demand situations (see Figures 4.4 and 4.5). In the absence of adult presence, chronic pain behaviors were noticeably infrequent. In fact, the data for crying in the clinic no-adult-present condition are very similar to what occurs during programmed extinction; that is, the behavior initially occurred at a very high rate, gradually decreased, increased to a high rate, and then decreased to zero percent for the majority of the remaining sessions. Perhaps more importantly, it was observed that when engaged in interesting activities with accompanying staff attention for these appropriate behaviors, pain complaints were reciprocally low.

Specifically, two types of baseline sessions were conducted in the clinic. In one, an adult was present in the room with the child and interacted with her. These baseline sessions were arranged so as to be analogous to the contingencies occurring during the patient's naptime in her bedroom, which had been identified by the nursing staff as a time of high frequency pain occurrence. Thus, the adult's attention in this condition was contingent upon the occurrence of the patient's pain behaviors. In the clinic, the adult attended to the child's pain responses saying, "I'm sorry it hurts. Show me where it hurts," and other such comforting statements. In the other type of baseline sessions, no adult was present with the child. At the beginning of this condition, the adult would leave the room, saying, "I'll be back in a few minutes. Why don't you rest awhile?" The child would then remain alone in the room for 5 minutes. During baseline sessions in the child's bedroom just prior to naptime, no instructions were given to the nursing staff except that they should put on the patient's knee extension splints in the usual manner, and place the patient in her crib. Baseline sessions in the physical therapy setting during the demand condition consisted of placing the child on a small four-step wooden staircase and asking her to descend the steps. If she did not respond, the patient was prompted with such statements as, "It's time to start down the steps. Come on now." If she refused to stand by herself, the therapist helped her up and continued to encourage her. In the no-demand condition, the therapist simply played with the child with her favorite toy.

Since the baseline assessment demonstrated that the chronic pain behaviors were influenced by socioenvironmental factors, treatment focused on rearranging the existing contingencies. A combination of an intrasubject multiple-baseline design across settings and a reversal design was employed to determine the functional effects of the behavioral program on the patient's pain behaviors. Multiple baselines were begun simultaneously in all three settings, with treatment implemented first in the physical therapy department, while baseline assessment continued in the clinic and bedroom. Shortly afterward, treatment began in the clinic setting and subsequently in the bedroom. Brief reversals back to baseline conditions were conducted in the clinic and physical therapy setting to further test the significance of the intervention.

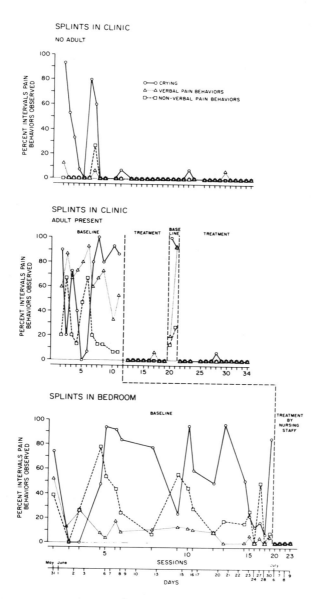

Fig. 4.4.    Percent of observation intervals in which chronic pain behaviors were noted in each of three situations.

Source: Reprinted with permission from J.W. Varni, C.A. Bessman, D.C. Russo, & M.F. Cataldo. Behavioral management of chronic pain in children: Case study. *Archives of Physical Medicine and Rehabilitation*, 1980, **61**, 375–379.

STEPS IN PHYSICAL THERAPY

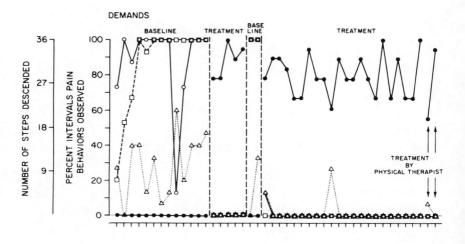

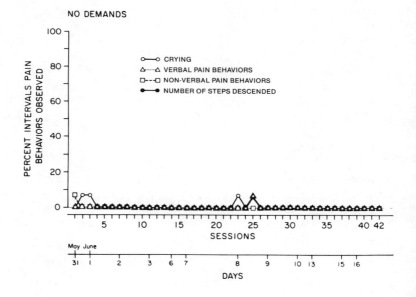

Fig. 4.5.   Number of steps descended and percent of observation intervals in which chronic pain behaviors were noted.

Source: Reprinted with permission from J.W. Varni, C.A. Bessman, D.C. Russo, & M.F. Cataldo. Behavioral management of chronic pain in children: Case study. *Archives of Physical Medicine and Rehabilitation*, 1980, **61**, 375–379.

In the clinic, treatment began with the adult verbalizing the following contingency to the child: "I'm going to put your splints on. If you don't cry, we can play for a while, and I'll give you some ice cream (cookies, etc.)." At the end of each minute in which no pain behaviors occurred, the adult reinforced the child with praise and a treat. Throughout the session, praise was given for periods of such "well" behaviors as helping to put on the splints, positive verbalizations, smiling, and the like, as well as the lack of pain behaviors (DRO schedule). Emission of pain behavior was placed on extinction (ignored), while the schedule of reinforcement was gradually changed so that the treat was offered at the end of the 5-minute session if no pain responses had been observed during that period (DRL schedule). At the beginning of treatment in the bedroom, the nursing staff was instructed to verbalize the contingency, "If you don't cry while I put your splints on, you can have some ice cream (cookies, etc.) when I'm finished." The nurse then placed the splints on the patient while giving praise for "well" behaviors, such as, "You're being so good. What a big girl you are. Don't you look nice." After the splints were secured, the nurse verbalized a second contingency: "If you don't cry during naptime, when you wake up you can have some more ice cream." The nurse then returned to her other duties, periodically checking for the emission of pain behaviors. At the end of the hour-long naptime, the nurse returned, praised the patient, and gave her a treat if no pain behaviors had occurred. Any pain responses made during naptime were ignored by the nursing staff, and no reinforcers were provided at the end of the hour. Finally, the treatment in physical therapy began with the therapist verbalizing the contingency to the child, "I want you to go down the steps by yourself. If you do, I'll give you an M&M." Praise was given continuously for each step taken, and any instance of pain behavior was ignored. The schedule of reinforcement was gradually changed so that the child was reinforced with a treat for descending the entire four-step sequence every third time, while social reinforcement continued on a continuous schedule.

The objective data on chronic pain and rehabilitative behaviors obtained throughout baseline and treatment conditions demonstrated the therapeutic effectiveness of the behavioral program (Figures 4.4 and 4.5). In addition, other clinically significant changes were observed. At the beginning of the study, the child's behaviors had severely disrupted her physical as well as emotional rehabilitation. Physical therapy was essentially terminated because of the patient's interfering pain behaviors. Two patterns emerged in her bedroom when the patient was placed in her crib with the knee extension splints on. First, the child would struggle until she had removed the splints, resulting in further contractures and the need for additional plastic surgery. Second, if she failed to remove the splints, her crying would intensify to the point of screaming. At times she would fall asleep exhausted and continue sobbing well into the naptime hour. Other times, she would continue screaming until the nursing staff removed her to a separate room for the remainder of the hour in consideration of the other children. Thus, pain behaviors during the pretreatment period resulted in the child being separated from the other children, interfering with the normalization and socialization processes important for a child with a history of prolonged hospitalization and suspected previous abuse. Following the behavioral intervention, a number of concomitant responses were noted. Whereas the child initially resisted splinting attempts, she subsequently began requesting to assist, saying, for example, "I'll do it. I want to help you." She began to make positive statements about her accomplishments instead of statements of pain and resistance to rehabilitation. Rather than seeking attention from her caregivers for pain behaviors, there was a shift to the utilization of "well" behaviors to attract social attention and praise.

Fordyce (1976), in his extensive work with adult chronic pain, has suggested that during periods of initial trauma and its resultant pain, the patient has many opportunities for the pairing of environmental stimuli to feelings of pain. Whether or not the subjective experience of pain abates over the course of time may be independent of the pain behaviors that the patient displays. While it is not possible to determine if the patient actually feels pain or simply displays the associated behaviors, in the present case no further pain displays were observed in the treatment environments after the onset of the behavioral program. As further suggested by Fordyce (1976), through learning the patient may actually come to experience pain in certain circumstances in excess of the accompanying physical basis for such pain, or even in the absence of a physical basis for perceived pain. In such cases, or in cases like the present one in which the pain behavior served the patient's immediate needs while hindering long-term rehabilitation, the behavioral program provides an essential component in the comprehensive management of pediatric chronic pain.

In acute cases, pain is an important symptom of underlying physical distress, requiring sympathy, empathy, and a detailed search for the sources of the pain and appropriate therapies. Continued expression of pain in chronic cases, however, may serve as a signal to closer investigate the conditions of the child's daily care and therapy environment. In pediatric chronic pain, therefore, attempts should be made not only to determine the possible underlying physical distress causing pain, but also the potential socioenvironmental influences on pain expression for the patient. Considerations should be given to the secondary gains of pain behavior, particularly if the result is to increase the attention of staff and to avoid rehabilitation. Such an analysis can serve as the basis for therapeutic strategies to decrease the use of pain expression as manipulative behavior.

As a cautionary note, it is essential to point out that this approach to chronic pain would not contraindicate empathy and concern expressed to the child by staff and parents, but would examine the extent of empathetic attention and its contingent relationship to chronic pain behaviors. Contingent empathy for all pain expression runs the risk of reinforcing and maintaining the pain expression to the detriment of the child. Care staff should delineate when and where contingencies for pain behavior are in the therapeutic interests of the patient. Particular situations where pain expression occurs should result in empathy, while others should result in alternative consequences including ignoring pain behavior and proving attention (and other reinforcers if necessary) for adhering to rehabilitation programs. Thus, as in the present case, the aim is not the total suppression of pain expression, since such communication often serves an essential personal and societal function, but rather the relatively greater expression of "well" behaviors in those situations where chronic pain behaviors interfere with the child's long-term rehabilitation and psychosocial adjustment. Such differential expression of emotion represents both a normal and adaptive developmental process.

## Pain Not Associated with Physical Injury or a Disease State

### Migraine and Tension Headaches

Pediatric headache represents an exemplary area demonstrating the necessity for an interdisciplinary assessment in determining the etiology and maintaining conditions of pain perception and pain complaints, and in subsequently selecting an appropriate treatment approach (Shinnar & D'Souza, 1981). For example, headache report may increase once the child discovers that this strategy successfully allows him or her to avoid aversive or negative school situations, such as an impending exam. What may develop is a self-perpetuating cycle whereby the child progressively falls further and further behind in school, subsequently setting the occasion for more negative school situations and resultant headache-avoidance behaviors. This does not imply that the child originally did not experience a headache or that her headaches do not continue to reoccur, but that the intensity and frequency of headache perception and complaint may be influenced by stress and other socioenvironmental factors. On the other hand, the chronic, recurrent headache complaint may be a symptom of a brain tumor or intracranial hemorrhage (Curless & Corrigan, 1976; Tomasi, 1979). Evidence of antecedent brain damage or brain dysfunction of possible etiological significance in pediatric recurrent headaches has ranged as high as 69 percent in one clinic sample (Millicap, 1978), whereas other investigators studying pediatric migraine and tension headaches point to socioenvironmental stress factors as the most frequent precipitating event (Bille, 1981; Brown, 1977; Moe, 1978; Shinnar & D'Souza, 1981).

Given the rather high prevalence rates of pediatric migraine and tension headaches [e.g., Deubner (1977), in studying a sample of 600 ten- to 20-year-olds, found that 22.1 percent of the girls and 15.5 percent of the boys reported migraine headaches], a successful biobehavioral treatment approach may impact on a significant number of children in pain.

Diamond (1979) described a three-stage pediatric migraine treatment program: (1) The first stage consisted of skin temperature biofeedback with autogenic phrases (e.g., suggestions of warmth and body heaviness/relaxation and guided imagery). The children were instructed to raise their hand temperature using the autogenic techniques, with feedback provided via a thermal biofeedback unit. (2) The second stage involved teaching the children progressive muscle relaxation exercises. (3) The third stage consisted of electromyographic (EMG) biofeedback, with surface electrodes placed across the frontalis muscle. Home practice sessions were encouraged, involving muscle relaxation and hand warming techniques learned during EMG and thermal biofeedback. Of 32 children under the age of 18 years diagnosed as having migraine headaches, 26 were reported to respond with good results, defined as a decrease in both the frequency and the severity of migraine headaches; three showed fair results, decreasing in either frequency or severity; two showed no response, and one patient was unavailable for follow-up.

Masek (1982) utilized a biobehavioral treatment package with 20 children, ages 6 to 12 years, diagnosed as demonstrating migraine headaches. A multiple-baseline across subjects design was used to evaluate the effectiveness of the program, with the children randomly assigned to one of four baseline conditions: 3, 6, 9, or 12 weeks of monitoring headache activity prior to starting treatment. Treatment consisted of frontalis EMG biofeedback training, meditative breathing, and behavioral management/parent training. Treatment effectiveness was determined by examining the daily headache diary, which provided data on headache frequency, duration of attacks, total hours of headache, intensity of pain, and medication usage. A total of 18 children experienced at least a 50 percent reduction in both total hours of headache per week and intensity of pain. A subsequent report by Fentress and Masek (1982) involved a controlled group design with children aged 8 to 12 years. The three groups were:

1. Treatment group receiving frontalis EMG biofeedback, meditative breathing training, and behavioral management/parent training;
2. Treatment group receiving the same treatment package as above, except without frontalis EMG biofeedback training and with the addition of progressive muscle relaxation training;
3. Waiting-list control group.

The results showed a statistically significant treatment effect for both treatment groups as compared to the control group on the measures: headache frequency, duration of attacks, total hours of headache, and intensity of pain. No effect was found for medication use, which was very low prior to biobehavioral treatment.

## Recurrent Abdominal Pain

Oster (1972) studied the prevalence rates of recurrent abdominal pain, headache, and limb pains in an 8-year longitudinal study of 18,162 school-age children and adolescents between 6 and 19 years of age. The prevalence of recurrent headaches was 20.6 percent; recurrent abdominal pain, 14.4 percent; and recurrent limb or "growing" pain, 15.5 percent, with a higher prevalence in all three categories of pain for girls than for boys. From a prognostic perspective, Christensen and Mortensen (1975) conducted a 28-year follow-up investigation of 34 patients who were initially diagnosed during childhood as evidencing recurrent abdominal pain (RAP) in comparison to a control group without childhood RAP. The average age of the clinical and control populations at follow-up was 35.9 and 36.4 years, respectively. At follow-up, 53 percent of the clinical group reported gastrointestinal pain consistent with a diagnosis of irritable colon syndrome, peptic ulcer/gastritis, and duodenal ulcer, as well as milder symptoms such as diarrhea, constipation, and meteorism (abdominal or intestinal distension by gas). Eighty-nine percent of the clinical group reported that these symptoms were provoked by stress. In contrast, only 29 percent of the control group reported gastrointestinal pain as adults. Nongastrointestinal pain symptoms were also more frequent among the clinical patients (32 percent) than among the controls (13 percent), with such complaints as migraine and tension headaches, back pain, and gynecological pain. There were no differences between the clinical and control groups in the incidence of abdominal pain in their children (average age, 8.5 and 9.3 years, respectively). However, in combining the two groups, 28 percent of those children whose parents were complaining of abdominal pain at the time of the follow-up evidenced RAP, whereas only 7 percent of those children whose parents had no abdominal pain at follow-up reported RAP.

Although pediatric chronic, recurrent abdominal pain may be a symptom of a spinal cord tumor (Buck & Bodensteiner, 1981; Eeg-Olofsson, Carlsson, & Jeppsson, 1982), chronic intermittent volvulus (Janik & Ein, 1979), lactose or sorbitol malabsorption (Hyams, 1982; Lebenthal, Rossi, Nord, & Branski, 1981; Wald, Chandra, Fisher, Gartner, & Zitelli, 1982), only an estimated 5 percent of childhood RAP has an organic etiology (Maddison, 1977).

Further, when compared to children not evidencing RAP, childhood RAP patients do *not* show a significant differential biobehavioral response to an acute laboratory induced stress (cold pressor stimulus) on autonomic (peripheral vasomotor and heart rate), somatic (forearm EMG), subjective (pain intensity and distress), and behavioral (facial expression) responses when recorded during baseline, stressor and recovery periods (Feuerstein, Barr, Francoeur, Houle, & Rafman, 1982). Rather, a high frequency of such potential socioenvironmental factors as emotional stress, parental abdominal pain complaints, and recurrent school absences have been implicated as causal factors of childhood RAP (Berger, Honig, & Liebman, 1977; Michener, 1981).

Significantly, in a long-term follow-up study of 161 children with RAP, approximately 20 percent underwent surgical or medical treatments of doubtful necessity: that is, no organic cause was evident (Stickler & Murphy, 1979). Thus, as in pediatric headache, an extensive interdisciplinary and comprehensive assessment is mandated prior to any intervention program.

The biobehavioral treatment of pediatric recurrent abdominal pain is relatively unexplored thus far. Sank and Biglan (1974) worked with a 10-year-old boy with a 2½-year history of recurrent abdominal pain. The child complained of severe pain episodes in the central abdominal region usually lasting 5 to 20 minutes, but occasionally as long as several hours. Abdominal pain episodes occurred at least once a day. Additionally, the patient reported at least a low level of abdominal pain at all times. Prior to the behavioral intervention, the child was absent 45 of the previous 72 school days (37.5 percent attendance rate). Typically, when the child reported a severe pain episode, his mother would give him aspirin or Maalox, take his temperature, stay with him, and often give him back rubs in an attempt to soothe him. On the days he stayed home from school because of pain, the child was allowed to read, watch television, and get out of bed when he felt better. His mother remained at home with him on these occasions, restricting her activities outside the home.

During a 7-day baseline, the patient recorded the frequency and duration of all severe pain episodes, and rated the intensity of total abdominal pain every half hour on a 10-point scale (1 = no pain, 10 = the most severe pain ever experienced). School attendance was also recorded. After baseline, a shaping program was established for the reinforcement of: (1) the gradual decrease in the frequency of severe pain episodes, (2) the gradual decrease in abdominal pain ratings below systematically lower criteria, and (3) a gradual increase in school attendance. Initially, the child received a point for every half day in which he had no severe pain episodes and an average pain rating below 5.5 (a level just below his mean baseline rating). As treatment progressed the criterion for pain ratings was gradually reduced to 3.5. Additionally, a point was given for every half day of school attendance, but he could not attend school unless he was below the pain rating criterion and had no severe pain episodes just prior to going to school. Each point was immediately exchanged for a nickel, which could then be later exchanged for items on a reinforcement list of favorite meals, toys, books, and family outings. When the child reported severe abdominal pain, he had to stay in bed for the rest of that half day. Although he could read school books, he was not allowed to read other materials, listen to the radio, or watch television. Gradually, the criteria for both the days of school attendance and the days without severe pain episodes were increased so that reinforcement (points) were provided for longer periods of "well" behavior. This reinforcement and shaping program resulted in no severe pain episodes during the last 15 weeks of treatment, daily pain ratings at 3.0, with school attendance increasing to 92 days out of the subsequent 107 post-treatment school days (86 percent attendance rate).

Miller and Kratochwill (1979) utilized a multiple-baseline design across home and school settings in the treatment of a 10-year-old girl with recurrent abdominal pain. The child described a vague dull pain in the epigastric and umbilical regions which had been recurrent for over a year. Each pain episode lasted from a few minutes to an hour. The child averaged approximately 1.5 pain episodes per day in spite of a 6-month course of Donnatal (a belladonna and phenobarbital elixir). When the child reported abdominal pain, her mother kept her home from school, resulting in frequent school absences. Additionally, when the child complained of abdominal pain, her mother would give her Donnatal and have her lie down, during which time the child would watch television, read, or play with toys. Food, drinks, and social attention were also provided on demand. Pain episodes did not occur when the child was asleep or when she was involved in play activities.

Within the multiple-baseline design across settings, the treatment program was initiated first in the home environment and subsequently in the school. When the child reported abdominal pain at home, she was placed in her room to "rest," with the curtains drawn, the light turned on, and the door almost closed (a contingent time-out procedure). She was allowed one or two books, but no television, toys, or games. Food was made available only during regular meal times. Regardless of when the abdominal pain episode occurred, the child was required to rest for the remainder of that day in her room. Subsequent treatment in the school setting also utilized a time-out procedure. After a gradual reduction in abdominal pain complaints during treatment, no abdominal pain complaints occurred during a one-year follow-up.

## Pain and Anxiety Associated with Medical and Dental Procedures

Even routine well-child examinations may be a source of distress for children, influenced by developmental factors, clinician behavior, and mother-child interactions (Heffernan & Azarnoff, 1971; Hyson, Snyder, & Andujar, 1982; Shaw & Routh, 1982). Although a preventive approach based on modeling in the school setting has been encouraging in reducing medical fears in a general pediatric population (Roberts, Wurtele, Boone, Ginther, & Elkins, 1981), intervention approaches with clinical populations have emphasized procedural and sensory information regarding the medical procedure (e.g., Johnson, Kirchhoff, & Endress, 1975) and relaxation/guided imagery training (e.g., Kohen, 1980).

### Injections

In an epidemiological study of common fears and phobias, Agras, Sylvester and Oliveau (1969) found a prevalence rate of 140 per 1000 of the general population at age 20 who reported injection phobias (phobia being defined as an irrational and/or disproportionate fear response). Field (1981) suggests that for children, the child's perception of an injection as a punishment must be taken into consideration when giving an injection. Fernald and Corry (1981) found that an empathic preparation that was supportive and child centered, and described the sensations, pain, fears, and crying that might occur during the injection, produced less crying, more cooperation, and fewer negative reactions than a directive preparation where the child was informed of the procedures that would occur but was told to be big, brave, not cry, and sit still. In the empathic preparation, the child was told, "I'm not doing this because you did anything wrong but just to help you get well." Further statements included, "You're probably feeling a little scared and it is going to hurt a little bit, but it won't last long. I don't mind if you cry because that's only natural." The directive preparation included statements such as, "I want you to stay still and not move because if you jerk your arm or flex, I may have to stick you again."

While the empathic preparation method appears to be a reasonable component in reducing children's anxiety associated with receiving injections, it does not directly teach the child a coping skill. *In vivo* systematic desensitization, combining relaxation training, modeling, and behavioral rehearsal, has been successfully utilized with adult patients with high levels of anxiety associated with injections (Ferguson, Taylor, & Wermuth, 1978; Kolko & Milan, 1980; Nimmer & Kapp, 1974; Taylor, Ferguson, & Wermuth, 1977; Turnage & Logan, 1974).

Ferguson, Taylor, and Wermuth (Ferguson et al., 1978; Taylor et al., 1977) described two adult patients with needle phobia, treated with a participant modeling approach consisting of the following components:

1. Instructions on the desensitization procedure and information about the fear object or situation which demonstrates that the fear is unfounded;
2. Response modeling where the clinician handles the feared object and interacts with it in a way that demonstrates that the patient's fear is unfounded;
3. Joint performance with the clinician, where the patient is encouraged to handle the fear object or enter the fear situation in a gradual, step-by-step fashion, starting with the least anxiety-provoking components;
4. Self-directed practice, where the patient is instructed to interact on her own with the fear objective or in the fear situation.

The participant modeling approach resulted in the successful treatment of both adult patients with severe needle phobia. Similar success with systematic desensitization and information on the irrationality of the fear response has been reported with other adult patients (Kolko & Milan, 1980; Nimmer & Kapp, 1974; Turnage & Logan, 1974).

With children, pleasant scene imagery, participant modeling, and *in vivo* systematic desensitization have been reported in nondata-based papers as a counteranxious response to needle phobias (Ayer, 1973; Dash, 1981; Katz, 1974). The empirical evaluation of these techniques with children who exhibit intense fear associated with injection and injection paraphernalia still needs to be conducted.

## Bone Marrow Aspirations and Lumbar Punctures

Conditioned anxiety in response to recurrent, painful medical procedures such as bone marrow aspirations, lumbar punctures, and venipunctures occurs frequently in childhood cancer patients (Jay, Ozolins, Elliott, & Caldwell, in press; Kellerman & Varni, 1982) (see Chapter 9). Katz et al. (1980) studied 115 children with cancer undergoing bone marrow aspirations in order to develop a reliable and valid measurement scale of behavioral distress. Given the difficulty in distinguishing between anxiety and acute pain since these terms refer to constructs, then behavioral distress has been defined as a general term encompassing behaviors of negative affect, including anxiety, fear, and acute pain (Katz et al., 1981). Katz et al. (1980) found that behavioral distress (e.g., crying, clinging, screaming, verbal statements of pain or fear) in response to bone marrow aspirations was virtually ubiquitous and did not habituate in the children studied, clearly suggesting the need for clinical intervention.

Ellenberg, Kellerman, Dash, Higgins, and Zeltzer (1980) worked with an adolescent girl with leukemia who manifested considerable behavioral distress to bone marrow aspirations. The patient received training in self-hypnosis which resulted in a significant decrease in self-reported pain and anxiety before, during, and after the procedure. A subsequent study by Kellerman, Zeltzer, Ellenberg, and Dash (1982) extended this intervention to a group of 16 adolescents with leukemia undergoing bone marrow aspirations and lumbar punctures, demonstrating significant reductions in both their self-reported anxiety and discomfort. Jay, Elliott, Ozolins, and Olson (1982) also reported the beneficial effects of a treatment package consisting of breathing exercises, imagery, filmed modeling, behavioral rehearsal, and reinforcement in reducing distress secondary to these medical procedures.

## Dental Procedures

The assessment of children's anxiety during dental procedures has included subjective, behavioral, and physiological measures. Venham, Bengston, and Cipes (1977) assessed the child's response to each dental visit using a combination of four measures: heart rate, rating scales of anxiety and uncooperative behavior, and a picture test (a projective self-report measure of anxiety). Each child had six dental visits: an examination visit, four visits involving restorative treatment, and a final visit to polish the restorations (fillings), clean the teeth, and apply topical fluoride. Each visit was divided into three periods corresponding to specific dental procedures. The three periods during the examination and polish visits were the mirror and explorer examination, the prophylaxis, and the application of topical fluoride. Dental treatment visits were divided into the mirror and explorer examination, the administration of local anesthesia, and the cavity preparation using the dental handpieces. The results showed no significant differences over the six visits on the pictures test; however, on the measures of anxiety and uncooperative behavior ratings and heart rate, it appeared that the children became increasingly anxious and uncooperative over the first four visits and then became increasingly more relaxed and cooperative over the fifth and sixth visits, suggesting unplanned or unsystematic *in vivo* (naturalistic exposure) desensitization to the dental stress. A subsequent study by Venham, Gaulin-Kremer, Munster, Bengston-Audia, and Cohan (1980) further documented the reliability and validity of the 6-point anxiety and uncooperative behavior rating scales, ranging from 0 (relaxed, smiling, willing and able to converse) to 5 (child out of contact with the reality of the threat; general loud crying, unable to listen to verbal communication, makes no effort to cope with threat; actively involved in escape behavior; physical restraint required) on the anxiety rating scale, and from 0 (total cooperation, best possible working conditions, no crying or physical protest) to 5 (general protest, no compliance or cooperation; physical restraint is required) on the uncooperative behavior rating scale.

Sheskin, Klein, and Lowental (1982) attempted to assess children's dental anxiety using a projective drawing test. The child was instructed to make a drawing of himself, the dentist, and the dental situation. The child received a standard sheet of white paper and six color pencils. The drawings were scored within two categories, 0 (no anxiety) and 1 (anxiety), along the dimensions: depicting the treatment situation, juxtaposition of the child's size as compared with the dentist's, drawing of the dentist, number of colors used, omission of parts of the body, and depicting dental instruments. The level of anxiety of each child's drawing was the sum of the score on the six dimensions (0 to 6 possible total). Additionally, the behavior of the children during dental treatment was scored using the Frankl Behavior Rating Scale. The correlation between the projective test and the behavior ratings was − 0.67, suggesting that the higher the anxiety score of the drawings, the lower the child's rated cooperation during the dental procedure.

Finally, Lindsay and Roberts (1980) developed a behavior checklist of children's obstructive behaviors during dental procedures, consisting of an interval recording of such behaviors as: choking/coughing, verbal complaints, stops/won't allow treatment, cries out at injection, strikes out with arms/legs, pushes away dentist, and restless. An estimate of the child's average amount of apprehensiveness was scored on a 10 cm visual analogue scale. Interobserver reliability coefficients were 0.94 for the ratings of the child's apprehensiveness and 0.86 for the mean number of obstructive activities per minute, indicating that both measures were characterized by high reliability.

In regard to intervention techniques for the management of children's anxiety during dental procedures, children cite extractions, restorative work, and the anesthetic injection as the most anxiety-provoking (Morgan, Wright, Ingersoll, & Seime, 1980). The primary anxiety reduction techniques utilized for children in dental situations have included components of filmed modeling, relaxation, and coping skills training. Melamed, Weinstein, Hawes, and Katin-Borland (1975) found the filmed modeling of a child successfully coping with a dental procedure as an effective preparation for children having no prior experience with the actual dental setting (see Chapter 5 for additional descriptions of filmed modeling as a preparation for surgery).

Parkin (1981) attempted to induce relaxation and refocusing of attention (distraction) in children as an anxiety reduction procedure using ambient music consisting of light orchestral popular music with slow, soothing rhythms. Ratings by observers of silent videotapes of the children on a visual analogue scale suggested that the children were less anxious when the music was playing.

The direct training in relaxation skills is most likely required for highly anxious dental patients. Lamb and Strand (1980) employed a brief audiotaped recording of standard progressive muscle relaxation exercises as a counteranxious response training procedure for patients undergoing dental treatment (cleaning, filling, or extraction), finding a significant decrease on a measure of state anxiety (see Spielberger, Gorsuch, & Lushene, 1970). Morse, Schacterle, Esposito, Furst, and Bose (1981) found that hypnosis in combination with local anesthesia was more effective than local anesthesia alone in endodontic patients as manifested by lower patient ratings on a dental anxiety questionnaire, increased salivary volume, increased salivary translucency, reduced salivary protein, and increased salivary pH.

Siegel and Peterson (1980, 1981) found that teaching specific coping skills and/or providing sensory information about the dental experience were both effective in reducing children's anxiety during dental treatment as manifested by lower levels of disruptive and uncooperative behaviors, lower ratings of anxiety and discomfort, and lower levels of physiological arousal (radial pulse rate). The children were taught to use several coping techniques in a 30-minute session prior to the dental treatment (anesthetic injection and restoration), consisting of relaxation, distracting (pleasant) imagery, and calming self-instructions. The sensory information provided the children included what to expect at the dentist's office, such as the sights, sounds, and sensations of the dental procedure; they also heard tape-recorded sounds of the dental equipment, such as the drill (this may be considered a form of *in vitro* desensitization).

Finally, Nocella and Kaplan (1982) studied 30 children between the ages of 5 and 13 years with prior dental experience. The majority of the children were scheduled for restorations, and the rest were scheduled for extractions or a combination of restorations and extractions. The children were randomly assigned to either a cognitive-behavioral (coping skills) group, an attention-control group, or a no-treatment control group. The children receiving the cognitive-behavioral treatment were taught a combination of coping strategies, including the identification of stimuli (events) which might evoke anxiety, deep breathing exercises, muscle relaxation, and positive self-instructions (e.g., "If I get scared or worried I tell myself to 'relax' and I let myself relax my whole body; I tell myself, this is a good dentist, I'm doing good, I can handle this, I'm doing terrific."). Additionally, the children were instructed to imagine their pending visit to the dentist utilizing their positive self-statements, deep breathing exercises, and the word "relax" to facilitate coping with procedural anxiety (*in vitro* desensitization). The cognitive-behavioral training session required only 15 minutes prior to the dental treatment. During the dental procedure, the children's behavior was recorded on a behavior checklist consisting of: facial grimaces, restlessness, moving arms and/or legs, sitting up, gripping chair, and verbalizations. The results demonstrated that the cognitive-behavioral treatment group evidenced significantly fewer disruptive behaviors during the dental procedures in comparison to both control groups.

# REFERENCES

Agras, S., Sylvester, D., & Oliveau, D. The epidemiology of common fears and phobias. *Comprehensive Psychiatry*, 1969, **10**, 151–156.

Ayer, W.A. Use of visual imagery in needle phobic children. *Journal of Dentistry for Children*, 1973, **40**, 41–43.

Barrios, B.A., & Shigetomi, C.C. Coping skills training: Potential for prevention of fears and anxieties. *Behavior Therapy*, 1980, **11**, 431–439.

Barrios, B.A., & Shigetomi, C.C. Coping-skills training for the management of anxiety: A critical review. *Behavior Therapy*, 1979, **10**, 491–522.

Baum, A., Grunberg, N.E., & Singer, J.E. The use of psychological and neuroendocrinological measures in the study of stress. *Health Psychology*, 1982, **1**, 217–236.

Berger, H.G., Honig, P.J., & Liebman, R. Recurrent abdominal pain: Gaining control of the symptom. *American Journal of Diseases of Children*, 1977, **131**, 1340–1344.

Bernstein, B.H., Singsen, B.H., Kent, J.T., Kornreich, H., King, K., Hicks, R., & Hanson, V. Reflex neurovascular dystrophy in childhood. *Journal of Pediatrics*, 1978, **93**, 211–215.

Bille, B. Migraine in childhood and its prognosis. *Cephalalgia*, 1981, **1**, 71–75.

Bonica, J.J. Neurophysiologic and pathologic aspects of acute and chronic pain. *Archives of Surgery*, 1977, **112**, 750–761.

Brown, J.K. Migraine and migraine equivalents in children. *Developmental Medicine and Child Neurology*, 1977, **19**, 683–692.

Buck, E.D., & Bodensteiner, J. Thoracic cord tumor appearing as recurrent abdominal pain. *American Journal of Diseases of Children*, 1981, **135**, 574–575.

Christensen, M.F., & Mortensen, O. Long-term prognosis in children with recurrent abdominal pain. *Archives of Diseases in Childhood*, 1975, **50**, 110–114.

Craig, K.D. Modeling and social learning factors in chronic pain. In J.J. Bonica, U. Lindblom, & A. Iggo (Eds.), *Advances in Pain Research and Therapy*. Vol. 5. New York: Raven Press, 1982.

Curless, R.G., & Corrigan, J.J. Headache in classical hemophilia: The risk of diagnostic procedures. *Child's Brain*, 1976, **2**, 187–194.

Dash, J. Rapid hypno-behavioral treatment of a needle phobia in a five-year-old cardiac patient. *Journal of Pediatric Psychology*, 1981, **6**, 34–42.

Dearborn, M.J., & Melamed, B.G. *The Self-Assessment Mannequin as a Measure of Emotional Reactions in Children*. Unpublished manuscript, 1982.

Degenaar, J.J. Some philosophical considerations on pain. *Pain*, 1979, **7**, 281–304.

Dennis, S.G., & Melzack, R. Pain-signalling systems in the dorsal and ventral spinal cord. *Pain*, 1977, **4**, 97–132.

Deubner, D.C. An epidemiologic study of migraine and headache in 10–20 year olds. *Headache*, 1977, **17**, 173–180.

Diamond, S. Biofeedback and headache. *Headache*, 1979, **19**, 180–184.

Dietrich, S.L. Medical management of hemophilia. In D.C. Boone (Ed.), *Comprehensive Management of Hemophilia*. Philadelphia: F.A. Davis, 1976.

Eeg-Olofsson, O., Carlsson, E., & Jeppsson, S. Recurrent abominal pains as the first symptom of a spinal cord tumor. *Acta Paediatrica Scandinavica*, 1981, **70**, 595–597.

Ellenberg, L., Kellerman, J., Dash, J., Higgins, G., & Zeltzer, L. Use of hypnosis for multiple symptoms in an adolescent girl with leukemia. *Journal of Adolescent Health Care*, 1980, **2**, 132–136.

Fabrega, H., & Tyma, S. Language and cultural influences in the description of pain. *British Journal of Medical Psychology*, 1976, **49**, 349–371.

Fentress, D., & Masek, B. Behavioral treatment of pediatric migraine. Paper presented at the Annual Meeting of the Association for Advancement of Behavior Therapy, Los Angeles, November 1982.

Ferguson, J.M., Taylor, C.B., & Wermuth, B. A rapid behavioral treatment for needle phobias. *Journal of Nervous and Mental Disease*, 1978, **166**, 294–298.

Fermaglich, D.R. Reflex sympathetic dystrophy in children. *Pediatrics*, 1977, **60**, 881–883.

Fernald, C.D., & Corry, J.J. Empathic versus directive preparation of children for needles. *Children's Health Care*, 1981, **10**, 44–47.

Feuerstein, M., Barr, R.G., Francoeur, T.E., Houle, M., & Rafman, S. Potential biobehavioral mechanisms of recurrent abdominal pain in children. *Pain*, 1982, **13**, 287–298.

Field, P.A. A phenomenological look at giving an injection. *Journal of Advanced Nursing*, 1981, **6**, 291–296.

Fordyce, W.E. *Behavioral Methods for Chronic Pain and Illness*. St. Louis: Mosby, 1976.

Fox, J.E., & Houston, B.K. Efficacy of self-instructional training for reducing children's anxiety in an evaluative situation. *Behaviour Research and Therapy*, 1981, **19**, 509–515.

Glennon, B., & Weisz, J.R. An observational approach to the assessment of anxiety in young children. *Journal of Consulting and Clinical Psychology*, 1978, **46**, 1246–1257.

Graziano, A.M., DeGiovanni, I.S., & Garcia, K.A. Behavioral treatment of children's fears: A review. *Psychological Bulletin*, 1979, **86**, 831–844.

Hatzenbuehler, L.C., & Schroeder, H.E. Desensitization procedures in the treatment of childhood disorders. *Psychological Bulletin*, 1978, **85**, 831–844.

Heffernan, M., & Azarnoff, P. Factors in reducing children's anxiety about clinic visits. *HSMHA Health Reports*, 1971, **86**, 1131–1135.

Hilgard, E.R. The alleviation of pain by hypnosis. *Pain*, 1975, **1**, 213–231.

Hyams, J.S. Chronic abdominal pain caused by sorbitol malabsorption. *Journal of Pediatrics*, 1982, **100**, 772–773.

Hyson, M.C., Snyder, S.S., & Andujar, E.M. Helping children cope with checkups: How good is the "good patient?" *Children's Health Care*, 1982, **10**, 139–144.

Janik, J.S., & Ein, S.H. Normal intestinal rotation with non-fixation: A cause of chronic abdominal pain. *Journal of Pediatric Surgery*, 1979, **14**, 670–674.

Jay, S.M., Elliott, C.H., Ozolins, M., & Olson, R.A. Behavioral management of children's distress during painful medical procedures. Paper presented at the Annual Meeting of the American Psychological Association, Washington, D.C., August 1982.

Jay, S.M., Ozolins, M., Elliott, C.H., & Caldwell, S. Assessment of children's distress during painful medical procedures. *Health Psychology*, in press.

Johnson, J.E., Kirchhoff, K.T., & Endress, M.P. Altering children's distress behavior during orthopedic cast removal. *Nursing Research*, 1975, **24**, 404–410.

Johnson, S.B., & Melamed, B.B. The assessment and treatment of children's fears. In B.B. Lahey & A.E. Kazdin (Eds.), *Advances in Clinical Child Psychology*. New York: Plenum Press, 1979.

Katz, E.R., Kellerman, J., & Siegel, S.E. Self-report and observational measurement of acute pain, fear, and behavioral distress in children with leukemia. Paper presented at the Annual Meeting of the Society of Behavioral Medicine, Chicago, March 1982.

Katz, E.R., Kellerman, J., & Siegel, S.E. Anxiety as an affective focus in the clinical study of acute behavioral distress: A reply to Schacham and Daut. *Journal of Consulting and Clinical Psychology*, 1981, **49**, 470–471.

Katz, E.R., Kellerman, J., & Siegel, D.E. Distress behavior in children with cancer undergoing medical procedures: Developmental considerations. *Journal of Consulting and Clinical Psychology*, 1980, **48**, 356–365.

Katz, E.R., Varni, J.W., & Jay, S.M. Cognitive-behavioral treatment of pediatric pain. In M. Hersen, R.M. Eisler, & P.M. Miller (Eds.), *Progress in Behavior Modification*. Vol 11. New York: Academic Press, in press.

Katz, R.C. Single session recovery from a hemodialysis phobia: A case study. *Journal of Behavior Therapy and Experimental Psychiatry*, 1974, **5**, 205–206.

Kellerman, J., & Varni, J.W. Pediatric hematology/oncology. In D.C. Russo & J.W. Varni (Eds.), *Behavioral Pediatrics: Research and Practice*. New York: Plenum Press, 1982.

Kellerman, J., Zeltzer, L., Ellenberg, L., & Dash, J. Hypnotic reduction of distress associated with adolescent cancer and treatment: I. Acute pain and anxiety due to medical procedures. Manuscript submitted for publication, 1982.

Klein, R.M., & Charlton, J.E. Behavioral observation and analysis of pain behavior in critically burned patients. *Pain*, 1980, **9**, 27–40.

Kohen, D.P. Relaxation/mental imagery (self-hypnosis) and pelvic examinations in adolescents. *Journal of Developmental and Behavioral Pediatrics*, 1980, **1**, 180–186.

Kolko, D.J., & Milan, M.A. Misconception correction through reading in the treatment of a self-injection phobia. *Journal of Behavior Therapy and Experimental Psychiatry*, 1980, **11**, 173–176.

Lamb, D.H., & Strand, K.H. The effect of a brief relaxation treatment for dental anxiety on measures of state and trait anxiety. *Journal of Clinical Psychology*, 1980, **36**, 270–274.

Lebenthal, E., Rossi, T.M., Nord, K.S., & Branski, D. Recurrent abdominal pain and lactose absorption in children. *Pediatrics*, 1981, **67**, 828–832.

Lehmann, H., Huntsman, R.S., Casey, R., Lang, A., Lorkin, P.A., & Comings, D.E. Sickle cell disease and related disorders. In J.W. Williams, E. Bentler, A.J. Ersler, & R.W. Rundles (Eds.), *Hematology*. New York: McGraw-Hill, 1977.

Lindsay, S.J.E., & Roberts, G.J. Methods for behavioral research on dentally anxious children. *British Dental Journal*, 1980, **149**, 175–179.

Maddison, T.G. Recurrent abdominal pain in children. *Medical Journal of Australia*, 1977, **1**, 708–710.

Marks, I.M. Anxiety states, phobic and obsessive-compulsive disorders: Clinical picture, differential diagnosis and management. *Progress in Neuro-Psychopharmacology*, 1981, **5**, 1979–186.

Masek, B.J. Behavioral medicine treatment of pediatric migraine. Paper presented at the Annual Meeting of the Society of Behavioral Medicine, Chicago, March 1982.

Melamed, B.G., & Siegel, L.J. Reduction of anxiety in children facing hospitalization and surgery by use of filmed modeling. *Journal of Consulting and Clinical Psychology*, 1975, **43**, 511–521.

Melamed, B.G., Weinstein, D., Hawes, R., & Katin-Borland, M. Reduction of fear-related dental management problems using filmed modeling. *Journal of The American Dental Association,* 1975, **90**, 822–826.

Melzack, R. Prolonged relief of pain by brief, intense transcutaneous somatic stimulation. *Pain,* 1975, **1**, 357–373.

Michener, W.M. An approach to recurrent abdominal pain in children. *Primary Care,* 1981, **8**, 277–283.

Miller, A.J., & Kratochwill, T.R. Reduction of frequent stomachache complaints by time out. *Behavior Therapy,* 1979, **10**, 211–218.

Millicap, J.G. Recurrent headaches in 100 children: Electroencephalographic abnormalities and response to Phenytoin (dilantin). *Child's Brain,* 1978, **4**, 95–105.

Moe, P.G. Headaches in children: Meeting the challenge of management. *Postgraduate Medicine,* 1978, **63**, 169–174.

Morgan, P.H., Wright, L.E., Ingersoll, B.D., & Seime, R.J. Children's perceptions of the dental experience. *Journal of Dentistry for Children,* 1980, **47**, 243–245.

Morse, D.R., Schacterle, G.R., Esposito, J.V., Furst, M.L., & Bose, K. Stress, relaxation and saliva: A follow-up study involving clinical endodontic patients. *Journal of Human Stress,* 1981, **7**, 19–26.

Newburger, P.E., & Sallan, S.E. Chronic pain: Principles of management. *Journal of Pediatrics,* 1981, **98**, 180–189

Nimmer, W.H., & Kapp, R.A. A multiple impact program for the treatment of injection phobias. *Journal of Behavior Therapy and Experimental Psychiatry,* 1974, **5**, 257–258.

Nocella, J., & Kaplan, R.M. Training children to cope with dental treatment. *Journal of Pediatric Psychology,* 1982, **7**, 175–178.

Oster, J. Recurrent abdominal pain, headache and limb pains in children and adolescents. *Pediatrics,* 1972, **50**, 429–436.

Parkin, S.F. The effect of ambient music upon the reactions of children undergoing dental treatment. *Journal of Dentistry for Children,* 1981, **48**, 430–432.

Parry, D.H., & Bloom, A.L. Failure of factor VIII inhibitor bypassing activity (Feiba) to secure hemostasis in hemophilic patients with antibodies. *Clinical Pathology,* 1978, **31**, 1102–1105.

Perry, S., & Heidrich, G. Management of pain during debridement: A survey of U.S. burn units. *Pain,* 1982, **13**, 267–280.

Richlin, D.M., Carron, H., Rowlingson, J.C., Sussman, M.D., Baugher, H., & Goldner, R.D. Reflex sympathetic dystrophy: Successful treatment by transcutaneous nerve stimulation. *Journal of Pediatrics,* 1978, **93**, 84–86.

Roberts, M.D., Wurtele, S.K., Boone, R.R., Ginther, L.J., & Elkins, P.E. Reduction of medical fears by use of modeling: A preventive application in a general population of children. *Journal of Pediatric Psychology,* 1982, **6**, 293–300.

Sank, L.I., & Biglan, A. Operant treatment of a case of recurrent abdominal pain in a 10-year-old boy. *Behavior Therapy,* 1974, **5**, 677–681.

Shacham, S., & Daut, R. Anxiety or pain: What does the scale measure? *Journal of Consulting and Clinical Psychology,* 1981, **49**, 468–469.

Shaw, E.G., & Routh, D.K. Effect of mother presence on children's reaction to aversive procedures. *Journal of Pediatric Psychology,* 1982, **7**, 33–42.

Sheskin, R.B., Klein, H., & Lowental, U. Assessment of children's anxiety throughout dental treatment by their drawings. *Journal of Dentistry for Children,* 1982, **49**, 99–106.

Shinnar, S., & D'Souza, B.U. The diagnosis and management of headaches in childhood. *Pediatric Clinics of North America,* 1981, **29**, 79–94.

Siegel, L.J., & Peterson, L. Maintenance effects of coping skills and sensory information on young children's response to repeated dental procedures. *Behavior Therapy,* 1981, **12**, 530–535.

Siegel, L.J., & Peterson, L. Stress reduction in young dental patients through coping skills and sensory information. *Journal of Consulting and Clinical Psychology*, 1980, **48**, 785–787.

Sokoloff, L. Biochemical and physiological aspects of degenerative joint diseases with special reference to hemophilic arthropathy. *Annals of New York Academy of Science*, 1975, **240**, 285–290.

Spielberger, C.D. *State-Trait Anxiety Inventory for Children: Preliminary Manual*. Palo Alto, CA: Consulting Psychologists Press, 1973.

Spielberger, C.D., Gorsuch, R., & Lushene, R. *The State-Trait Anxiety Inventory*. Palo Alto, CA: Consulting Psychologists Press, 1970.

Stickler, G.B., & Murphy, D.B. Recurrent abdominal pain. *American Journal of Diseases of Children*, 1979, **133**, 486–94.

Stilz, R.J., Carron, H., & Sanders, D.B. Reflex sympathetic dystrophy in a 6-year-old: Successful treatment by transcutaneous nerve stimulation. *Anesthesia and Analgesia*, 1977, **56**, 438–441.

Swezey, R.L. *Arthritis: Rational Therapy and Rehabilitation*. Philadelphia: Saunders, 1978.

Taylor, C.B., Ferguson, J.M., & Wermuth, B.M. Simple techniques to treat medical phobias. *Postgraduate Medical Journal*, 1977, **53**, 28–32.

Thelen, M.H., Fry, R.A., Fehrenback, P.A., & Frautschi, N.M. Therapeutic videotape and film modeling: A review. *Psychological Bulletin*, 1979, **86**, 701–720.

Tomasi, L.G. Headaches in children. *Comprehensive Therapy*, 1979, **5**, 13–19.

Turnage, J.R., & Logan, D.L. Treatment of a hypodermic needle phobia by in vivo systematic desensitization. *Journal of Behavior Therapy and Experimenatl Psychiatry*, 1974, **5**, 67–69.

Ultee, C.A., Griffioen, D., & Schellekens, J. The reduction of anxiety in children: A comparison of the effects of systematic desensitization in vitro and systematic desensitization in vivo. *Behaviour Research and Therapy*, 1982, **20**, 61–67.

Varni, J.W. Self-regulation techniques in the management of chronic arthritic pain in hemophilia. *Behavior Therapy*, 1981, **12**, 185–194. (a)

Varni, J.W. Behavioral medicine in hemophilia arthritic pain management: Two case studies. *Archives of Physical Medicine and Rehabilitation*, 1981, **62**, 183–187. (b)

Varni, J.W., Bessman, C.A., Russo, D.C., & Cataldo, M.F. Behavioral management of chronic pain in children: Case study. *Archives of Physical Medicine and Rehabilitation*, 1980, **61**, 375–379.

Varni, J.W., & Gilbert, A. Self-regulation of chronic arthritic pain and long-term analgesic dependence in a hemophiliac. *Rheumatology and Rehabilitation*, 1982, **22**, 171–174.

Varni, J.W., Gilbert, A., & Dietrich, S.L. Behavioral medicine in pain and analgesia management for the hemophilic child with factor VIII inhibitor. *Pain*, 1981, **11**, 121–126.

Varni, J.W., Katz, E.R., & Dash, J. Behavioral and neurochemical aspects of pediatric pain. In D.C. Russo & J.W. Varni (Eds.), *Behavioral Pediatrics: Research and Practice*. New York: Plenum Press, 1982.

Varni, J.W., Kellerman, J., & Dash, J. Assessment and management of pediatric pain. In T.J. Coates (Ed.), *Behavioral Medicine: A Practical Handbook*. Champaign, Illinois: Research Press, 1983.

Venham, L., Bengston, & Cipes, M. Children's response to sequential dental visits. *Journal of Dental Research*, 1977, **56**, 454–459.

Venham, L.L., Gaulin-Kremer, E., Munster, E., Bengston-Audia, D., & Cohan, J. Interval rating scales for children's dental anxiety and uncooperative behavior. *Pediatric Dentistry*, 1980, **2**, 195–202.

Wald, A., Chandra, R., Fisher, S.E., Gartner, J.C., & Zitelli, B. Lactose malabsorption in recurrent abdominal pain of childhood. *Journal of Pediatrics*, 1982, **100**, 65–68.

Wakeman, R.J., & Kaplan, J.Z. An experimental study of hypnosis in painful burns. *American Journal of Clinical Hypnosis*, 1978, **21**, 3–12.

Wasserman, R.R., Oester, Y.T., Oryshkevich, R.S., Montgomery, M.M., Poske, R.M., & Ruksha, A. Electromyographic, electrodiagnostic, and motor nerve conduction observations in patients with rheumatoid arthritis. *Archives of Physical Medicine and Rehabilitation*, 1968, **49**, 90–95.

Wernick, R.L., Jaremko, M.E., & Taylor, P.W. Pain management in severely burned adults: A test of stress inoculation. *Journal of Behavioral Medicine*, 1981, **4**, 103–109.

Wettrell, G., Hallbook, T., & Hultquist, C. Reflex sympathetic dystrophy in two young females. *Acta Paediatrica Scandinavica*, 1979, **68**, 923–924.

White, J.R. Effects of a counterirritant on perceived pain and hand movements in patients with arthritis. *Physical Therapy*, 1973, **53**, 956–960.

Zeltzer, L.K., Dash, J., & Holland, J.P. Hypnotically induced pain control in sickle cell anemia. *Pediatrics*, 1979, **64**, 533–536.

# 5

# Preparation for Hospitalization and Surgery

The hospitalized child experiences a number of stressful situations, for example, maternal separation, physical pain, a disruption in daily living, and an interruption in psychosocial and cognitive development (Hodapp, 1982). Particularly in young children, maternal separation is a primary stressor, with age and the prehospitalization maternal-child relationship suggested as additional significant factors in the child's adjustment to hospitalization (Goslin, 1978). An increasing number of hospitals nationally have developed pediatric preparation programs, employing a wide variety of techniques, such as printed materials (coloring books, written instructions, information booklets), audiovisual materials (slides, film strips, videotapes), models and miniatures (dolls, puppets, medical supplies), group discussion, and hospital tours (Azarnoff & Woody, 1981; Peterson & Ridley-Johnson, 1980). However, as recently reviewed by Melamed, Robbins, and Graves (1982), while it is generally agreed that some type of preparation is helpful for most children, the specific advantages and disadvantages of each technique for each child requires further empirical determination. Nevertheless, a statement may be made regarding the empirical findings on preparation procedures, identifying the generally accepted and most effective interventions. In evaluating these studies, the first concern is with the biobehavioral assessment of therapeutic effects.

## BIOBEHAVIORAL ASSESSMENT

The multidimensional assessment of children's reactions to hospitalization and surgery have generally included measurement of behavioral and physiological parameters. The pattern of the relationship between the various biobehavioral responses assessed provides the optimal strategy for determining the child's reaction to hospitalization and surgery (Melamed et al., 1982).

## Behavioral Assessment

The effects of hospitalization on children's behavior have been generally divided into inhospital and posthospital behavior (King & Ziegler, 1981). A number of motor behaviors have been identified that are proposed to reflect anxiety and adjustment to the hospital setting (Glennon & Weisz, 1978; Tesler & Savedra, 1981; Tureman & Johnson, 1980). Cormier (1979) studied 32 hospitalized children, observing each child by means of a 45-item behavior checklist, utilizing a time-sampling observation procedure. The major categories observed were: (1) the child's behaviors, e.g., smile, laugh, play, grimace, flinch, whimper, cry; (2) the location of the child, e.g., bed, wheelchair; (3) the child's activity, e.g., sleeping, eating, undergoing a medical procedure; (4) the adult(s) involved, e.g., nurse, physician, parent; and (5) the adult-child interaction, e.g., holding, rocking, medical content, nonmedical content. In addition to the time-sampling procedure observations, a list of 32 global measures was also completed on each child in an attempt to provide descriptors of behaviors which are characteristically cited in the literture to define psychological upset to hospitalization (e.g., restlessness, passivity, disruptiveness, negativism, irritableness, depressed, anxious, withdrawn). These data were divided into three factors:

1. Children in Factor I were characterized by friendliness, cooperative behavior, smiling, playing, verbalizing, but had limited relationship with family members;
2. Children in Factor II were withdrawn and passive, exhibiting limited verbalization and frequent self-stimulatory behaviors;
3. Children in Factor III were irritable, complaining, and aggressive, prone to excessive periods of crying and whimpering.

Vernon, Schulman, and Foley (1966) developed an assessment instrument to measure posthospitalization behavior, consisting of 28 items which were scored by the child's parent on a 5-point scale from "much less than before" to "much more than before." Factor analyses on 387 children resulted in six types of children's responses following hospitalization: (1) general anxiety and regression, (2) separation anxiety, (3) anxiety about sleep, (4) eating disturbance, (5) aggression toward authority, and (6) apathy-withdrawal.

## Physiological Assessment

A number of parameters have been suggested as measures of physiological reactions to hospitalization, including nausea, vomiting, changes in blood pressure, pulse rate, flushing, sweaty palms, disturbed sleep, and irregular breathing patterns (Melamed et al., 1982; Skipper & Leonard, 1968). Additionally, Melamed et al. (1982) suggest that postoperative physical recovery factors may be instructive, including vomiting, swelling, length of recovery, use of pain medication, reports of pain, time until first voiding, eating of solids, and wound healing. These parameters may be potentially affected by psychological factors and may provide a physiological assessment of various preparation techniques. Finally, neuroendocrinological measures of increased catecholamine (epinephrine and norepinephrine) levels through either plasma or urine samples have been found to be associated with stress situations (see Baum, Grunberg, & Singer, 1982, for review) and may provide a further measure of reaction to and coping with the stresses of hospitalization and surgery.

## PREPARATION TECHNIQUES

### Anesthesia Induction

Meyers and Muravchick (1977) studied the posthospitalization behavior of 85 children who were anesthetized for elective minor surgery of the head and neck. Thirty-seven other children who had been hospitalized but did not undergo anesthesia or surgery were the hospital control group. A standardized written questionnaire containing 46 items relating to specific behavior problems in nine categories was mailed to the parents of all children within the first month after discharge from the hospital. Parents were asked to indicate whether a problem was occurring, and if so, whether with greater, the same, or less frequency than preoperatively. The nine categories were:

1. Fears—of hospital, doctors, nurses, animals, shots, strangers
2. Regressive behavior—return to incontinence, baby talk, excessive clinging
3. Anger—discipline problems, biting, offensive language
4. Depression—listlessness, disinterest
5. Disturbance of social or peer interacting—social problems, hurting peers
6. Compulsions—repeated facial or body movements
7. Disturbance of sleeping habits—nightmares, insomnia
8. Disturbance of eating habits—amount and type of food eaten
9. Disturbance in speech—change in speech patterns.

The data indicated that children who were merely hospitalized exhibited as many behavioral problems as those who were hospitalized and underwent anesthesia for minor, nondisfiguring surgical operations, suggesting that hospitalization, irrespective of surgery, can itself be problematic. Further, the data demonstrated that an asleep anesthetic induction procedure resulted in significantly less children with behavioral problems than an awake induction.

Beeby and Hughes (1980) studied the behavior of 344 unsedated children in the anesthetic room prior to ear, nose, or throat surgery. The major finding was the influence of the child's age; children age 7 years and older exhibited fewer behavioral problems (e.g., apprehension, crying). This study points out the importance of considering age factors when determining the success of intervention programs.

## Modeling

Melamed and Siegel (1975) studied the effectiveness of filmed modeling in reducing the emotional reactions of 60 children between the ages of 4 and 12 years who were hospitalized for elective surgery for the first time. In order to assess the multidimensional parameters indicative of anxiety, a number of self-report, behavioral, and physiological measures were taken. Three measures were taken to assess trait anxiety, a relatively stable measure of an individual's anxiety proneness (Spielberger, 1973). These measures were an Anxiety Scale, the Children's Manifest Anxiety Scale, and the Human Figure Drawing Test. Situational or state anxiety was assessed by the Palmer Sweat Index, the Hospital Fears Rating Scale, and the Observer Rating Scale of Anxiety. The Palmer Sweat Index is a plastic impression method that enumerates the active sweat gland activity of the hand, providing a measure of transitory physiological arousal. The Hospital Fears Rating Scale is a 25-item self-report measure. Each child rated her degree of fear for each item on a fear thermometer that ranged from 1 (not afraid at all) to 5 (very afraid). The Observer Rating Scale of Anxiety consisted of 29 categories of verbal and skeletal behaviors designed to measure behavioral manifestations of anxiety in children. Examples of the items included crying, trembling hands, stutters, and talks about hospital fears, separation from mother, or going home. A time-sampling procedure was used in which an observer indicated the presence or absence of each response category on the behavior checklist during specified time periods. Finally, the child's mother completed the Behavior Problem Checklist, a 55-item rating scale of behavior problems frequently observed in children in the home and school settings.

The modeling film portrayed a 7-year-old child who hesitatingly approaches the hospital accompanied by his parents. He is shown going through the admission process and the preoperative blood test, during which he displays some anxiety. The child narrates the film to enhance the likelihood of imitation. He is shown talking with the surgeon and the anesthesiologist about what he should expect during surgery. The anesthesia induction in the operating room is depicted, since the child, though premedicated, is awake. He wakes up with some discomfort in the recovery room, but is tended by a caring nurse. His parents are at his bedside when he returns from surgery. His departure from the hospital is the final scene. Thus, this child provides a peer model who is observed overcoming his own fear and acquiring mastery of the situation, hypothesized to be an effective method for reducing fear in a child observer.

The results showed a significant reduction of preoperative (night before) and postoperative (3 to 4 weeks postsurgery examination) fear arousal in the film prepared group as compared to a standard prepared control group. Also, the parents of the control group reported a significant increase in the frequency of behavior problems in the children who had not been film prepared; the prepared children did not show an increase or decrease in behavior problems from pre- to posthospitalization. The effect of immediate physical recovery from the operation was obtained on a global postoperative recovery questionnaire evaluating time of first liquids, solid foods, nausea, vomiting, and amount of pain medication. This questionnaire showed a tendency for the film prepared group to exhibit fewer postsurgical complications than the standard prepared group. A subsequent study by Melamed, Meyer, Gee, and Soule (1976) showed that children 7 years and older appeared to benefit from seeing the film one week in advance of actual hospitalization, whereas the younger children needed more immediate preparation. These data suggest that the age of the child must be considered in deciding the optimal time for film preparation of children prior to surgery. Finally, it is important to point out that these results reflect the *added* therapeutic effects of the modeling film in addition to the standard preoperative preparation at the hospital, which included talks with the surgeon and/or anesthesiologist, a playroom visit with the child-life worker, demonstrations of the masks, anesthesia induction procedures, and observation of a photograph album depicting other children at various stages of their hospital experience.

Ferguson (1979) also prepared children 3 to 7 years of age using film modeling. The self-report measures included the Hospital Fears Rating Scale utilized by Melamed and Siegel (1975), and a Mood Adjective Checklist, divided into six mood scales (anger, happiness, fear, depression, psychological well-being, and lethargy). The physiological measure involved muscle tension as reflective of anxiety, with the attachment of surface electrodes at the trapezius muscle providing the measure of electromyographic (EMG) activity. The behavioral measures included The Observer Rating Scale of Anxiety designed by Melamed and Siegel (1975), and the Post-Hospitalization Behavior Rating Scale developed by Vernon et al. (1966). The results showed that viewing a peer modeling film was associated with a decrease in the children's hospital-specific physiological anxiety response at the preoperative measure. Additionally, the children displayed a significantly lower incidence of undesirable posthospitalization behavior in comparison to a control group receiving standard preparation. Thus, the sum of these three studies point to the efficacy of film modeling as an additional component of the preparation of children for hospitalization and surgery.

## Cognitive-Behavioral Coping Procedures

Peterson and Shigetomi (1981) assessed the effectiveness of combining cognitive-behavioral coping procedures with filmed modeling in comparison to coping only, modeling only, and information only controls. Sixty-six children, ages 2.5 to 10.5 years (average age of 5.5 years) who were anticipating elective tonsillectomies, were studied. None of the children had experienced previous surgery or had been hospitalized within a year of admission.

The preoperative information procedure consisted of a narrated story of a typical hospital stay from admission to discharge while a puppet pantomimed the activities. The parents' continued role in helping the child prepare for hospitalization was noted. The blood test, preoperative medications, postoperative discomforts, and the necessity for fluid consumption were stressed. This narrative lasted approximately 15 minutes. After the verbal presentation, the children viewed the film previously developed by Melamed and Siegel (1975). The cognitive-behavioral coping procedure consisted of three components: (1) cue-controlled deep muscle relaxation, (2) distracting mental imagery, and (3) comforting self-instruction. The children first heard a technique described, watched the puppet Big Bird perform it, and then were helped to practice it. The children were trained in deep muscle relaxation by stretching and tensing their muscles, then relaxing them completely. After the children had practiced the relaxation technique, the cue word *calm* and slow deep breathing were introduced. Children practiced the sequence of stretching, relaxing, and saying the word *calm* to themselves during exhalation.

The technique of imaginal distraction (guided imagery) was then introduced. The children were asked to imagine a scene that was quiet and made them feel happy. The scenes of lying by a stream in the mountains or being on a sunny beach were suggested, but the children were asked to pick a scene of their own, with the help of their parents. Parents and children were encouraged to make the scene as positive and as vivid as possible by imagining temperatures, smells, sounds, and sights. Finally, the childern were given two comforting self-instructional phases: "I will be all better in a little while," and "Everything is going to be all right." The children were encouraged to say the phrases out loud and then just to think them. Occasions on which to use the techniques, such as during injections and during postoperative pain, as well as the importance of practice with the parent's encouragement were stressed.

The study assessed several self-report, observational, behavioral, and physiological parameters. The Faces Scale (Venham, Bengston, & Cipes, 1977) and The Hospital Fears Rating Scale (Melamed & Siegel, 1975) were given before and after surgery. The child was also asked to indicate how much anxiety she was experiencing on a 5-point scale. During blood tests, the child was rated by the laboratory technician on three 5-point Likert-type scales measuring how anxious the child seemed, how cooperative he was, and how well he tolerated the procedure. Additionally, the parent and nurse each rated the child before and after surgery on two 5-point scales measuring how anxious and how cooperative the child was. The parent and nurse also completed a behavior checklist of 16 maladaptive behaviors typical of anxious hospitalized children. Each parent was asked to mark two 10-point scales describing how confident and how calm the child was both before and after surgery, as well as to rate the hospital experience from 1 (worse than I expected) to 5 (better than I expected). Finally, the child's pulse and temperature were taken by the nurse the night before, the morning after, and the afternoon after surgery. The parent was also asked to record the amount of liquid and food consumption in one-half cup units postsurgery during the first 10 hours, and the time in minutes to first postsurgical voiding. The results indicated that the children receiving the cognitive-behavioral coping techniques training plus the modeling film were more calm and cooperative during invasive procedures than the children receiving cognitive-behavioral coping training or the modeling film alone. A 1-year follow-up indicated that the parents most often selected distracting imagery over relaxation or self-instruction as the most effective of the cognitive-behavioral coping techniques (Peterson & Shigetomi, 1982).

## Parent-Child Relationship and Preparation

Increasing maternal participation in the hospitalization of young children has received growing support in recent years in the literature (Roskies, Mongeon, & Gagnon-Lefebure, 1978). However, Vardaro (1978) found a highly significant positive correlation between anxiety in the mother regarding the hospitalization of her young child for elective surgery and anxiety in the child. Such a relationship between anxiety in the parent and anxiety in the child suggests the need for child *and* parental preparation.

Skipper and Leonard (1968) proposed that the mother is a prime factor in determining whether changes in the child's emotions and behavior will be detrimental or beneficial to his hospitalization and recovery. They reasoned that if the mother is affected by severe stress herself, her ability to aid her child may be reduced. Further, in her interactions with her child this anxiety may be communicated to the child and actually increase the child's emotional reaction. On the other hand, if the mother were able to manage her own stress and be calm, confident, and relaxed, this emotional message might instead be communicated to her child and ease his distress. Skipper and Leonard (1968) hypothesized that the child's stress might be reduced indirectly by reducing the stress of the mother. The primary intervention in this study was the accurate communication of information to the mother regarding all aspects of the child's hospitalization and surgery. The data suggest that the reduction in the mother's stress positively affected psychosocial and physiological measures taken on the child.

Wolfer and Visintainer (1975) studied the effectiveness of preparation and stress-point supportive care in minimizing stress and assisting the child in coping through the provision of accurate information about sequences of events, sensory experiences, role expectations and appropriate responses, previews of procedures through play techniques, and supportive care given by a specific nurse at critical points (stress points) both pre- and postoperatively. Six stress points were identified: (1) admission, (2) shortly before the blood test, (3) late in the afternoon the day before the operation, (4) shortly before the preoperative medications, (5) before transport to the operating room, and (6) upon return from the recovery room. Information about what to expect and how to respond shortly before these events, along with support and reassurance during the events, was considered stress-point nursing care (the preparation intervention). This preparation and support was integrated for both the parent and child. For the mothers, the preparation attempted to provide individualized attention, to explore and clarify their feelings and thoughts, to provide accurate information and appropriate reassurance, and to explain how the mother could help care for her child. For the child, information included the time of the procedure, who would do it and how, why it was done, how it would end, and what could be expected after it was completed. The sensations and emotions the child might experience were described and demonstrated, e.g., the cold sensation and smell of the alcohol, the pressure and smell of the anesthesia mask. Any misconceptualizations were clarified in age-appropriate terms. Behavioral rehearsal included practicing the specific behaviors needed for a blood test and anesthesia induction.

The multidimensional assessment for the child included:

1. *Behavioral Ratings,* a 5-point manifest anxiety scale designed to reflect the emotional state of the child at a given point, in terms of verbal and nonverbal expressions of fear, anxiety, or anger, from 1 (calm appearance, no crying, no verbal protest), 3 (some temporary whimpering and/or mild verbal protest), to 5 (agitated, intense crying or screaming and/or strong verbal protest), and a 5-point cooperation scale indicating the degree to which the child cooperated with a procedure, from 1 (active participation in and assistance with the procedure), 3 (mild or initial resistance or passive participation without assistance), to 5 (extreme resistance, strong avoidance, and the necessity to restrain the child.
2. *Physiological measures,* the ease of fluid intake on a 4-point scale, pulse rates (as a measure of physiological arousal accompanying fear, anxiety, or general emotional distress), recovery room medication, and time to first voiding.
3. *Posthospital Behavior Questionnaire* (Vernon et al., 1966).
   For the parent, five measures were taken: (1) 5-point manifest anxiety scale; (2) 5-point coping and cooperation scale; (3) self-rating of anxiety; (4) self-rating of satisfaction with the care; and (5) self-rating of the adequacy of the information given.

The results of the study demonstrated significant differences between the experimental group and a control group of children and parents on ratings of anxiety behavior, cooperation with procedures, pulse rate before and after painful procedures, resistance to induction, time to first voiding, posthospital adjustment, and parental anxiety and satisfaction with information and care. A subsequent study by Visintainer and Wolfer (1975) further supported the effectiveness of a combination of systematic preparation, rehearsal, and supportive care conducted prior to each stressful procedure. Additionally, Wolfer and Visintainer (1979) tested the stress-reducing effects of written and illustrated materials which were designed to prepare children for hospitalization for minor surgery *prior to* hospitalization, incorporating information and procedures from their earlier studies. This home-preparation (prehospitalization) method resulted in success similar to the inhospital-preparatory approach.

Finally, Zabin and Melamed (1980) developed a 14-item parent's questionnaire, finding that the disciplinary methods utilized by parents regarding their children's approach to fearful situations may affect the children's reaction to hospitalization for surgery. Parents who reported using positive reinforcement, modeling, and persuasion as ways of encouraging their child to deal with fearful situations had children who were low in anxiety during the hospitalization. The parents who reported using punishment, force, or reinforcement of dependency had children who evidenced higher anxiety reactions during hospitalization. These data suggest the possibility of administering this questionnaire prior to hospitalization to identify those children who may be at risk for developing an anxiety reaction related to hospitalization and surgery, subsequently indicating an even greater effort directed toward preparation and coping skills training.

# EMERGENCY HOSPITALIZATION AND PEDIATRIC INTENSIVE CARE UNITS

The vast majority of studies on pediatric preparation for hospitalization and surgery have typically involved children admitted for minor elective surgery. However, emergency admissions are the most common form of hospitalization for young children, containing not only the usual stresses of elective hospitalization on an intensified scale, but other adverse factors such as lack of preparation and extremely high anxiety in both the child and parents (Roskies, Bedard, Gauvreau-Guilbault, & Lafortune, 1975). Additionally, children with serious illness may be expected to exhibit more intense agitation, distress, and behavioral depression (Hollenbeck, Susman, Nannis, Strope, Hersh, Levine, & Pizzo, 1980) (see Chapter 9 under protective environments). Infants with serious illness who are hospitalized in a pediatric intensive care unit (PICU) may also subsequently experience a disruption in the development of parent-child relationships (Allen, McGrade, Affleck, & McQueeney, 1982).

As reviewed by Cataldo, Jacobs, and Rogers (1982), children hospitalized in PICUs may experience a number of undesirable biobehavioral effects. In the PICU, children may be isolated from parents, exposed to a number of children with life-threatening illnesses or injuries, witness critical medical interventions, and experience a number of necessary but painful medical procedures. The children are typically connected to a number of vital-signs monitoring equipment, receive fluids intravenously, and are restrained from moving freely in their beds. Cataldo et al. (1982) proposed a behavioral analysis of the PICU, identifying the environmental events that affect the child's behavior and the functional relationship between these events and the child's behavior. Cataldo et al. (1982) further proposed that events such as separation, unfamiliarity, and painful and frightening procedures are likely to be especially aversive to children. Such aversive contingencies may result in a behavioral sequelae of conditioned response suppression and learned helplessness (see Cataldo et al., 1982, for review). In reviewing the basic animal and human research literature, Cataldo et al. (1982) found that in situations in which strong, unpredictable, unavoidable, and inescapable aversive stimulation is programmed, appetitive and goal-oriented behavior is suppressed, avoidance and escape behavior may cease, and adverse biological reactions increase (e.g., increase in gastric secretions and catecholamine levels). Further, the basic literature indicates that these aversive-related reactions may be mitigated by providing a biobehaviorally stronger positive stimulus and by making the occurrence of aversive events more predictable.

Cataldo, Bessman, Parker, Pearson, and Rogers (1979) observed 99 children in a PICU, recording six patient behaviors and three behaviors of caregivers. The behaviors recorded were: (1) waking state, e.g., alert, awake, asleep; (2) position, e.g., sitting, lying; (3) verbalizations from the child; (4) verbalizations to the child; (5) attention/eye contact; (6) affective state, e.g., smiles, laughs, cries, whines, neutral (no overt behavioral response); (7) number and type of people within close proximity to the bedside, e.g., doctors, nurses, parents, child life workers, and (8) activity, e.g., play, reading, being read to, watching television. The first part of the study by Cataldo et al. (1979), which only involved behavioral assessment, revealed that the children did not verbalize 82 percent of the time observed, did not attend to anything in the room 37 percent of the time, were not engaged in any activity 54 percent of the time, and the predominant affect was judged to be neutral (58 percent of the observations). Cataldo et al. (1982) suggested that such neutral affect and noninteraction is characteristic of aversive stimulation research findings as described in the conditioned response suppression and learned helplessness literature.

In the second part of the study by Cataldo et al. (1979), an attempt was made to mitigate these effects by providing positive stimulation through play with toys and interactions with a child life teacher. The effect of providing even a brief, planned play-related activity for these children on a PICU was to increase positive child behaviors, i.e., increased attention (eye contact) and social interaction. A subsequent study by Pearson, Cataldo, Tureman, Bessman, and Rogers (1980) further supported these initial findings. In sum, the PICU represents a situation where medical procedures are conducted frequently and on the basis of the child's medical status, not her overt behaviors. Child behaviors typically attended to, such as crying, screaming, and complaining of pain and discomfort, are not successful in avoiding and escaping the aversive aspects of critical medical care, resulting in a decrease in these behaviors (extinction), leading to conditioned response suppression and learned helplessness (i.e., neutral affect, no eye contact with activities on the unit, and little verbal interaction). While the aversiveness of the essential medical procedures may not be reduced, positive interactions may be programmed so as to provide a contrast and may subsequently mitigate the overall aversive biobehavioral effects of the PICU.

# REFERENCES

Allen, D.A., McGrade, B.J., Affleck, G., & McQueeney, M. The predictive validity of neonatal intensive care nurses' judgements of parent-child relationships: A nine-month follow-up. *Journal of Pediatric Psychology,* 1982, **7**, 125–134.

Azarnoff, P., & Woody, P.D. Preparation of children for hospitalization in acute care hospitals in the United States. *Pediatrics,* 1981, **68**, 361–368.

Baum, A., Grunberg, N.E., & Singer, J.E. The use of psychological and neuroendocrinological measurements in the study of stress. *Health Psychology,* 1982, **1**, 217–236.

Beeby, D.G., & Hughes, J.O.M. Behavior of unsedated children in the anesthetic room. *British Journal of Anaesthesia,* 1980, **52**, 279–281.

Cataldo, M.F., Bessman, C.A., Parker, L.H., Pearson, J.E., & Rogers, M.C. Behavioral assessment for pediatric intensive care units. *Journal of Applied Behavior Analysis,* 1979, **12**, 83–97.

Cataldo, M.F., Jacobs, H.E., & Rogers, M.C. Behavioral/environmental considerations in pediatric inpatient care. In D.C. Russo and J.W. Varni (Eds.), *Behavioral Pediatrics: Research and Practice.* New York: Plenum Press, 1982.

Cormier, P.P. Identification of typologies derived from child behaviors in the hospital as predictors of psychology upset. *Journal of Pediatric Nursing and Mental Health Services,* 1979, **5**, 28–35.

Ferguson, B.F. Preparing young children for hospitalization: A comparison of two methods. *Pediatrics,* 1979, **64**, 656–664.

Glennon, B., & Weisz, J.R. An observational approach to the assessment of anxiety in young children. *Journal of Consulting and Clinical Psychology,* 1978, **46**, 1246–1257.

Goslin, E.R. Hospitalization as a life crisis for the preschool child: A critical review. *Journal of Community Health,* 1978, **3**, 321–346.

Hodapp, R.M. Effects of hospitalization of young children: Implications of two theories. *Children's Health Care,* 1982, **10**, 83–86.

Hollenbeck, A.R., Susman, E.J., Nannis, E.D., Strope, B.E., Hersh, S.P., Levine, A.S., & Pizzo, P.A. Children with serious illness: Behavioral correlates of separation and isolation. *Child Psychiatry and Human Development,* 1980, **11**, 3–11.

King, J., & Ziegler, S. The effects of hospitalization on children's behavior: Review of the literature. *Children's Health Care,* 1981, **10**, 20–28.

Melamed, B.G., Meyer, R., Gee, C., & Soule, L. The influence of time and type of preparation on children's adjustment to hospitalization. *Journal of Pediatric Psychology,* 1976, **1**, 31–37.

Melamed, B.G., Robbins, R.L., & Graves, S. Preparation for surgery and medical procedures. In D.C. Russo & J.W. Varni (Eds.), *Behavioral Pediatrics: Research and Practice.* New York: Plenum Press, 1982.

Melamed, B.G., & Siegel, L.J. Reduction of anxiety in children facing hospitalization and surgery by use of filmed modeling. *Journal of Consulting and Clinical Psychology,* 1975, **43**, 511–521.

Meyers, E.F., & Muravchick, S. Anesthesia induction technics in pediatric patients: A controlled study of behavioral consequences. *Anesthesia and Analgesia,* 1977, **56**, 538–542.

Pearson, J.E., Cataldo, M.F., Tureman, A., Bessman, C.H., & Rogers, M.C. Pediatric intensive care unit patients: Effects of play intervention on behavior. *Critical Care Medicine,* 1980, **8**, 64–67.

Peterson, L., & Ridley-Johnson, R. Pediatric hospital response to survey on prehospital preparation for children. *Journal of Pediatric Psychology,* 1980, **5**, 1–7.

Peterson, L., & Shigetomi, C. One-year follow-up of elective surgery child patients receiving preoperative preparation. *Journal of Pediatric Psychology,* 1982, **7**, 43–48.

Peterson, L., & Shigetomi, C. The use of coping techniques to minimize anxiety in hospitalized children. *Behavior Therapy,* 1981, **12**, 1–14.

Roskies, E., Bedard, P., Gauvreau-Guilbault, H., & Lafortune, D. Emergency hospitalization of young children: Some neglected psychological considerations. *Medical Care,* 1975, **13**, 570–581.

Roskies, E., Mongeon, M., & Gagnon-Lefebure, B. Increasing maternal participation in the hospitalization of young children. *Medical Care,* 1978, **16**, 765–777.

Skipper, J.K., & Leonard, R.C. Children, stress, and hospitalization: A field experiment. *Journal of Health and Social Behavior,* 1968, **9**, 275–287.

Spielberger, C.D. *State-Trait Anxiety Inventory for Children.* Palo Alto, CA.: Consulting Psychologists Press, 1973.

Tesler, M., & Savedra, M. Coping with hospitalization: A study of school-age children. *Pediatric Nursing,* 1981, **7**, 35–38.

Tureman, C.A., & Johnson, P.A. Observing and recording behaviors of hospitalized children. *Australasian Nursing Journal,* 1980, **9**, 27–29.

Vardaro, J.A. Preadmission anxiety and mother-child relationships. *Journal of the Association for the Care of Children in Hospitals,* 1978, **7**, 8–15.

Venham, L., Bengston, D., & Cipes, M. Children's response to sequential dental visits. *Journal of Dental Research,* 1977, **56**, 454–459.

Vernon, D.T.A., Schulman, J.L., & Foley, J.M. Changes in children's behavior after hospitalization: Some dimensions of response and their correlates. *American Journal of Diseases of Children,* 1966, **111**, 581–593.

Visintainer, M.A., & Wolfer, J.A. Psychological preparation for surgical pediatric patients: The effect on children's and parents' stress responses and adjustment. *Pediatrics,* 1975, **56**, 187–202.

Wolfer, J.A., & Visintainer, M.A. Prehospital psychological preparation for tonsillectomy patients: Effects on children's and parents' adjustment. *Pediatrics,* 1979, **64**, 646–655.

Wolfer, J.A. & Visintainer, M.A. Pediatric surgical patients' and parents' stress responses and adjustment as a function of psychologic preparation and stress-point nursing care. *Nursing Research,* 1975, **24**, 244–255.

Zabin, M.A., & Melamed, B.G. Relationship between parental discipline and children's ability to cope with stress. *Journal of Behavioral Assessment,* 1980, **2**, 17–38.

# Part III

## Prevention, Health Maintenance, and Therapeutic Adherence

# 6
# Prevention and Therapeutic Adherence

## PREVENTIVE MEDICINE

Preventive medicine encompasses all aspects of health-related behaviors concerned with the prevention or reduction of disease, including the identification and modification of health-related behaviors which may result in illness and further disability after the onset of illness (Breslow & Somers, 1977; Masek, Epstein, & Russo, 1981). Preventive medicine may be categorized into three dimensions (Clark, 1967): (1) *Primary prevention* refers to efforts designed to prevent the occurrence of disease, for example, through immunization against infectious diseases and modification of eating, diet, and exercise patterns in the prevention of cardiovascular disease; (2) *Secondary prevention* refers to the early detection and treatment of disease so as to prevent increased morbidity and mortality, for example, through regular physical examinations for the early detection and treatment of coronary heart disease and cancer through such diagnostic measures as serum cholesterol levels and blood pressure readings, breast palpation and mammography, Pap test; and (3) *Tertiary prevention* refers to rehabilitative efforts designed to prevent further morbidity which may be associated with chronic disease and disabilities, for example, through the enhancement and maintenance of the activities of daily living and functional independence in patients with rheumatoid arthritis. Thus, preventive medicine includes the identification of biobehavioral factors (e.g., obesity, improper diet, sedentary lifestyle, stress, elevated cholesterol levels) and the modification of health-related behaviors (e.g., eating, exercise, diet, and stress-reduction behaviors).

Historically, preventive efforts have been directed primarily toward infectious diseases. With the prevention and treatment of infectious diseases now generally well managed through biomedical science and technology, the focus has shifted toward the prevention of noninfectious chronic diseases (Breslow & Somers, 1977). Since many of the proposed risk factors associated with the prevention of two major chronic diseases (cardiovascular disease and cancer) are a function of health-related behaviors (eating, diet, exercise, smoking, and

113

stress-related behaviors), biobehavioral techniques may significantly contribute to health enhancement and maintenance and the prevention of these chronic diseases in children and adolescents (Brown, 1980; Haggergy, 1977; Williams, Carter, Arnold, & Wynder, 1979), particularly when viewed from the perspective that many health-related behaviors are initially learned and developed during childhood and adolescence (Hamburg & Brown, 1978; Marks, 1980).

The systematic application of biobehavioral techniques in pediatric preventive medicine should consider the relationship between children's health beliefs and health-related behaviors (Weisenberg, Kegeles, & Lund, 1980), the empirical evaluation of risk factors, the identification of antecedents and consequences of health-related behaviors, the determination of the unit of intervention (e.g., the child, family, school), and be concerned with the motivation for and long-term maintenance of behavior change (Lund, Kegeles, & Weisenberg, 1977; Masek et al., 1981). In all aspects of preventive medicine, the modification of risk factors and health-related behaviors requires adherence to a healthy lifestyle, and when indicated, to prescribed therapeutic regimens. Thus, therapeutic adherence represents an essential component of preventive medicine (Kasl, 1975).

# THERAPEUTIC ADHERENCE AND NONCOMPLIANCE

Interest in therapeutic adherence has greatly increased in the past 25 years, primarily because modern biomedical science has provided the patient with therapy worth adhering to. It may be suggested that improving adherence to therapeutic regimens will produce as great an impact upon disability and death as the development of new treatment techniques and may result in greater cost effectiveness in the provision of health care services. Patient noncompliance with prescribed therapeutic regimens seriously undermines the effectiveness of therapy in both preventive and curative situations and results in unnecessary morbidity, mortality, and cost. For instance, the effectiveness of a treatment program may be misjudged, with undetected noncompliance leading to unnecessary additional diagnostic tests, alternative treatments, increased or additional medications, and even eventual hospitalization.

The term *compliance* has been criticized because of its connotation of medical professional dominance and the "patient-as-defaulter" (Stimson, 1974). Thus, the term *adherence* has been suggested by some authors as less judgmental and as implying greater participation by the patient. In this text, the term *adherence* will generally be used to describe the correct and appropriate performance of recommended health-related behaviors, whereas the term *noncompliance* will be used to describe the incorrect and inappropriate performance or nonperformance of recommended health-related behaviors. Noncompliance with therapeutic regimens includes medication noncompliance, failure to keep appointments, failure to follow therapeutic recommendations, and nonparticipation in health maintenance activities (Masek, 1982). Adherence to therapeutic regimens encompasses a broad spectrum of health-related behaviors, including correct consumption of prescribed medications, appropriate eating, diet, and exercise patterns, and avoidance of risk behaviors such as smoking, alcohol, and drug abuse (Glanz, 1980; Mayo, 1978; Shope, 1981).

Reviews of the literature have indicated that noncompliance with therapeutic regimens represents a serious problem facing the health care system, with noncompliance in the adult population averaging over 40 percent and ranging from 4 to 92 percent (Marston, 1970). While average noncompliance to therapeutic regimens in the pediatric population has generally been reported to be somewhat less prevalent, it nevertheless is considered a widespread and major concern in pediatrics (Litt & Cuskey, 1980; Masek & Jankel, 1982; Mattar & Yaffe, 1974). This prevalence of noncompliance may have a profound and detrimental effect on the quality of comprehensive pediatric care in the prevention and treatment of illnesses, resulting in greater patient morbidity and higher costs as prescribed medications, recommended health actions, and health services are incorrectly utilized. This incorrect utilization is exemplified by the "errors" found in adherence to prescribed medication regimens.

Five errors or patterns of medication noncompliance have been delineated: (1) complete failure to take the precise medication; (2) improper taking of medication because of misunderstanding of the proper dosage intervals; (3) a pattern of missed doses; (4) increasing or reducing the dose or daily number of doses; (5) taking medication for the wrong purpose, taking outdated or discontinued drugs, and taking more medications than the clinician is aware of (Dunbar & Stunkard, 1979; Litt & Cuskey, 1980). Similar noncompliance patterns may be identified for other health-related behaviors, such as not following a weight management program completely, incorrectly following a diet program by over- or undereating or over- and underexercising and by taking diet pills without the clinician's knowledge. An awareness and assessment by the clinician of these noncompliance patterns is necessary to accurately measure and monitor treatment efficacy, safety, and side effects (Dunbar & Agras, 1980).

Before discussing the specific factors associated with noncompliance and the intervention strategies for improving therapeutic adherence, the essential issue of measurement parameters must first be considered.

## Measurement of Adherence and Noncompliance

Assessment of therapeutic adherence and noncompliance has included both direct and indirect measures (see Dunbar & Agras, 1980; Dunbar & Stunkard, 1979; Litt & Cuskey, 1980; Rapoff & Christophersen, 1982, for reviews). Direct measures include biochemical assessments of medications or related metabolic by-products, as well as direct observation of patient behavior by the clinician or family member. Indirect measures include various forms of self-report, pill counts, and clinician ratings of adherence.

## Patient Self-report

Two types of patient self-reporting of adherence may be delineated: (1) verbal report during patient interview, and (2) self-monitoring, which includes the process of daily self-observation and self-recording on a recording form of adherence behaviors by the patient. The patient interview has traditionally been the most commonly utilized measure of adherence by the clinician, although its validity is limited by the interviewing skills of the clinician and the patient's willingness/ability to accurately remember and report noncompliance. Typically, the patient interview method has been found to result in an underreporting of noncompliance and an overreporting of adherence.

The process of self-monitoring reduces some of the inherent problems with the interview method in that it emphasizes that the specific health-related behaviors be observed and recorded when they occur in the patient's natural environment, subsequently circumventing the memory or recall of adherence/noncompliance required by the interview method. Self-monitoring is best utilized as an assessment procedure when the patient is reinforced by the clinician for the *accuracy* of the self-recorded data rather than for specific health-related behavior change. The focus on accuracy rather than behavior change may reduce the demand characteristics to overreport adherence inherent in the clinician-patient interview process. Additionally, the calculated percent of correctly completed self-monitoring data sheets returned to the clinician may also serve as an adherence measure. Self-monitoring is discussed further in the section on intervention strategies.

## Treatment Outcome

Treatment outcome does *not* represent a valid measure of adherence/noncompliance. The tendency to use treatment outcome as an adherence measure is based on the faulty assumption that patient improvement is associated with a high degree of adherence, and conversely, that lack of patient improvement is associated with some degree of noncompliance. Some limitations of this assumption include the facts that patients may improve for reasons other than the prescribed regimen, that an incorrect regimen was initially prescribed, and that spontaneous disease remission may occur, to name but a few extraneous variables unrelated to adherence.

## Biochemical Analysis

Biochemical assessment provides a direct measurement of the metabolic by-products of a medication or diet-related change, the medication itself, or a marker (e.g., riboflavin or phenol red) added to a medication, through an analysis of the pertinent serum, urine, saliva, and breath assays. However, biochemical measures are limited as a sole determinant of adherence because of individual variations in the absorption, metabolism, and excretion of biochemical substances (Vesell, 1974), which produce biochemical assays that may be unrelated to the performance of specific adherence behaviors. Additionally, a patient may adhere to a medication regimen the day or two before a clinic appointment, resulting in a positive biochemical assay, yet this measure would not necessarily reflect adherence throughout the interval between clinic appointments.

*Pill Counts*

The pill count ideally specifies the ratio of pills consumed to the amount that should have been consumed within a designated time interval. The measurement requires that the number of pills in the medication bottle or dispenser be counted before and periodically during the prescribed medication regimen time period. In general, the pill count method tends to overestimate adherence. Methodological problems in assessing adherence through pill counts include the fact that the patient may deliberately leave unused medications at home or forget to return all or a portion of the unused medication, may share the medication with a family member or friend, or simply discard the pills in the amount prescribed just prior to the clinic appointment. Further, the pill count does not delineate the medication consumption pattern, that is, consumption may be inconsistent, resulting in overdoses and underdoses during particular time intervals between clinic appointments.

*Clinician Ratings*

Clinician estimates tend to overestimate adherence and are the least accurate and least reliable adherence assessment, with ratings typically being little better than chance estimates. Further, accuracy is not associated with the degree of clinical experience, the amount of contact with the patient, or with the clinician's confidence in his judgment. Thus, clinician ratings should not be considered a reliable or valid measurement of adherence and noncompliance.

*Direct Observation*

Direct observation of patient health-related behaviors may be made by the clinician and family members. The clinician may periodically observe and record the patient's performance of the component skills required for the prescribed regimen in the clinic setting so as to determine memory and recall of the correct regimen. If the patient cannot correctly perform the regimen in front of the clinician, it seems unlikely that the regimen is being performed correctly in the patient's natural environment. Another clinician's direct observation is the percent of attendance at scheduled appointments. While not specifically related to adherence to the prescribed regimen itself, it does provide an additional measure of adherence and noncompliance, particularly a measure of the most severe degree of noncompliance, that is, treatment dropout by complete nonattendance at scheduled clinic appointments. Parental monitoring and recording of child health-related behaviors can be an invaluable source of adherence measurement in the patient's natural environment. Additionally, the percent of correctly completed parental monitoring data sheets returned to the clinician by the parent provides one measure of the parent's adherence behaviors.

### Summary

Since reliance on any one measurement parameter is inadequate, the optimal assessment strategy for adherence and noncompliance should include a systematic integration of interview material, self-monitoring data, biochemical analyses, pill counts, parental or other family member monitoring, and direct observations by the clinician. The intercorrelations between these various measures will provide a more accurate data base for determining adherence and noncompliance.

## Factors Affecting Adherence and Noncompliance

In the past, investigations on therapeutic adherence and noncompliance have sought to determine the patient characteristics that might result in noncompliance. More recently, comprehensive and multidimensional analyses of noncompliance have suggested a multitude of factors that may result in lack of adherence. These analyses have also resulted in the identification of factors that are amenable to systematic modification so as to improve adherence. However, before addressing the issue of intervention programs for enhancing adherence, a general overview of factors that have been studied in the past will be presented. These factors have been typically analyzed in terms of the characteristics of the patient, family, clinician, clinic, illness, and treatment regimen (see Dunbar & Agras, 1980; Dunbar & Stunkard, 1979; Litt & Cuskey, 1980; Mayo, 1978; Shope, 1981, for reviews).

### Patient Characteristics

The sociodemographic variables that have been investigated for their potentially contributing effect on noncompliance have included age, sex, socioeconomic status, race, education, religion, marital status, and occupation. On the whole, these sociodemographic variables do not have any independent correlation with patient adherence. Whenever a correlation has been found, other factors were also involved. For example, comprehension and recall of the regimen may be associated with age and educational level. Thus, by themselves, these sociodemographic variables have not been demonstrated to differentiate between adherent and noncompliant patients. Furthermore, these sociodemographic variables are not subject to modification; it is more appropriate to look to factors that might be changed so as to improve adherence, such as the complexity of the regimen.

*Family Characteristics*

Although such family characteristics as socioeconomic status, number of people living at home, history of family illness, and communication problems have been investigated in relation to noncompliance, the clearest pattern to emerge is that family support and involvement have been associated with greater adherence. This is especially true in the pediatric population, where parental involvement may serve to cue and reinforce adherence.

*Clinician Characteristics*

One of the most consistent findings on clinician characteristics is that adherence is greater when the patient receives care from the same clinician over time. Additional clinician characteristics that have been found to be associated with better adherence include a warm and empathic manner and an active interaction with patients in planning their regimen.

*Clinic Characteristics*

In the clinic setting, a consistent relationship has been found between waiting time and adherence; longer waiting time is associated with a higher incidence of missed clinic appointments. Four factors have been found to increase waiting time: the block scheduling system, clinician lateness, patient lateness, and patient no-shows. The first two factors are directly within the control of the clinic setting through providing a specific time and clinician for each patient appointment and maintaining an on-time schedule. The second two factors may be affected by an appointment reminder system, such as a telephone call or postcard sent near the time of the scheduled clinic appointment. Additionally, a warm, positive, and personalized approach by the entire clinic staff has been suggested as another factor in enhancing appointment adherence.

*Illness Characteristics*

Greater noncompliance has been found to be associated with regimens in the treatment of longer duration illnesses, asymptomatic conditions, and in the prevention of future illness. Greater adherence has been associated with short-er duration illnesses, symptomatic conditions, and illnesses that limit daily activity.

*Treatment Regimen Characteristics*

The most important single determinant of therapeutic adherence has consis-tently been found to be the complexity of the treatment regimen. More complex regimens result in greater noncompliance. This includes multiple dose medication regimens and regimens that require considerable alteration in the patient's established daily lifestyle, such as changes in eating, diet, exercise, and other personal habits. Also of considerable importance is the required length of time the prescribed regimen must be followed. Longer duration regimens result in progressively greater noncompliance. Other factors found to be of less singular importance in noncompliance include the side effects of the regimen and the irregularity of the routine required by the regimen.

*Summary*

As cogently stated by Zifferblatt (1975), "Even if certain characteristics were significantly correlated with noncompliance, influencing them might be quite difficult. It is one thing to identify education, age, gender, personality, or attitude as a significant determinant of noncompliance, and quite another to change these factors [p. 174]." In sum, efforts may be most parsimoniously directed toward the identification of *modifiable* factors.

## Intervention Strategies for Improving Therapeutic Adherence

Although a rather large literature exists for documenting the extent of the noncompliance problem in health care, a relatively small number of studies have addressed the issue of what strategies may improve therapeutic adher-ence. However, by extrapolating the findings from the analyses of *modifiable* factors associated with noncompliance and the research and clinical findings from the applied behavioral sciences (Zifferblatt, 1975), a set of logical inter-vention strategies may be generated (see Becker & Maiman, 1980; Dunbar & Agras, 1980; Dunbar & Stunkard, 1979; Litt & Cuskey, 1980; Mayo, 1978; Masek & Jankel, 1982; Rapoff & Christophersen, 1982; Shope, 1981 for reviews). Table 6.1 contains a summary outline of the intervention strategies for improving therapeutic adherence as described below.

*Patient Education*

Patient education may be best viewed as a necesssary but insufficient condition for improving therapeutic adherence. Simply providing information without

Table 6.1.   Strategies for Improving Therapeutic Adherence.

| Dimension | Intervention Strategies |
|---|---|
| Patient Education | (1) Provide specific instructions on the regimen itself<br>(2) Dispense the information over time<br>(3) Organize the information into discrete categories<br>(4) Combine both verbal and written instructions<br>(5) Measure comprehension and recall through verbal and written questions |
| Treatment Regimen | (1) Decrease the complexity and/or use shaping<br>(2) Decrease the duration and/or maintain long-term monitoring<br>(3) Decrease the number of lifestyle changes and/or use shaping<br>(4) Decrease the inconvenience by tailoring to the patient's daily activities<br>(5) Decrease the cost by prescribing generic medication and aiding in third-party reimbursement |

| Functional Analysis | Antecedents | → | Health-Related Behaviors | → | Consequences |
|---|---|---|---|---|---|
| | (1) Self-monitoring<br>(2) Daily routine<br>(3) Building in reminders<br>(4) Clinic characteristics | | (1) Diet, exercise, regimens<br>(2) Medication regimens<br>(3) Stress-reduction regimens<br>(4) Appointment-keeping | | (1) Self-reinforcement<br>(2) Family reinforcement<br>(3) Clinician reinforcement<br>(4) Contingency contract |

teaching the pediatric patient and her parents the specific skills to effect health-related behavior change will most likely not result in lasting therapeutic adherence. Additionally, providing information about the illness itself may be of limited value in improving adherence; providing specific instructions regarding the prescribed treatment regimen itself has been found to facilitate correct adherence. Further, it must not be assumed that simply presenting information will result in pediatric patient and/or parent comprehension. For the pediatric patient, cognitive developmental level must be considered as discussed in Chapter 2. For the parent, misunderstanding and lack of comprehension and recall is also an issue. Lack of accurate recall or forgetting has been found to increase in direct proportion to the amount of information given by the clinician. The following instructional strategies are suggested for enhancing comprehension and recall: (1) provide specific instructions on the regimen itself; (2) dispense the information over time; (3) organize the information into specific categories; (4) combine both verbal and written instructions; (5) measure comprehension and recall through both verbal and written questions.

However, even if patients know what they are supposed to do, additional strategies are needed to optimize the potential for their adhering to the treatment regimen.

## Treatment Regimen

Although there may be incidences where a particular treatment regimen cannot be modified, whenever possible the following regimen characteristics should be altered to facilitate therapeutic adherence.

**Regimen Complexity.** An attempt should be made to simplify the treatment plan as much as therapeutically feasible. For instance, reducing the number of prescribed daily administrations and/or different medications by requiring fewer but larger doses, prescribing medications designed for once-a-day oral administration, prescribing medication combinations in single tablets, and synchronizing doses of different medications into temporally simultaneous administration. If complex medication regimens are necessary and/or numerous alterations in daily lifestyle are required for optimal clinical effects (e.g., major changes in diet, exercise, smoking, stress patterns), the gradual introduction of the component parts of the complex regimen through behavioral shaping procedures is the recommended implementation strategy. In this shaping approach, the regimen would be divided into a series of health-related behaviors in the order of greatest to least difficult. The easiest or simplest step would first be required. With demonstrated success at this step, the next most difficult step would be incorporated into the regimen. Through this shaping sequence, the complete regimen would be attained as the patient achieved successful adherence at each successive component step. In this way, the patient would have the opportunity to gradually change her lifestyle to optimally fit the regimen, as opposed to potentially being overwhelmed initially, possibly resulting in a greater probability of some degree of noncompliance.

**Regimen duration.** Adherence has been found to decrease over time with long-term regimens. Consequently, when possible, an attempt should be made to reduce the length of therapy. However, when this is not clinically feasible, then regularly scheduled follow-up visits may serve to prompt and maintain adherence by providing a systematic monitoring of patient behavior. Additionally, when clinically feasible, the complexity of the regimen should be gradually reduced over time so as to increase the probability of long-term patient adherence.

**Lifestyle changes, inconvenience, and cost.** Intuitively, financial cost may be seen as a barrier to optimal adherence for many patients. Whenever possible, the financial cost should be minimized by prescribing generic medication, the judicious prescription of medications, encouraging the patient to compare prices at different pharmacies, and aiding the patient in securing third-party reimbursement. Additionally, an attempt should be made to minimize the inconvenience to the patient by tailoring the regimen to the patient's daily lifestyle. Once again, a shaping approach may be used to gradually introduce the regimen into the patient's activities of daily living (ADL) routine, fitting the health-related behaviors into this ADL scheme where they would have a high probability of performance with minimal barriers to their performance. A functional analysis, as described next, can facilitate this process.

*Functional Analysis*

A functional analysis of therapeutic adherence attempts to delineate the socioenvironmental situations and temporal cues that may influence the occurrence or nonoccurrence of health-related behaviors, that is, to identify the functionally related antecedents and consequences of health-related behaviors. The initial step is to specify the health-related behaviors that require modification (e.g., adherence to diet, exercise, medication, and smoking-reduction regimens). The next step consists of identifying the antecedents of these health-related behaviors and determining the naturally occurring consequences for these health-related behaviors. With the information from this functional analysis, an intervention plan can be developed for rearranging the socioenvironmental situations and temporal cues so as to functionally influence the occurrence or nonoccurrence of these health-related behaviors.

***Antecedents of Adherence.***   The first step in identifying the antecedents of the target health-related behaviors in the patient's natural environment (e.g., home, school, work), is to instruct the patient in self-monitoring and/or parental monitoring for the younger child. Self-monitoring and parental monitoring consist of the recording on a behavior checklist of the occurrence of the target health-related behaviors and the situations governing their performance. A food and beverage intake record is an example of such a behavior checklist, identifying not only the foods and beverages consumed, but also the times, people, and situations (e.g., viewing television) associated with the eating or drinking behaviors (see Chapter 7). Additionally, self- and parental monitoring facilitate the identification of those socioenvironmental situations and temporal cues in the patient's daily routine that may enhance the probability that the target health-related behaviors will occur (e.g., exercising early in the morning, taking a medication before lunch and dinner). Reminders may be built into the daily routine, such as placing the medication bottle on the kitchen table, inserting jogging into a chain of morning behaviors (e.g., get up, wash face, go jogging, take shower, eat breakfast, brush teeth, go to school/work).

Finally, the clinic setting can be arranged to set-up the antecedents for appointment-keeping, such as providing a positive and well-organized environment, providing specific appointment times with the same clinician, and using telephone or postcard reminders as prompts just prior to the scheduled appointment.

*Consequences of Adherence.* After conducting an analysis of the naturally occurring reinforcement and punishment consequences contingent on health-related behaviors, an intervention plan may be implemented to rearrange these consequences so as to promote appropriate health-related behaviors and increase adherence to the prescribed treatment regimens. Contingent reinforcement should optimally be designed to include a combination of self-reinforcement, family reinforcement, and clinician reinforcement. The reinforcement paradigm consists of providing tokens (e.g., points, stars, smiling faces, poker chips) contingent on the correct performance of a health-related behavior. These tokens are then exchanged for designated reinforcers from a reinforcement list. In self-reinforcement, the patient has control over the utilization of the reinforcement list, whereas in family reinforcement, the parents control the access to the reinforcers. The key to successful self- or family reinforcement is that the reinforcers only be made available *contingent* on the correct performance of adherent behaviors (see Chapter 3 for a detailed discussion of contingent reinforcement procedures).

Finally, the clinician characteristics of a warm and empathetic manner may serve as social reinforcers when contingent on adherent behavior. Additionally, the clinician may formally arrange a reciprocal agreement with the pediatric patient and/or parent through behavioral or contingency contracting. In the contingency contract, both the clinician and the pediatric patient/parent mutually agree on a treatment goal, specifying the reciprocal obligations of each party in attempting to achieve the treatment goal, and the time line for the achievement of the treatment goal. As a bilateral agreement, the contingency contract spells out the contingent consequences that will occur if and only if one party engages in a particular action in which case the other party will respond reciprocally (see Epstein & Wing, 1979, for review). For instance, the clinician may agree to be on time for clinic appointments with the patient if the patient agrees to bring in his self-monitoring data. Further, the clinician and the parent may work with the older child and adolescent in developing a contingency contract whereby the patient agrees to engage in certain health-related behaviors, and the parent then allows the adolescent to go to a movie or the younger child more time to play outside with friends. Thus, contingency contracting provides a clear written specification of target health-related behaviors and the contingencies that will be available for their performance. As proposed by Lewis and Michnich (1977), the contingency contract works as an adherence enhancing intervention by:

(1) clarification of the relative responsibilities of both provider and consumer in achieving an agreed-upon goal by explicit exchange of information about what is required in the act of treatment by the patient; and (2) a perceived (or real) transfer of power from provider to consumer that affects certain health-related expectancies.

Thus, as summarized by Becker and Maiman (1980), the contingency contract offers the following advantages:

(1) a written outline of behavioral expectations is created; (2) the patient becomes involved in the decision-making process concerning the regimen, and thus has an opportunity to discuss potential problems and solutions; (3) formal commitment to the program is elicited; and (4) the reward/reinforcement components create incentives for achieving compliance goals.

Table 6.2 contains a sample contingency contract.

*Summary*

As outlined in Table 6.1, intervention strategies for improving therapeutic adherence should include an integrated multicomponent program consisting of

Table 6.2.    Contingency Contract Sample (Older Children and Adolescent Patients).

| *Patient Behavior* | *Parent Behavior* | *Clinician Behavior* |
| --- | --- | --- |
| (1) Take two medication tablets at 9 a.m., 12 p.m., 3 p.m., 6 p.m. | (1) Allow 15 minutes extra television viewing time for each incidence of medication adherence | (1) Be on time for clinic appointments |
| (2) Swim 20 laps and perform 10 minutes of stretching exercises each afternoon | (2) Provide 10 token points for each incidence of exercise adherence in exchange for reinforcers on reinforcement list | (2) Provide 5 token points for each incidence of exercise adherence in exchange for earning previously donated baseball, basketball, zoo tickets |

I understand my responsibilities and agree to fulfill my part of this mutually negotiated contract from 4/15/83 to 6/15/83, at which time the contract will be renegotiated.

Date: _____

_____     _____     _____
Patient Signature              Parent Signature              Clinician Signature

three major dimensions: (1) the patient education instructional method, (2) the therapeutic regimen implementation, and (3) the functional analysis of the antecedents and consequences functionally related to adherence and noncompliance. Specific applications of these components are illustrated in the next chapter and throughout the text.

# REFERENCES

Becker, M.H., & Maiman, L.A. Strategies for enhancing patient compliance. *Journal of Community Health,* 1980, **6**, 113–135.

Breslow, L., & Somers, A.R. The lifetime health-monitoring program: A practical approach to preventive medicine. *New England Journal of Medicine,* 1977, **296**, 601–608.

Brown, J.B. Child health maintenance. *Nurse Practitioner,* 1980, **5**, 33–43.

Clark, D.W. A vocabulary for preventive medicine. In D.W. Clark & B. MacMahon (Eds.), *Preventive Medicine.* Boston: Little, Brown, 1967.

Dunbar, J.M., & Agras, W.S. Compliance with medical instructions. In J.M. Ferguson & C.B. Taylor (Eds.), *Comprehensive Handbook of Behavioral Medicine.* Vol. 3. New York: Spectrum Publications, 1980.

Dunbar, J.M., & Stunkard, A.J. Adherence to diet and drug regimen. In R. Levy, B. Rifkind, & B. Dennis (Eds.), *Nutrition, Lipids, and Coronary Heart Disease.* New York: Raven Press, 1979.

Epstein, L.H., & Wing, R.R. Behavioral contracting: Health behaviors. *Clinical Behavior Therapy Review,* 1979, **1**, 1–22.

Glanz, K. Compliance with dietary regimens: Its magnitude, measurement, and determinants. *Preventive Medicine,* 1980, **9**, 787–804.

Haggerty, R.J. Changing lifestyles to improve health. *Preventive Medicine.* 1977, **6**, 276–289.

Hamburg, D.A., & Brown, S.S. The science base and social context of health maintenance: An overview. *Science,* 1978, **200**, 847–849.

Kasl, S.V. Issues in patient adherence to health care regimens. *Journal of Human Stress,* 1975, **1**, 5–17.

Lewis, C.E., & Michnich, M. Contracts as a means of improving patient compliance. In I. Barofsky (Ed.), *Medication Compliance: A Behavioral Management Approach.* Thorofare, N.J.: Charles B. Slack, 1977.

Litt, I.F., & Cuskey, W.R. Compliance with medical regimens during adolescence. *Pediatric Clinics of North America,* 1980, **27**, 3–15.

Lund, A.K., Kegeles, S.S., & Weisenberg, M. Motivational techniques for increasing acceptance of preventive health measures. *Medical Care,* 1977, **15**, 678–692.

Marks, A. Aspects of biosocial screening and health maintenance in adolescents. *Pediatric Clinics of North America,* 1980, **27**, 153–161.

Marston, M.V. Compliance with medical regimens: A review of the literature. *Nursing Research,* 1970, **19**, 312–323.

Masek, B.J. Compliance and medicine. In D.M. Doleys, R.L. Meredith, & A.R. Ciminero (Eds.), *Behavioral Medicine: Assessment and Treatment Strategies.* New York: Plenum Press, 1982.

Masek, B.J., Epstein, L.H., & Russo, D.C. Behavioral perspectives in preventive medicine. In S.M. Turner, K.S. Calhoun, & H.E. Adams (Eds.), *Handbook of Clinical Behavior Therapy.* New York: John Wiley & Sons, 1981.

Masek, B.J., & Jankel, W.R. Therapeutic adherence. In D.C. Russo & J.W. Varni (Eds.), *Behavioral Pediatrics: Research and Practice.* New York: Plenum Press, 1982.

Mattar, M.E., & Yaffe, S.J. Compliance of pediatric patients with therapeutic regimens. *Postgraduate Medicine,* 1974, **56**, 181–188.

Mayo, N.E. Patient compliance: Practical implications for physical therapists. *Physical Therapy,* 1978, **58**, 1083–1090.

Rapoff, M.A., & Christophersen, E.R. Improving compliance in pediatric practice. *Pediatric Clinics of North America,* 1982, **29**, 339–357.

Shope, J.T. Medication compliance. *Pediatric Clinics of North America,* 1981, **28**, 5–21.

Stimson, G.V. Obeying doctor's orders: A view from the other side. *Social Science and Medicine,* 1974, **8**, 97–104.

Vesell, E.S. Factors causing interindividual variations of drug concentrations in blood. *Clinical Pharmacology and Therapeutics,* 1974, **16**, 135–148.

Weisenberg, M., Kegeles, S.S., & Lund, A.K. Children's health beliefs and acceptance of a dental preventive activity. *Journal of Health and Social Behavior,* 1980, **21**, 59–74.

Williams, C.L., Carter, B.J., Arnold, C.B., & Wynder, E.L. Chronic disease risk factors among children: The "Know Your Body" study. *Journal of Chronic Diseases,* 1979, **32**, 505–513.

Zifferblatt, S.M. Increasing patient compliance through the applied analysis of behavior. *Preventive Medicine,* 1975, **4**, 173–182.

7

# Eating, Exercise, and Diet Modification: Cardiovascular Disease, Obesity, Anorexia Nervosa, Bulimia

There are a number of pediatric disorders in which eating, exercise, and diet behaviors are instrumental in the prognosis and course of the condition, for example, insulin-dependent juvenile diabetes mellitus and end-stage renal disease (see Chapter 11). Additionally, eating, exercise, and diet modification is primarily involved in the prevention and treatment of cardiovascular disease, obesity, anorexia nervosa, and bulimia. The plan of this chapter is to provide a brief overview of these four areas where eating, exercise, and diet modification is indicated, followed by a detailed description of a comprehensive program for modifying these biobehavioral patterns in children.

## CARDIOVASCULAR DISEASE

Two emerging areas of investigation in pediatric cardiology are the early identification and treatment of juvenile hypertension and the primary prevention of risk factors of potential predictive significance in the development of cardiovascular disease (see Coates & Masek, 1982, for review). Despite advances in biomedical science and technology, cardiovascular-related deaths continue to be the leading cause of mortality in the United States. At present, an American child has a one in five risk of developing clinical evidence of coronary heart disease before sixteen years of age. In the pediatric population, the primary prevention of atherosclerosis through eating, exercise, and diet modification appears warranted.

### Atherosclerosis

Recent evidence indicates that the atherosclerotic process begins in childhood, but only becomes clinically evident in adulthood (see Voller & Strong, 1981 for review). A number of prospective studies on adults have shown definite associations between specific socioenvironmental, biochemical, physiologic, genetic, and pathologic conditions and the development of atherosclerosis, most notably coronary heart disease. The major risk factors are: hypercholesterolemia, hypertension, and smoking, while obesity, physical inactivity, hyperglycemia, psychosocial stress (Type A behavior) and family history have a lesser influence (Margolis, 1977). Modifiable risk factors (smoking, hypertension, hypercholesterolemia, obesity, hyperglycemia, psychosocial stress, physical inactivity) may be effected by changes in lifestyle (nonsmoking behavior, alterations in diet, i.e., reductions in caloric intake, saturated fats, salt, simple sugars, animal protein, increased fiber, and an increase in aerobic exercise).

Longitudinal studies on adults have shown that there is a gradient of risk for coronary heart disease that is associated with the serum concentration of cholesterol, the level of blood pressure, and the amount of obesity. Epidemiological, autopsy, and animal studies support this relationship between elevated serum cholesterol and the incidence of coronary heart disease, with further evidence now demonstrating a positive association of dietary cholesterol with serum cholesterol and coronary disease. Hypercholesterolemia is one form of hyperlipoproteinemia. The major classes of lipoproteins include both low density lipoproteins (LDL) and high density lipoproteins (HDL). Several studies have reported increased LDL levels in patients with atherosclerotic disease, and an inverse relationship between HDL level and increased coronary risk, suggesting a protective role of HDL against coronary heart disease.

Dietary cholesterol and saturated fats are both key factors in the development of atherosclerosis. Increasing amounts of dietary saturated fats are found to elevate the serum cholesterol level while polyunsaturated fats decrease it. Cholesterol restriction and an alteration of the polyunsaturated to saturated fats ratio in adults results in significant decreases in the serum cholesterol level. Thus, diet modification (see Dwyer, 1980) can be instrumental in decreasing serum cholesterol level. Further, physical activity in adults has been shown to increase HDL levels (Hartung, Foreyt, Mitchell, Vlasek & Gotto, 1980), potentially serving a protective role against coronary heart disease.

Large scale studies on children have indicated that a considerable number of school-age children evidence the risk factors which in adults are associated with coronary heart disease (Beaglehole, Trost, Tamir, Kwiterovich, Glueck, Insull, & Christensen, 1980; Frerichs, Srinivasan, Webber, & Berenson, 1976; Lauer, Connor, Leaverton, Reiter, & Clarke, 1975). Studies of arterial pathology in children and young adults dying of unrelated disease and war injuries have shown that fatty intimal lesions are present in the aortas of children as young as three years of age, and that by age 20, raised atherosclerotic lesions significant to the development of clinical atherosclerotic disease have already begun to appear in coronary arteries (Voller & Strong, 1981).

If primary prevention is to be effective, then it must be begun early in life. Diet has been demonstrated to be a significant determinant of serum lipid and lipoprotein levels in children (Morrison, Larsen, Glatfelter, Boggs, Burton, Smith, Kelly, Mellies, Khoury, & Glueck, 1980). It can be expected that without systematic intervention, children identified as evidencing the cardiovascular risk factors of elevations in serum lipids, lipoproteins, blood pressure, and obesity will continue to do so into adulthood (Frerichs, Webber, Vorrs, Srinivasan, & Berenson, 1979). The interrelationships between nutrient intake (dietary cholesterol, total carbohydrate, saturated and polyunsaturated fat, and total calories) of parents and their children (Laskarzewski, Morrison, Khoury, Kelly, Glatfelter, Larsen, & Glueck, 1980) strongly suggest the necessity of parent training in the prevention of pediatric atherosclerosis. Further, school-based programs (Brownell & Kaye, 1982; Coates, Jeffery & Slinkard, 1981; Williams, Carter, Arnold, & Wynder, 1979) and adolescent treatment groups (Coates, Jeffery, Slinkard, Killen, & Danaher, 1982) may also provide child and adolescent cardiovascular risk factor education on a potentially large scale.

Williams et al. (1979) described the first phase of a large scale longitudinal school-based primary disease prevention program in a sample of school children (ages 10 to 15 years), designed to reduce specific disease risk factors by means of a multidimensional, behaviorally oriented health education intervention primarily focused on antismoking and weight/cholesterol control. The program entitled "Know Your Body," combined screening for relevant risk factors (total cholesterol, physical fitness test, height/weight ratio, blood pressure, skinfold thickness), discussion of this screening's findings with the child in the form of a personal "Health Passport," provision in the classroom of a behaviorally oriented health education curriculum emphasizing healthier everyday habits, particularly better nutrition, avoiding cigarettes, and exercising daily, and specific peer-oriented intervention activities aimed at antismoking and weight/cholesterol control. Preliminary findings from the second year suggested that the rate of increase in the selected risk factors were significantly retarded in the intervention schools in comparison to the control schools.

Coates et al. (1981) designed a comprehensive school-based program, entitled the "Heart Healthy Program," for elementary school children to: (1) increase the consumption of complex carbohydrates and decrease the consumption of saturated fat, cholesterol, sodium, and sugar; (2) increase the level of habitual physical activity; and (3) generalize these lifestyle changes to other family members. The overall program and classroom lessons were designed using informative instruction, participatory classroom activities, personal goal setting, parent handouts, systematic feedback, and reinforcement. Evaluation of the program was conducted using direct observation of eating and physical activity patterns, as well as paper-and-pencil measures of knowledge and health attitudes. The results indicated substantial positive changes in eating behavior at school, knowledge about heart health, food preferences, and family eating patterns as reported by the children's parents. Observed changes in exercise were minimal and were related to seasonal sports activities. The authors suggest that future programs to increase student physical activity might encourage increases in already existing vigorous playground activities rather than a specialized exercise program (e.g., rather than the Parcourse exercise stations that were used in their study).

Coates et al. (1982) designed a weight loss program for obese adolescents within a group treatment approach to teaching behavioral self-management of weight. Weight loss skills were taught using a combination of videotape demonstrations, modeling, role-playing, and group discussions. The sequence of topics covered were: self-observation and caloric goals, what to eat, when and where to eat, exercise, food portions, self-instructions, situational control, self-talk and imagery, social control, and general problem-solving skills. Although the role of exercise in weight loss was discussed, the emphasis of the program was on caloric restriction to achieve weight loss. The adolescents were instructed on the caloric values of food and instructed to choose predominantly low calorie food to lose weight. The adolescents were further instructed to keep daily diaries of foods eaten and activities performed and to calculate the caloric equivalents of each. A daily caloric intake necessary to achieve a weight loss of 1 to 2 pounds per week was selected. Additionally, the advantages for cardiovascular health of physical activity and of diets higher in complex carbohydrates and polyunsaturated fats and lower in cholesterol, sugar, and saturated fats were discussed.

The authors point out that teaching weight loss skills to adolescents is not difficult. Rather, finding ways to optimize adherence to the weight loss program long enough to realize benefits seems to be central to short- and long-term success. Consequently, to enhance motivation, the patients or their parents had to be willing to deposit an amount of money equal to 15 weeks of their allowance or 50 percent of their earnings from part-time employment to be used in the incentive plan during the program. These deposits were returned during the program contingent on weight loss or habit change. The group that received reinforcement for weight loss and came to the clinic five times per week was the only group to lose significant amounts of weight during the treatment program, maintained over a 6-month follow-up. Additionally, clinically and statistically significant changes in recommended directions in blood presssure, total cholesterol, high density and low density lipoproteins, and triglycerides were correlated with changes in weight. The results suggest how difficult it can be to change an obese lifestyle even as young as during the adolescent years. Intervention in the preadolescent years, when eating and exercise patterns may be more easily modifiable and parental support may be more meaningful, seems to be indicated.

## Hypertension

Adult epidemiologic studies have demonstrated that hypertension is a significant coronary risk factor. As with serum cholesterol level, there does not appear to be a simple critical level. Rather, hypertension represents a continuum of risk for coronary heart disease, with the greater the blood pressure the greater the risk of an atherosclerotic event. The pathogenesis of the observed accelerated atherosclerosis seen in patients with hypertension appears to be related to the distending pressure of the blood within the vessel which exerts shearing force and damage to the intima (Voller & Strong, 1981). Experimental work suggests that increased pressure exerts a lateral force on the arterial walls and promotes a deposition of lipid within the intima.

Earlier reports suggested that most hypertension in children was secondary, with essential primary hypertension occurring only rarely. Secondary hypertension may be caused by renal, endocrine, vascular, metabolic, and neurologic dysfunction, as well as drug-related causes (Londe, 1978). However, more recent studies indicate that hypertensive children often do not show an underlying secondary cause, and that children ranking high in blood pressure among their peers are likely to continue this high ranking (see Voors, Webber, & Berenson, 1978, for review). Although blood pressures in the general population do not track as well during childhood (Clarke, Schrott, Leaverton, Connor, & Lauer, 1978), juvenile hypertension does track well, with reported persistent elevated systolic and/or diastolic pressures above the mean for age and sex (Goldring, Hernandez, Choi, Lee, Londe, Lindgren, & Burton, 1979). Further, the level of blood pressure in adolescence in general is closely related to hypertension in adulthood, suggesting that adult essential hypertension may find its origins during childhood and adolescence (Kilcoyne, 1978; Voors et al., 1978).

Factors associated with juvenile hypertension include obesity, extreme levels of sodium intake, and elevated serum triglyceride concentration (Goldring et al., 1979; Voors et al., 1978). Although normal blood pressure values for childhood have been suggested, there still remains some controversy regarding measurement technique and criterion blood pressure levels (Adams & Landeau, 1981). However, it is generally agreed that routine measurement of blood pressures in children and adolescents should be an integral part of comprehensive care (Lauer, Clarke, & Rames, 1978).

Regarding hypertension management, extreme elevations or acute increases in blood pressure indicate the need for a pharmacologic approach (Pruitt, 1981), whereas mildly or moderately hypertensive patients may best be managed through lifestyle modifications such as alterations in diet and salt restriction (Lauer et al., 1978; Ruley, 1978). Increasing the amounts of sodium in the diet causes the blood pressure to increase, at least in some individuals, whereas potassium has the opposite effect of decreasing blood pressure. While fresh fruits and vegetables are generally quite low in sodium and high in potassium content, frozen or canned foods generally have substantially elevated sodium content and low potassium content. This further suggests the potential of diet modification as a variable in hypertension management. Early intervention is once again indicated, since hypertensive children not only face an increased risk of coronary heart disease later in life, but may also suffer significant morbidity and mortality during later childhood and early adult years (Hulse, Taylor, & Dillon, 1979; Voller & Strong, 1981).

## Coronary-Prone Behavior

There is evidence in adult patients that the coronary-prone or Type A behavior pattern, characterized by a drive to achieve, a sense of time urgency, aggressiveness, and a competitive nature, is independently associated with an increased risk of coronary heart disease (Blumenthal, Williams, Kong, Schanberg, & Thompson, 1978). Recent studies suggest that this behavior pattern may have its origin in childhood, not as a genetically determined trait (Matthews & Krantz, 1976), but as a learned pattern through parental child-rearing practices and parental modeling (Coates & Masek, 1982; Matthews, 1977). Children classified as Type A resemble Type A adults when compared on physiological responses to stress (Lawler, Allen, Critcher, & Standard, 1981). Given that chronic sympathetic nervous system overactivity has been implicated as a factor capable of elevating and maintaining high serum cholesterol levels in adults independent of dietary measures, the regular practice of relaxation techniques may be clinically significant (Cooper & Aygen, 1979). Regular exercise may also serve a stress-reducing function, but is as yet an uninvestigated area with children and adolescents.

## Physical Inactivity

Although the direct effect of physical inactivity on the development of atherosclerosis remains unclear, there is little doubt that the physical conditioning obtained from regular exercise exerts a beneficial effect on other major coronary risk factors and thus exerts an indirect influence on the incidence of cardiovascular disease (Fogle & Verdesca, 1975; Folkins & Sime, 1981; Fraioli, Moretti, Paolucci, Alicicco, Crescenzi, & Fortunio, 1980; Hartung et al., 1980; Hollmann, Rost, & Liesen, 1980). The hemodynamic consequences of proper physical conditioning should improve the ability of the cardiovascular system to tolerate stress and beneficially improve weight, hypertension, HDL, and hypertriglyceridemia (Voller & Strong, 1981).

If physical activity is to be successful in the prevention of cardiovascular disease, appropriate exercise habits must be developed in early childhood. Such a long-term lifestyle change requires attention to the issues of therapeutic adherence and motivation, a problem clearly seen with adults in regards to regular exercise (Dishman & Ickes, 1981; Reid & Morgan, 1979). Behavioral techniques (contingency contracting, stimulus control, family reinforcement, self-reinforcement) have shown some initial success in increasing exercise behavior with adults (Epstein, Wing, Thompson, & Griffin, 1980; Keefe & Blumenthal, 1980; Wysocki, Hall, Iwata, & Riordan, 1979) and children (Allen & Iwata, 1980; Greenan, Powell, & Varni, 1983). Large scale physical education and reinforcement procedures in school-based programs may be ultimately of greatest benefit (Brownell & Kaye, 1982; Coates et al., 1981).

## Smoking

Cigarette smoking has been shown to be a significant factor independent of the other coronary risk factors in both the development and acceleration of the atherosclerotic process (Voller & Strong, 1981). Although the exact mechanisms by which smoking affects the atherosclerotic process are still unclear, it has been suggested that nicotine causes a release of norepinephrine and epinephrine, which in turn results in intimal damage and increased thrombus formation, or that carboxyhemoglobin concentration in heavy smokers may be elevated sufficiently to cause tissue hypoxia, which enhances the progression of the atherosclerotic lesion.

Adoption of the smoking habit typically occurs during adolescence, with over a third of all adolescents reporting cigarette smoking (Hunter, Webber, & Berenson, 1980). Further surveys suggest that adolescents are more likely to acquire the smoking habit if one or more of their parents or older sibling smoke and are influenced by peer smoking, suggesting the importance of modeling, imitation, and vicarious reinforcement in the development of this pattern (Hymowitz, 1980). Primary prevention of adoption of the cigarette smoking habit in childhood and adolescence appears clearly indicated when the disappointing results of adult smoking-cessation programs are considered (Chassin, Presson, Bensenberg, Corty, Olsharsky, & Sherman, 1981).

Since prevention of the smoking habit in childhood may prove to be more useful than attempts to intervene later in adulthood, various school-based prevention programs for children have recently been developed (Evans, 1976; Hurd, Johnson, Pechacek, Bast, Jacobs, & Leupker, 1980; Perry, Killen, Slinkard, & McAlister, 1980; McAlister, Perry, Killen, Slinkard, & Maccoby, 1980; McAlister, Perry, and Maccoby, 1979). A particularly interesting strategy in both the primary prevention and modification of smoking behavior of children and adolescents is the emphasis on immediate rather than long-term physiological effects of smoking and skill training in coping with the social pressures to smoke (Botvin, Eng, & Williams, 1980; Evans, Rozelle, Mittelmark, Hansen, Bane, & Havis, 1978; Hurd et al., 1980; Perry, Killen, Telch, Slinkard, & Danaher, 1980).

# OBESITY

Obese and overweight children and adolescents are at a considerably greater risk for adulthood obesity than their nonobese peers (see Coates & Thoresen, 1978, for review). An estimated 80 percent of overweight children become overweight adults (Mobbs, 1970), while Zack, Harlan, Leaverton, and Coronoi-Huntley (1979) found that childhood fatness was the most predictive factor for adolescent fatness. These studies clearly signal the importance of early treatment of obesity in the pediatric population.

Existing evidence strongly supports the notion of a multifactorial origin of childhood obesity (Vuille & Mellbin, 1979), including such factors as distinctive eating styles consisting of eating food faster than nonobese peers, food preferences, and leaving less food on the plate (Ballard, Gipson, Guttenberg, & Ramsey, 1980; Geller, Keane, & Scheirer, 1981; Jeffrey, Lemnitzer, Hickey, Hess, McLellarn, & Stroud, 1980; Keane, Geller, & Scheirer, 1981), and a far less active lifestyle than nonobese peers (Epstein & Wing, 1980; Waxman & Stunkard, 1980). In pediatric weight management interventions, particular attention must be directed toward the measurement of weight in consideration of height/age status or growth charts (Weil, 1977), with close supervision of a rational modification in diet to assure proper nutrition for the rapidly growing child and adolescent (Dwyer, 1980).

A number of studies have indicated the potential of behavioral techniques in controlling infant, childhood, and adolescent obesity through the modification of eating, exercise, and diet patterns (Aragona, Cassady, & Drabman, 1975; Coates & Thoresen, 1981; Cohen, Gelfand, Dodd, Jensen, & Turner, 1980; Epstein, Wing, Steranchak, Dickson, & Michelson, 1980; Gross, Wheeler, & Hess, 1976; Kingsley & Shapiro, 1977; Pisacano, Lichter, Ritter, & Siegel, 1978; Weiss, 1977; Wheeler & Hess, 1976). As reviewed by Brownell & Stunkard (1978), these initial studies hold considerable promise in the management of pediatric obesity. Two recent studies exemplify the current biobehavioral approach to weight management in children (Epstein et al., 1980) and adolescents (Coates & Thoresen, 1981).

Epstein et al. (1980) compared a family-based behavioral treatment group with a family-based nutrition education group for children and their mothers. The inclusion criteria for the child were: 6 to 12 years of age, greater than 20 percent above ideal weight according to American Child Health Association height-weight tables, no medical problems that would contraindicate weight loss, and at least one parent who would be willing to actively participate in the program. Six families were assigned to the behavioral treatment group and seven families were assigned to the nutritional education comparison group. Both groups were provided information on calorie-counting, basic nutrition, and exercise. Additionally, the behavioral treatment group received instructions on self-monitoring, changing specific eating behaviors, prompts, social reinforcement and a contingency contract for weekly weight loss of 1 pound for both the child and the parent (the parent participants averaged 48 percent overweight), self-monitoring of daily calorie and weight measures by the child, and reduction of high-caloric foods by the child.

The results showed that at the 3-month follow-up, the behavioral treatment group averaged a 13 percent overweight loss compared to a 5 percent overweight loss for the nutrition education comparison group. Also, a positive relationship was found between parent and child weight loss for the behavioral treatment group, suggesting active participation by the parents in the weight loss program. Epstein et al. (1980) suggest that the changes in parental health habits may profoundly influence their children's health habits through the modeling process and may further enhance weight control for obese children. For the pediatric population, active parental involvement is clearly necessary to optimize the potential impact on weight control through eating, exercise, and diet modification. Through parent training, the parents can be taught to not only serve as healthy models for their children, but also to prompt and reinforce appropriate weight-related behaviors by their children within a self-management approach (Epstein, Wing, Koeske, Andrasik, & Ossip, 1981). A related study by Epstein et al. (1982) suggested the utility of promoting children's lifestyle exercise as a way to increase energy expenditure and long-term weight control through a parent training/child self-management approach.

Coates and Thoresen (1981) intensely studied the behavior and weight changes in three obese adolescents, 128, 71, and 73 percent overweight, respectively (ages 16, 16, and 15 years, respectively). The 16 year olds served as treatment subjects, while the 15 year old served as a placebo control subject to control for the potential reactive effects of therapist contact and observation. The study was designed to examine the relationships between treatment strategies, changes in eating behaviors and home environments, and weight loss. The treatment program consisted of teaching the adolescents specific skills for altering eating and exercise behaviors (e.g., self-monitoring, stimulus control, lower calorie foods, self-instructions, self-reinforcement) and teaching family members specific procedures for supporting and encouraging their children's use of appropriate eating behaviors (e.g., parents establishing a token exchange point system).

The dependent measures in the study consisted of weight, percent overweight, self-report measures, and observations in the home by the experimenters. The self-report measure, The Daily Energy Diary, provided information on six measures: average meal duration, number of places at home where food was eaten, the times of food intake, the activities associated with eating (e.g., television viewing), the number of minutes of exercise, and the average hunger rating (on a scale of 0 = not hungry to 3 = extremely hungry). The Eating Analysis and Treatment Schedule form was designed to be used by the observers in the adolescents' home at mealtimes to gather data on the physical environment (e.g., a list of the foods in the cupboards, refrigerator, and freezer), and on the adolescents' eating behaviors during the meals.

The results showed that in a 14-week period, the treatment subjects lost 20 and 11.5 pounds, respectively, while the control subject gained 5 pounds. Further, the self-report and observer data indicated behavioral and environmental changes. However, each adolescent showed different patterns of change, even though both received identical instructions. These differential behavioral changes strongly indicate the need to systematically assess therapeutic adherence.

The biobehavioral assessment and management of adherence by children, adolescents, and their parents to the prescribed eating, exercise, and diet regimens clearly requires further research (Becker, Maiman, Kirscht, Haefner, & Drachman, 1977; Glanz, 1980; Johnson, Wildman, & O'Brien, 1980; Stalonas, Johnson, & Christ, 1978), particularly since the greatest noncompliance has been associated with both long-term and complex regimens, two major characteristics of weight control programs (Dunbar & Stunkard, 1979). Thus a systematic assessment of therapeutic adherence factors must be an integral part of weight management programs for childhood and adolescent obesity.

If adherence to the prescribed eating, exercise, and diet regimen is not systematically assessed, weight loss as measured during the clinic visit may be a result of inappropriate eating, exercise, and diet behaviors, such as fasting, excessive exercise, unhealthy diet, or even self-induced vomiting and the use of cathartics (see following section on bulimia). Thus, weight loss *per se* cannot be the sole determinant of therapeutic adherence within the biobehavioral perspective; rather, weight loss and behavioral parameters must both be systematically assessed. This biobehavioral assessment of therapeutic adherence may be particularly important in working with obese adolescents given the recent findings on the relatively high prevalence of bulimia in this age group.

## ANOREXIA NERVOSA

Primary anorexia nervosa may be defined as an excessive desire to attain an idealized body shape, associated with a weight loss at least 20 percent below height/age standards, which is not secondary to other psychopathology or physical illness. Anorexia nervosa is a complex biobehavioral disorder, with an onset typically during adolescence and predominantly in females. It may include such clinical symptoms as an aberrant eating pattern (fasting, binging, vomiting), overly restricted diet, excessive exercise, social skills deficit, "weight phobia," amenorrhea, endocrine disturbances, body image distortion, and maladaptive family transactions (Casper, Offer, & Ostrov, 1981; Hsu, 1980; Strober, Goldenberg, Green, & Saxon, 1979; Walsh, 1982; Yager, 1982). In

anorexia nervosa, eating, exercise, and diet modification is an essential component of a comprehensive treatment approach.

The treatment of anorexia nervosa may be broadly divided into an initial
short-term intervention phase aimed primarily at recovering a healthy nutritional status and normalizing weight so as to reduce the life-threatening
condition, and a long-term intervention phase aimed at preventing nutritional
and weight gain relapse and promoting psychosocial adjustment (Hsu, 1980;
Stunkard & Mahoney, 1976). Currently, the initial short-term intervention
phase has been successfully investigated and applied; however, long-term
nutritional maintenance (adherence) and psychosocial adjustment have in
general been elusive, regardless of the treatment modality (Hsu, 1980).

Eating, exercise, and diet modification in anorexia nervosa have been conducted within the short-term intensive inpatient hospitalization model (Agras,
Barlow, Chapin, Abel, & Leitenberg, 1974; Munford, 1980), with increasing
attention now being directed toward the long-term maintenance of normal
eating, exercise, and diet patterns posthospitalization (Ferguson, 1981;
Hauserman & Lavin, 1977; McGlynn, 1980; Pertschuk, Edwards, & Pomerleau, 1978), often within the context of structured family therapy (Leibman,
Minuchin, & Baker, 1974). A limitation of most of these studies has been the
lack of a systematic assessment of adherence to the prescribed eating, exercise,
and diet regimen. This is a particularly significant problem, since some patients
with anorexia nervosa may maintain an adequate weight gain while engaging in
idiosyncratic or maladaptive eating, exercise, and diet habits (Rosen, 1980).
Considerable empirical work remains to be conducted in anorexia nervosa
before a specific comprehensive treatment approach can be recommended.


# BULIMIA

Bulimia is similar to anorexia nervosa in that the patient strives to attain an
idealized body shape, with the onset of this biobehavioral disorder occurring
typically during adolescence and predominantly in females. In contrast to
anorexia nervosa, however, these patients are usually of normal or slightly over
normal weight. Bulimia literally means "ox hunger" or a voracious appetite,
characterized by a rapid consumption of large amounts of food in a short
period of time. These binge-eating episodes are invariably followed by self-
induced vomiting and/or purging (purgatives or cathartics) in an attempt to
counteract the effects of overeating and prevent a weight gain (Mitchell, Pyle,
& Eckert, 1981; Russell, 1979). Bulimia as a symptom complex was initially
identified in patients with anorexia nervosa. Casper, Eckert, Halmi, Goldberg,
and Davis (1980) studied the eating habits of 105 hospitalized female patients
with anorexia nervosa, finding that 53 percent had achieved weight loss by
consistently fasting, whereas 47 percent periodically resorted to binging and

vomiting. Whereas the fasting patients more often denied hunger, the bulimic patients admitted more frequently to a strong appetite and tended to be older. Casper et al. (1980), in analyzing their findings, suggested that patients with bulimia represent a subgroup among patients with anorexia nervosa.

Russell (1979) suggested that this variant of anorexia nervosa be termed bulimia nervosa. Russell (1979) provided an extensive description of 30 patients whose symptoms resembled anorexia nervosa, but did not conform fully to its diagnostic criteria. These patients were in common with true anorexia nervosa in that they were determined to keep their weight below a self-determined threshold. However, in contrast to true anorexia nervosa, they tended to be heavier and more likely to menstruate regularly (28 of the 30 patients were females with an average age of 19 years old at the onset of the disorder). All 30 patients were selected on two criteria: an irresistible urge to overeat followed by self-induced vomiting and/or purging and a morbid fear of becoming fat ("weight phobia"). In addition to self-induced vomiting and/or purging to prevent weight gain subsequent to a binge, some patients alternated overeating with periods of eating abstinence and/or excessive exercise.

Casper et al. (1980) reported that bulimic patients discovered that consumption of carbohydrates in sweets or ice cream and the activities associated with the eating process, such as biting, chewing, and swallowing, had an emotionally soothing effect and provided a mechanism for the relief of distressing thoughts and emotions such as frustration, tension, emptiness, and boredom, independent of hunger sensations. Russell (1979) further found that bulimic patients frequently overate as a sequence to ingesting even a small amount of a favorite food, especially foods that the patients considered fattening such as carbohydrate-rich foods. There was often found to be an all-or-none pattern to the sequence of overeating, excessive exercise, and overly restricted diet patterns, related to intense feelings of becoming fat, with overeating tending to be a solitary and secretive habit. Thus, eating, exercise, and diet modification, as in anorexia nervosa, is an essential component of an overall comprehensive treatment approach. Of particular significance, recent findings have indicated that bulimia is by no means confined to patients with anorexia nervosa.

Hawkins and Clement (1980) investigated binge-eating in a sample of normal weight and overweight male and female college undergraduates, none of whom were ostensibly displaying mental health problems. The initial sample comprised 182 females and 65 males, while the replication sample contained 73 females and 45 males. An additional clinical sample of 26 overweight college females (mean excess weight of 40 percent) from a weight control program were studied for comparison. A 19-item questionnaire was developed to measure behavioral and attitudinal parameters of bulimia, with binge-eating defined as uncontrolled, excessive eating.

The frequency of self-reported occurrences of binge-eating for the initial classroom sample showed that 79 percent of the undergraduate females, and 49 percent of the undergraduate males reported binge-eating episodes. The same pattern of results were found for the replication sample. Binges were also reported as frequently among the overweight sample as among the normal weight females. One-third of the male and female normal weight subjects in the initial sample reported binging at least once per week, compared with 40 percent of the overweight subjects. The duration of the binge episodes for 90 percent of the subjects was less than one hour in duration. Only nine students, all women, eight of whom were of normal weight, reported that they had ever induced vomiting after a binge. Three-quarters of the students indicated that their binge-eating tendencies began between the age of 15 to 20 years (the mean of the sample was 20 years). For both sexes, the severity of reported binge-eating was positively correlated with the degree of dieting concern, and in females, with a negative physical self-image.

Herman and Mack (1975) had previously speculated that extreme dieting concern may characterize a chronic deprivational state wherein individuals are trying to maintain their body weight below a biologically determined "set point," and are able to sustain this relative deprivation precisely because of the restraint they habitually exhibit. Hawkins and Clement (1980) speculate that the efforts to maintain body weight below this equilibrium level (in pursuit of the idealized body shape) through restrained eating or strict dieting may increase the susceptibility to loss of control binge-eating episodes. Gray's (1977) findings that almost one-half of a sample of college male and female subjects displayed some body image distortion further supports the potential prevalence of precipitating conditions for bulimic behavior. Paradoxically, it appears that the more severe binge-eating problems are coincident with more stringent attempts at restrained eating behavior, with binge-eating episodes frequently precipitated by life stress events (Hawkins & Clement, 1980).

The biobehavioral treatment of bulimia has included the modification of eating, exercise, diet and vomiting/purgative patterns through self-regulation, reinforcement, contingency contracting, systematic desensitization, and parent training techniques (Geller, Kelly, Traxler, & Marone, 1978; Linden, 1980; Monti, McCrady, & Barlow, 1977; Rosen & Leitenberg, 1982). However, further empirical investigation is required with larger population samples.

# EATING, EXERCISE, AND DIET MODIFICATION TECHNIQUES

A programmatic study by Killam, Apodaca, Manella, and Varni (1983) provides a comprehensive methodological approach to the management of pediatric eating, exercise, and diet behaviors. The specific techniques will be discussed below in detail, while the study population and results will be presented in Chapter 8.

## Biobehavioral Assessment

Prior to beginning the group biobehavioral intervention, all the children underwent a problem-oriented record (POR) evaluation by the interdisciplinary health team. A pediatric nurse practitioner performed a complete physical examination and a history which included information regarding

Table 7.1.    Food and Beverage Intake Record.

Name:                              Date:

Completed by:

|  | TIME | FOOD EATEN | HOW MUCH? | DOING WHAT? |
|---|---|---|---|---|
| 1st MEAL | | | | |
| SNACK(S) | | | | |
| 2nd MEAL | | | | |
| SNACK(S) | | | | |
| 3rd MEAL | | | | |
| SNACK(S) | | | | |

Table 7.2.  Exercise Chart.

Name:

Completed by:

Week of:

| EXERCISE | Sunday | Monday | Tuesday | Wednesday | Thursday | Friday | Saturday |
|----------|--------|--------|---------|-----------|----------|--------|----------|
|          |        |        |         |           |          |        |          |
|          |        |        |         |           |          |        |          |
|          |        |        |         |           |          |        |          |
|          |        |        |         |           |          |        |          |
|          |        |        |         |           |          |        |          |
|          |        |        |         |           |          |        |          |

Key:  X = number of times;  min = minutes;  hr = hour

previous attempts at weight control, the presence of overweight among other family members, any special problems with nutrition (e.g., any food intolerances), and identification of the family member responsible for food preparation. A physical therapist performed sensory and motor testing and gathered information regarding the child's level of independence with activities of daily living. A psychosocial assessment battery was administered by a medical social worker to identify any psychosocial adjustment and behavior problems.

The children were weighed on the same scale in the clinic during the POR evaluation and subsequent treatment and follow-up sessions (skin fold thickness was also measured). Due to the emphasis of the program on long-term changes in eating, exercise, and diet behaviors rather than on weight loss *per se* (particularly in children who may "grow into" their weight), the children were not required to weigh themselves at home. Height measurements were obtained at the POR evaluation, the first and last treatment sessions, and at all follow-up sessions. Percent overweight was calculated by determining the ideal weight (50th percentile) for height per National Center for Health Statistics Standards (1976) and dividing the pounds overweight by the ideal weight.

Baseline information on eating, exercise, and diet habits was collected during the first two weeks of the program. Time of food and beverage intake, type and amount, and any associated activity (e.g., television viewing, playing, reading) were recorded on a daily food record (Table 7.1). Exercise was recorded daily on an exercise record (Table 7.2). Questionnaires were devised to test the parents' knowledge of basic nutritional information and parents' and children's knowledge regarding exercise and its role in weight control. These were administered during the first session to identify goals for instruction.

As the treatment program progressed, the children (generally with the help of their parents) continued to keep food intake and exercise records. Later, a self-evaluation form was introduced which required a rating by the children on the appropriateness of their eating, exercise, and diet behaviors for the day (Table 7.3). Parents were asked throughout the program to keep reinforcement charts at home which specified the desired eating, exercise, and diet behaviors and helped identify when reinforcement was earned (see Table 12.1).

To assess therapeutic adherence, data were compiled on the number of completed recording forms in relation to the number assigned. In addition, the number of treatment and follow-up sessions attended by each family member was recorded. As a subjective measure of adherence, a questionnaire was administered at the second follow-up session (Table 7.4). This questionnaire described 21 behaviors related to weight control that had been introduced during the program. The parents rated the items according to the change in frequency of occurrence of the behaviors on a + 3 (greatly increased) to a − 3 (greatly decreased) 7-point scale.

Table 7.3.    Self-Evaluation Record.

Name:

Completed by:

| DATE | APPROPRIATE EATING PATTERN | | APPROPRIATE DIET PATTERN | | APPROPRIATE EXERCISE PATTERN | |
|---|---|---|---|---|---|---|
| | YES | NO | YES | NO | YES | NO |
| | | | | | | |
| | | | | | | |
| | | | | | | |
| | | | | | | |
| | | | | | | |
| | | | | | | |
| | | | | | | |
| | | | | | | |
| | | | | | | |
| | | | | | | |
| | | | | | | |
| | | | | | | |
| | | | | | | |
| | | | | | | |
| | | | | | | |
| | | | | | | |
| | | | | | | |
| | | | | | | |
| | | | | | | |
| | | | | | | |
| | | | | | | |
| | | | | | | |

Table 7.4.    Adherence Questionnaire.

We would like to get an idea of any changes in your home that have occurred as a result of the weight control program. We have listed some behaviors involved in weight control. Think about whether these occur with *more* frequency ("increased") or *less* frequency ("decreased") or whether no change has occurred and circle the corresponding number.

|  | Greatly decreased | Moderately decreased | Slightly decreased | No change | Slightly increased | Moderately increased | Greatly increased |
|---|---|---|---|---|---|---|---|
| 1. Parent food shops on a full stomach instead of when hungry. | −3 | −2 | −1 | 0 | 1 | 2 | 3 |
| 2. Parent shops from a list—no "impulse" buying. | −3 | −2 | −1 | 0 | 1 | 2 | 3 |
| 3. Parent buys more low-calorie foods. | −3 | −2 | −1 | 0 | 1 | 2 | 3 |
| 4. Parent buys fewer high-calorie foods. | −3 | −2 | −1 | 0 | 1 | 2 | 3 |
| 5. If high-calorie foods are bought, they are bought in smaller portions. | −3 | −2 | −1 | 0 | 1 | 2 | 3 |
| 6. If high-calorie foods are bought, they are bought in a form that requires more preparation. | −3 | −2 | −1 | 0 | 1 | 2 | 3 |
| 7. High-calorie foods are kept out of sight. | −3 | −2 | −1 | 0 | 1 | 2 | 3 |
| 8. Low calorie foods are kept where child has easy access to them. | −3 | −2 | −1 | 0 | 1 | 2 | 3 |
| 9. Child separates eating from other activities. | −3 | −2 | −1 | 0 | 1 | 2 | 3 |
| 10. Child eats only in one place at home. | −3 | −2 | −1 | 0 | 1 | 2 | 3 |
| 11. Meals and snacks are scheduled instead of spontaneous. | −3 | −2 | −1 | 0 | 1 | 2 | 3 |
| 12. Portion sizes are smaller. | −3 | −2 | −1 | 0 | 1 | 2 | 3 |
| 13. Second helpings are harder to get to. | −3 | −2 | −1 | 0 | 1 | 2 | 3 |
| 14. Child puts down utensils between bites. | −3 | −2 | −1 | 0 | 1 | 2 | 3 |
| 15. Child has slower rate of eating. | −3 | −2 | −1 | 0 | 1 | 2 | 3 |
| 16. Child stops eating before feeling full. | −3 | −2 | −1 | 0 | 1 | 2 | 3 |
| 17. Child exercises at least 3 times per week. | −3 | −2 | −1 | 0 | 1 | 2 | 3 |
| 18. Child evaluates food intake and exercise at the end of each day. | −3 | −2 | −1 | 0 | 1 | 2 | 3 |
| 19. Child eats fewer high-calorie foods. | −3 | −2 | −1 | 0 | 1 | 2 | 3 |
| 20. Child eats more low-calorie foods. | −3 | −2 | −1 | 0 | 1 | 2 | 3 |
| 21. Parents use praise and other reinforcement to increase desired behavior. | −3 | −2 | −1 | 0 | 1 | 2 | 3 |

Table 7.5.    Social Validity Questionnaire.

Your response to these questions will help us evaluate the effectiveness of the program. We would like to hear your ideas about how it may be improved. Please circle the number that best expresses your feelings about *every* question. Then, add comments as desired. THANK YOU!!!

| | No, strongly | No, moderately | No, mildly | Uncertain | Yes, mildly | Yes, moderately | Yes, strongly |
|---|---|---|---|---|---|---|---|
| 1. Did the program help your child with weight control?<br>Comments: _____ | −3 | −2 | −1 | 0 | 1 | 2 | 3 |
| 2. Did the program meet your expectations as to its content?<br>Comments: _____ | −3 | −2 | −1 | 0 | 1 | 2 | 3 |
| 3. Have you learned any new techniques from the program?<br>Comments: _____ | −3 | −2 | −1 | 0 | 1 | 2 | 3 |
| 4. If so, can these techniques be helpful with other family members?<br>Comments: _____ | −3 | −2 | −1 | 0 | 1 | 2 | 3 |
| 5. Has anyone in the family beside your child lost weight during the program?<br>If so, how much? _____ | −3 | −2 | −1 | 0 | 1 | 2 | 3 |
| 6. Do you feel this type of program is a good way to improve weight control in your child?<br>Comments: _____ | −3 | −2 | −1 | 0 | 1 | 2 | 3 |
| 7. Did the staff teach the material in each lesson so it was easily understood?<br>Comments: _____ | −3 | −2 | −1 | 0 | 1 | 2 | 3 |
| 8. Was the time required (2 hours, 8 weeks) reasonable?<br>Comments: _____ | −3 | −2 | −1 | 0 | 1 | 2 | 3 |
| 9. Was the scheduling (day and time) convenient?<br>If not, what would have been better? _____ | −3 | −2 | −1 | 0 | 1 | 2 | 3 |
| 10. Were the home assignments reasonable?<br>Comments: _____ | −3 | −2 | −1 | 0 | 1 | 2 | 3 |
| 11. Were the videotapes and slides shown helpful?<br>Comments: _____ | −3 | −2 | −1 | 0 | 1 | 2 | 3 |
| 12. Was the book assigned (*Slim Chance in a Fat World*) helpful?<br>Comments: _____ | −3 | −2 | −1 | 0 | 1 | 2 | 3 |
| 13. Were the group discussions (personal comments, problems, ideas) helpful?<br>Comments: _____ | −3 | −2 | −1 | 0 | 1 | 2 | 3 |
| 14. Were the recording charts useful? | −3 | −2 | −1 | 0 | 1 | 2 | 3 |
| Food record? | −3 | −2 | −1 | 0 | 1 | 2 | 3 |
| Exercise record? | −3 | −2 | −1 | 0 | 1 | 2 | 3 |
| Self-evaluation record? | −3 | −2 | −1 | 0 | 1 | 2 | 3 |
| Reward chart?<br>Comments: _____ | −3 | −2 | −1 | 0 | 1 | 2 | 3 |

Please add any other comments or ideas you have:

A final assessment tool used was a social validity questionnaire administered at the first follow-up session (Table 7.5). Two dimensions of social validity were addressed: social appropriateness (i.e., acceptability of the treatment procedures) and social importance (i.e., satisfaction with the results). The parents rated 14 items on a $+3$ (yes, strongly) to $-3$ (no, strongly) 7-point scale.

## Treatment Program

The children and at least one of their parents met with a pediatric nurse practitioner, a physical therapist, and a medical social worker for weekly two-hour group sessions over eight weeks. During the first hour of each session, the children and their parents remained together for instruction on selected aspects of diet, exercise, and specific behavioral techniques for altering eating habits, and for discussion of the previous week's home assignments. During the second hour, the children left with the physical therapist and were instructed on various exercise and sports activities. The parents remained with the pediatric nurse practitioner and medical social worker and were instructed on specific behavioral parenting skills and additional nutritional information. Each parent purchased a copy of a behavioral weight control manual to facilitate the learning process (Stuart & Davis, 1978). Throughout, the emphasis was on the children's self-regulation of eating, exercise, and diet behaviors, rather than weight change *per se*.

Nutritional instruction included discussions of the four basic food groups, servings required, nutrients available, and considerations of calorie value and cost. Ideas for low calorie snacking were introduced early in the program and discussed throughout. The parents were encouraged to share ideas for low calorie food preparation and substitutions of low for high calorie foods. Several types of raw vegetables new to the children were brought in for them to sample to increase their awareness of alternatives to high calorie snacks.

In order to further increase the children's awareness of the caloric densities of specific foods, a method suggested by Epstein, Masek, and Marshall (1978) was developed. Foods were divided into red, yellow, and green groups, corresponding to high, medium, and low caloric density, respectively and were explained in relationship to the colors of a traffic light. "Green" foods could be eaten freely, caution was required for "yellow" foods, and "red" foods signalled "stop!". Pictures of specific foods in each group were pasted on large bright posters in each of these colors. In addition, red, yellow, and green colored sheets with the appropriate foods listed according to each food group were distributed (Table 7.6). These verbal and written instructions were incorporated into every treatment session.

Basic exercise physiology and exposure to a variety of exercise activities were incorporated into the program via slides and videotape presentations accompanied by instructions from the physical therapist. Information regarding the

Table 7.6.    Color-coded Food Groups.

---

## GREEN

---

*Fruit-Vegetable Group*
Asparagus
Bean sprouts
Broccoli
Cabbage
Cauliflower
Celery
Chinese pea pods
Cucumbers
Greens
Lettuce
Pickles-dill or sour
Radishes
String beans
Summer squash
Zucchini

*Miscellaneous*
Bouillon or broth
Consomme
Chewing gum (sugarless)
D-Zerta gelatin
Iced tea with lemon and/or sugar
    substitute
Kool-aid or lemonade (made with sugar
    substitute)
Soft drinks (diet)
Tomato juice
V-8 juice
Zero salad dressing*

*Zero Salad Dressing

½ cup tomato or V-8 juice
2 Tbsp vinegar or lemon juice
1 Tbsp minced onion
    Salt/pepper/herbs as desired

Add if desired: minced parsley, green pepper, horseradish, dry mustard, etc.

---

## YELLOW

---

*Milk Group*
Cottage cheese, low-fat
Milk, non-fat or low-fat
Yoghurt (plain)
Cheese

*Meat* Group*
Beans
Beef (lean cut-fat removed)
Bologna
Chicken (broiled, baked)
Eggs
Fish
Frankfurter
Ham (fat removed)
Hamburger (lean)
Lentils
Lamb (fat removed)
Liver
Peas (dried split)
Shellfish

Tuna (packed in water)
Turkey
* Cooked without frying or batter

*Bread-Cereal Group*
Bagel
Breads (except sweet breads)
Crackers
Dry cereal (non-sugared)
Hot cereal
Pasta
Rice
Tortilla

*Miscellaneous*
Fruit juices
Jam, jelly (dietetic, low sugar)
Popcorn (unbuttered)
Pretzels
Salad dressings (dietetic)

Table 7.6.    Color-coded Food Groups (continued).

*Fruit\*-Vegetable Group*

| Apple | Beets |
|---|---|
| Berries | Brussel sprouts |
| Cherries | Carrots |
| Grapes | Corn |
| Melon | Eggplant |
| Orange | Mushrooms |
| Peach | Peas |
| Pear | Peppers |
| Pineapple | Potato |
| Plum | Tomato |
| Watermelon | |

\*Fresh or packed only in natural juices

*RED*

*Milk Group*
Cottage cheese (regular)
Cream
Ice cream
Ice milk
Sour cream
Whole milk

*Meat Group*
Cheese\*
Fried and/or battered meat/fish
Meats cut relatively fat and/or with fat
  not removed
Nuts and nut butters
Pork

*Fruit\*\*-Vegetable Group*

| Banana | Avocado |
|---|---|
| Prunes | Lima beans |
| Raisins | Pickles, sweet |
| | Sweet potato |

\*Cheese is a "red" food in the meat
  group because serving size is 3 oz, not
  1 oz as in milk group

\*\*Plus all canned in sugar or syrup

*Bread-Cereal Group*
Biscuit
Bun
Cake
Coffee cake
Cookies
Danish pastry
Doughnut
Pancake
Pie
Waffle

*Miscellaneous*
Candy
Chocolate milk
Fats (butter, margarine, etc.)
Jam, jelly
Mayonnaise
Potato chips
Salad dressings (regular bottled)
Soft drinks
Syrup

effects of exercise and caloric expenditure upon weight management as well as physical fitness was presented in lecture-discussion format with the parents and their children. The children participated in four one-hour exercise sessions in which they performed warm-up exercises, strengthening and stretching exercises, aerobics, and relaxation techniques. These activities were individually adapted to accommodate each child's physical ability. The exercises were discussed with the parents and used as a guideline for the child's home exercise program. Subsequent to the exercise sessions, the children were instructed in sports activities.

The behavioral techniques emphasized included stimulus control, specific changes in eating behaviors, and reinforcement of the prescribed eating, exercise, and diet patterns. The stimulus control techniques focused on the management of the antecedents of eating behaviors. Antecedent stimuli management included (for the parents) shopping on a full stomach, buying items only from a prepared list, increasing the purchase of low calorie foods, reduced buying of high calorie foods, and buying in the smallest portions requiring the most preparation. It was suggested that the parents reduce portion size at each meal, make normal portions appear larger by placing on smaller dishes, and make second helpings harder to obtain by serving food in the kitchen instead of family-style. In addition, the parents were asked to keep problem foods out of reach and sight of the children and to make low calorie foods of various types readily available in special drawers or shelves. The children were asked to separate eating from other activities and to eat only in one place at home and one place at school and to schedule all meals and snacks.

The children were encouraged to put down eating utensils after every bite, slow the eating rate by other means (such as conversation) to make the meal last at least twenty minutes, and to stop eating before they felt full. It was explained by pictures that a sensation of fullness occurred not because food was present in the stomach, but because food was absorbed and its "message" reached the brain. Hence, it was shown that a sense of fullness occurred 10 to 15 minutes after eating was completed. The children and their parents were encouraged to delay desserts, for example, for this amount of time.

The management of the consequences of successful eating and exercise was a joint effort of both the parent and child. A reinforcement list of special activities (e.g., being read a story, painting, trips to the zoo) was developed by each parent/child pair under the guidance of the therapist. In addition, it was stressed to the parents that social reinforcement (praise, attention) was equally if not more important than material reinforcers. A reinforcement chart was developed to aid parents in reinforcing desired behaviors. Reinforcement was contingent on gradual approximations of the targeted behavioral repertoire (shaping). Thus, the children were initially reinforced for simply recording their food and beverage intake after a 1-week baseline; subsequently self-recording of exercise behaviors was reinforced. Next, small changes in eating behaviors were reinforced, followed by the addition of reinforcement for small changes in exercise behaviors. By the half way point of the treatment sessions, the children were being reinforced for the self-monitoring and the self-regulation of eating and exercise patterns. Before the self-evaluation phase was introduced, the children were asked to circle foods on their self-recording charts with red, yellow, and green pens (according to the previously introduced color-code system) to facilitate the identification and teaching of appropriate diet and eating patterns. Finally, during the last several treatment sessions, they were reinforced for limiting the intake of "red" foods. By the end of the eight weeks of treatment, the food, beverage, and exercise records were phased out, and reinforcement was contingent on the correct self-evaluation of eating, exercise, and diet patterns.

During the first half of each follow-up session, the children were weighed, their progress was discussed, with feedback provided on problem areas, and social reinforcement was contingent on adherence to the treatment regimens. The children were encouraged to continue using the self-evaluation record daily. After the analysis of the adherence data, the children engaged in sports activities which appeared to be reinforcing for them (e.g., bowling, horseback riding, basketball). The specifics of the results of this program are presented in Chapter 8.

## REFERENCES

Adams, F.H., & Landau, E.M. What are healthy blood pressures for children? *Pediatrics,* 1981, **68**, 268–270.

Agras, W.S., Barlow, D.H., Chapin, H.N., Abel, G.G., & Leitenberg, H. Behavior modification of anorexia nervosa. *Archives of General Psychiatry,* 1974, **30**, 279–286.

Allen, L.D., & Iwata, B.A. Reinforcing exercise maintenance using existing high-rate activities. *Behavior Modification,* 1980, **4**, 337–354.

Aragona, J., Cassady, J., & Drabman, R.S. Treating overweight children through parental training and contingency contracting. *Journal of Applied Behavior Analysis,* 1975, **8**, 269–278.

Ballard, B.D., Gipson, M.T., Guttenberg, W., & Ramsey, K. Palatability of food as a factor influencing obese and normal-weight children's eating habits. *Behaviour Research and Therapy,* 1980, **18**, 598–600.

Beaglehole, R., Trost, D.C., Tamir, I., Kwiterovich, P., Glueck, C.J., Insull, W., & Christensen, B. Plasma high-density lipoprotein cholesterol in children and young adults: The lipid research clinics program prevalence study. *Circulation,* 1980, **62**, 83–92.

Becker, M.H., Maiman, L.A., Kirscht, J.P., Haefner, D.P., & Drachman, R.H. The Health Belief model and prediction of dietary compliance: A field experiment. *Journal of Health and Social Behavior,* 1977, **18**, 348–366.

Blumenthal, J.A., Williams, R.B., Kong, Y., Schanberg, S.M., & Thompson, L.W. Type A behavior pattern and coronary atherosclerosis. *Circulation,* 1978, **58**, 634–639.

Botvin, G.J., Eng, A., & Williams, C.L. Preventing the onset of cigarette smoking through life skills training. *Preventive Medicine,* 1980, **9**, 135–143.

Brownell, K.D., & Kaye, F.S. A school-based behavior modification, nutrition education, and physical activity program for obese children. *American Journal of Clinical Nutrition,* 1982, **35**, 277–283.

Brownell, K.D., & Stunkard, A.J. Behavioral treatment of obesity in children. *American Journal of Diseases of Children,* 1978, **132**, 403–412.

Casper, R.C., Eckert, E.K., Halmi, K.A., Goldberg, S.C., & Davis, J.M. Bulimia: Its incidence and clinical importance in patients with anorexia nervosa. *Archives of General Psychiatry,* 1980, **37**, 1030–1035.

Casper, R.C., Offer, D., & Ostrov, E. The self-image of adolescents with acute anorexia nervosa. *Journal of Pediatrics,* 1981, **98**, 656–661.

Chassin, L., Presson, C.C., Bensenberg, M., Corty, E., Olsharsky, R.W., & Sherman, S.J. Predicting adolescents' intentions to smoke cigarettes. *Journal of Health and Social Behavior,* 1981, **22**, 445–455.

Clarke, W.R., Schrott, H.G., Leaverton, P.E., Connor, W.E., & Lauer, R.M. Tracking of blood lipids and blood pressure in school age children: The Muscatine study. *Circulation,* 1978, **58**, 626–634.

Coates, T.J., Jeffery, R.W., & Slinkard, L.A. Heart healthy eating and exercise: Introducing and maintaining changes in health behaviors. *American Journal of Public Health,* 1981, **71**, 15–23.

Coates, T.J., Jeffery, R.W., Slinkard, L.A., Killen, J.D., & Danaher, B.G. Frequency of contact and monetary reward in weight loss, lipid changes, and blood pressure reduction with adolescents. *Behavior Therapy,* 1982, **13**, 175–185.

Coates, T.J., & Masek, B.J. Pediatric cardiology: Congenital disorders and preventive cardiology. In D.C. Russo & J.W. Varni (Eds.), *Behavioral Pediatrics: Research and Practice.* New York: Plenum Press, 1982.

Coates, T.J., & Thoresen, C.E. Behavior and weight changes in three obese adolescents. *Behavior Therapy,* 1981, **12**, 383–399.

Coates, T.J., & Thoresen, C.E. Treating obesity in children and adolescents: A review. *American Journal of Public Health,* 1978, **68**, 143–151.

Cohen, E.A., Gelfand, D.M., Dodd, D.K., Jensen, J., & Turner, C. Self-control practices associated with weight loss maintenance in children and adolescents. *Behavior Therapy,* 1980, **11**, 26–37.

Cooper, M.J., & Aygen, M.M. A relaxation technique in the management of hypercholestrolemia. *Journal of Human Stress,* 1979, **5**, 24–27.

Dishman, R.K., & Ickes, W. Self-motivation and adherence to therapeutic exercise. *Journal of Behavioral Medicine,* 1981, **4**, 421–438.

Dunbar, J.M., & Stunkard, A.J. Adherence to diet and drug regimen. In R. Levy, B. Rifkind, B. Dennis, & N. Ernst (Eds.), *Nutrition, Lipids, and Coronary Heart Disease.* New York: Raven Press, 1979.

Dwyer, J. Diets for children and adolescents that meet the dietary goals. *American Journal of Diseases of Children,* 1980, **134**, 1073–1080.

Epstein, L.H., Masek, B.J., & Marshall, W.R. A nutritionally based school program for control of eating in obese children. *Behavior Therapy,* 1978, **9**, 766–778.

Epstein, L.H., & Wing, R.R. Aerobic exercise and weight. *Addictive Behaviors,* 1980, **5**, 371–388.

Epstein, L.H., Wing, R.R., Koeske, R., Andrasik, F., & Ossip, D.J. Child and parent weight loss in family-based behavior modification programs. *Journal of Consulting and Clinical Psychology,* 1981, **49**, 674–685.

Epstein, L.H., Wing, R.R., Koeske, R., Ossip, D., & Beck, S. A comparison of lifestyle change and programmed aerobic exercise on weight and fitness changes in obese children. *Behavior Therapy,* 1982, **13**, 651–665.

Epstein, L.H., Wing, R.R., Steranchak, L., Dickson, B., & Michelson, J. Comparison of family-based behavior modification and nutrition education for childhood obesity. *Journal of Pediatric Psychology,* 1980, **5**, 25–36.

Epstein, L.H., Wing, R.R., Thompson, J.K., & Griffin, W. Attendance and fitness in aerobics exercise: The effects of contract and lottery procedures. *Behavior Modification,* 1980, **4**, 465–479.

Evans, R.I. Smoking in children: Developing a social psychological strategy of deterrence. *Preventive Medicine,* 1976, **5**, 122–127.

Evans, R.I., Rozelle, R.M., Mittelmark, M.B., Hansen, W.B., Bane, A.L., & Havis, J. Deterring the onset of smoking in children: Knowledge of immediate physiological effects and coping with peer pressure, media pressure, and parent modeling. *Journal of Applied Social Psychology,* 1978, **8**, 126–135.

Ferguson, J.M. The behavioral treatment of anorexia nervosa. In J.M. Ferguson & C.B. Taylor (Eds.), *Comprehensive Handbook of Behavioral Medicine.* Vol. 2. New York: Spectrum, 1981.

Fogle, R.K., & Verdesca, A.S. The cardiovascular conditioning effects of a supervised exercise program. *Journal of Occupational Medicine,* 1975, **17**, 240–246.

Folkins, C.H., & Sime, W.E. Physical fitness training and mental health. *American Psychologist,* 1981, **36**, 373–389.

Fraioli, F., Moretti, C., Paolucci, D., Alicicco, E., Crescenzi, F., & Fortunio, G. Physical exercise stimulates marked concomitant release of β-endorphin and adrenocorticotropic hormone (ACTH) in peripheral blood in man. *Experientia,* 1980, **36**, 987–989.

Frerichs, R.R., Srinivasan, S.R., Webber, L.S., & Berenson, G.S. Serum cholesterol and triglyceride levels in 3,446 children from a biracial community: The Bogalusa heart study. *Circulation,* 1976, **54**, 302–309.

Frerichs, R.R., Webber, L.S., Voors, A.W., Srinivasan, S.R., & Berenson, G.S. Cardiovascular disease risk factor variables in children at two successive years: The Bogalusa heart study. *Journal of Chronic Diseases,* 1979, **32**, 251–262.

Geller, S.E., Keane, T.M., & Scheirer, C.J. Delay of gratification, locus of control, and eating patterns in obese and nonobese children. *Addictive Behaviors,* 1981, **6**, 9–14.

Geller, M.I., Kelly, J.A., Traxler, W.T., & Marone, F.J. Behavioral treatment of an adolescent female's bulimic anorexia: Modification and immediate consequences and antecedent conditions. *Journal of Clinical Child Psychology,* 1978, **7**, 138–141.

Glanz, K. Compliance with dietary regimens: Its magnitude, measurement, and determinants. *Preventive Medicine,* 1980, **9**, 787–804.

Goldring, D., Hernandez, A., Choi, S., Lee, J.Y., Londe, S., Lindgren, F.T., & Burton, R.M. Blood pressure in a high school population: II. Clinical profile of the juvenile hypertensive. *Journal of Pediatrics,* 1979, **95**, 298–304.

Gray, S.H. Social aspects of body image: Perception of normalcy of weight and affect of college undergraduates. *Perceptual and Motor Skills,* 1977, **45**, 1035–1040.

Greenan, E., Powell, C., & Varni, J.W. Adherence to therapeutic exercise by children with hemophilia. Manuscript submitted for publication, 1983.

Gross, I., Wheeler, M., & Hess, K. The treatment of obesity in adolescents using behavioral self-control. *Clinical Pediatrics,* 1976, **15**, 920–924.

Hartung, G.H., Foreyt, J.P., Mitchell, R.E., Vlasek, I., & Gotto, A.M. Relationship of diet to high-density-lipoprotein cholesterol in middle-aged marathon runners, joggers, and inactive men. *New England Journal of Medicine,* 1980, **302**, 357–361.

Hauserman, N., & Lavin, P. Post-hospitalization continuation treatment of anorexia nervosa. *Journal of Behavior Therapy and Experimental Psychiatry,* 1977, **8**, 309–313.

Hawkins, R.C., & Clement, P.F. Development and construct validation of a self-report measure of binge eating tendencies. *Addictive Behaviors,* 1980, **5**, 219–226.

Herman, C.P., & Mack, D. Restrained and constrained eating. *Journal of Personality,* 1975, **43**, 647–660.

Hollman, W., Rost, R., & Liesen, H. The importance of sport and physical training in preventive cardiology. *Journal of Sports Medicine,* 1980, **20**, 5–12.

Hsu, L.K.G. Outcome of anorexia nervosa: A review of the literature. *Archives of General Psychiatry,* 1980, **37**, 1041–1046.

Hulse, J.A., Taylor, D.S.I., & Dillon, M.J. Blindness and paraplegia in severe childhood hypertension. *Lancet,* 1979, **1**, 553–556.

Hunter, S.M., Webber, L.S., & Berenson, G.S. Cigarette smoking and tobacco usage behavior in children and adolescents: Bogalusa heart study. *Preventive Medicine,* 1980, **9**, 701–712.

Hurd, P.D., Johnson, C.A., Pechacek, T., Bast, L.P., Jacobs, D.R., & Luepker, R.V. Prevention of cigarette smoking in seventh grade students. *Journal of Behavioral Medicine,* 1980, **3**, 15–27.

Hymowitz, N. Teenage smoking: A medical responsibility. *Journal of Developmental and Behav-*

*ioral Pediatrics.* 1980, **1**, 164–172.

Jeffrey, D.B., Lemnitzer, N.B., Hickey, J.S., Hess, M.J., McLellarn, R.W., & Stroud, J.M. The development of a behavioral eating test and its relationship to a self-report food attitude scale in young children. *Behavioral Assessment,* 1980, **2**, 87–98.

Johnson, W.G., Wildman, H.E., & O'Brien, T. The assessment of program adherence: The Achilles' Heel of behavioral weight reduction? *Behavioral Assessment,* 1980, **2**, 297–301.

Keane, T.M., Geller, S.E., & Scheirer, C.J. A parametric investigation of eating styles in obese and nonobese children. *Behavior Therapy,* 1981, **12**, 280–286.

Keefe, F.J., & Blumenthal, J.A. The life fitness program: A behavioral approach to making exercise a habit. *Journal of Behavior Therapy and Experimental Psychiatry,* 1980, **11**, 31–34.

Kilcoyne, M.M. Natural history of hypertension in adolescence. *Pediatric Clinics of North America,* 1978, **25**, 47–53.

Killam, P.E., Apodaca, L., Manella, K.J., & Varni, J.W. Behavioral pediatric weight rehabilitation for children with myelomeningocele. *MCN: American Journal of Maternal Child Nursing,* 1983, **8**, in press.

Kingsley, R.C., & Shapiro, J. A comparison of three behavioral programs for the control of obesity in children. *Behavior Therapy,* 1977, **8**, 30–36.

Laskarzewski, P., Morrison, J.A., Khoury, P., Kelly, K., Glatfelter, L., Larsen, R., & Glueck, C. Parent-child nutrient intake interrelationships in school children ages 6 to 19: The Princeton school district study. *American Journal of Clinical Nutrition,* 1980, **33**, 2350–2355.

Lauer, R.M., Clarke, W.R., & Rames, L.K. Blood pressure and its significance in children. *Postgraduate Medical Journal,* 1978, **54**, 206–210.

Lauer, R.M., Connor, W.E., Leaverton, P.E., Reiter, M.A., & Clarke, W.R. Coronary heart disease risk factors in school children: The Muscatine study. *Journal of Pediatrics,* 1975, **86**, 697–706.

Lawler, K.A., Allen, M.T., Critcher, E.C., & Standard, B.A. The relationship of physiological responses to the coronary-prone behavior pattern in children. *Journal of Behavioral Medicine,* 1981, **4**, 203–216.

Leibman, R., Minuchin, S., & Baker, L. An integrated treatment program for anorexia nervosa. *American Journal of Psychiatry,* 1974, **131**, 432–436.

Linden, W. Multi-component behavior therapy in a case of compulsive binge-eating followed by vomiting. *Journal of Behavior Therapy and Experimental Psychiatry,* 1980, **11**, 297–300.

Londe, S. Causes of hypertension in the young. *Pediatric Clinics of North America,* 1978, **25**, 55–65.

Margolis, S. Physician strategies for the prevention of coronary heart disease. *Johns Hopkins Medical Journal,* 1977, **141**, 170–176.

Matthews, K.A. Caregiver-child interactions and the Type A coronary-prone behavior pattern. *Child Development,* 1977, **48**, 1752–1756.

Matthews, K.A., & Krantz, D.S. Resemblances of twins and their parents in Pattern A behavior. *Psychosomatic Medicine,* 1976, **38**, 140–144.

McAlister, A.L., Perry, C., Killen, J., Slinkard, L.A., & Maccoby, N. Pilot study of smoking, alcohol and drug abuse prevention. *American Journal of Public Health,* 1980, **70**, 719–721.

McAlister, A.L., Perry, C., & Maccoby, N. Adolescent smoking: Onset and prevention. *Pediatrics,* 1979, **63**, 650–658.

McGlynn, F.D. Successful treatment of anorexia nervosa with self-monitoring and long distance praise. *Journal of Behavior Therapy and Experimental Psychiatry,* 1980, **11**, 283–286.

Mitchell, J.E., Pyle, R.L., & Eckert, E.D. Frequency and duration of binge-eating episodes in patients with bulimia. *American Journal of Psychiatry,* 1981, **138**, 835–836.

Mobbs, J. Childhood obesity. *International Journal of Nursing Studies,* 1970, **7**, 3–18.

Monti, P.M., McCrady, B.S., & Barlow, D.H. Effect of positive reinforcement, informational feedback, and contingency contracting on a bulimic anorexic female. *Behavior Therapy,* 1977, **8**, 258–263.

Morrison, J.A., Larsen, R., Glatfelter, L., Boggs, D., Burton, K., Smith, C., Kelly, K., Mellies, M.J., Khoury, P., & Glueck, C.J. Interrelationships between nutrient intake and plasma lipids and lipoproteins in school children aged 6 to 19: The Princeton school district study. *Pediatrics,* 1980, **65,** 727–734.

Munford, P.R. Haloperidol and contingency management in a case of anorexia nervosa. *Journal of Behavior Therapy and Experimental Psychiatry,* 1980, **11,** 67–71.

National Center for Health Statistics: NCHS Growth Charts, 1976. Monthly Vital Statistics Report. Vol. 25, No. 3, Supp. (HRA) 76–1120. Rockville, Maryland: Health Resources Administration, 1976.

Perry, C.L., Killen, J., Slinkard, L.A., & McAlister, A.L. Peer teaching and smoking prevention among junior high students. *Adolescence,* 1980, **15,** 277–281.

Perry, C., Killen, J., Telch, M., Slinkard, L.A., & Danaher, B.G. Modifying smoking behavior of teenagers: A school-based intervention. *American Journal of Public Health,* 1980, **70,** 722–725.

Pertschuk, M.J., Edwards, N., & Pomerleau, O.F. A multiple-baseline approach to behavioral intervention in anorexia nervosa. *Behavior Therapy,* 1978, **9,** 368–376.

Pisacano, J.C., Lichter, H., Ritter, J., & Siegel, A.P. An attempt at prevention of obesity in infancy. *Pediatrics,* 1978, **61,** 360–364.

Pruitt, A.W. Pharmacologic approach to the management of childhood hypertension. *Pediatric Clinics of North America,* 1981, **28,** 135–144.

Reid, E.L., & Morgan, R.W. Exercise prescription: A clinical trial. *American Journal of Public Health,* 1979, **69,** 591–595.

Rosen, J.C., & Leitenberg, H. Bulimia nervosa: Treatment with exposure and response prevention. *Behavior Therapy,* 1982, **13,** 117–124.

Rosen, L.W. Modification of secretive or ritualized eating behavior in anorexia nervosa. *Journal of Behavior Therapy and Experimental Psychiatry,* 1980, **11,** 101–104.

Ruley, E.J. Compliance in young hypertensive patients. *Pediatric Clinics of North America,* 1978, **25,** 175–182.

Russell, G. Bulimia nervosa: An ominous variation of anorexia nervosa. *Psychological Medicine,* 1979, **9,** 429–448.

Stalonas, P.M., Johnson, W.G., & Christ, M. Behavior modification for obesity: The evaluation of exercise, contingency management, and program adherence. *Journal of Consulting and Clinical Psychology,* 1978, **46,** 463–469.

Strober, M., Goldenberg, I., Green, J., & Saxon, J. Body image disturbance in anorexia nervosa during the acute and recuperative phase. *Psychological Medicine,* 1979, **9,** 695–701.

Stuart, R.R., & Davis, B. *Slim Chance in a Fat World: Behavioral Control of Obesity.* Champaign, Ill.: Research Press, 1978.

Stunkard, A.J., & Mahoney, M.J. Behavioral treatment of the eating disorders. In H. Leitenberg (Ed.), *Handbook of Behavior Modification and Behavior Therapy.* Englewood Cliffs, N.J.: Prentice-Hall, 1976.

Voller, R.D., & Strong, W.B. Pediatric aspects of atherosclerosis. *American Heart Journal,* 1981, **101,** 815–836.

Voors, A.W., Webber, L.S., & Berenson, G.S. Epidemiology of essential hypertension in youth: Implications for clinical practice. *Pediatric Clinics of North America,* 1978, **25,** 15–27.

Vuille, J.C., & Mellbin, T. Obesity in 10-year-olds: An epidemiologic study. *Pediatrics,* 1979, **64,** 564–572.

Walsh, B.T. Endocrine disturbances in anorexia nervosa and depression. *Psychosomatic Medicine,* 1982, **44,** 85–91.

Waxman, M., & Stunkard, A.J. Caloric intake and expenditure of obese boys. *Journal of Pediatrics,* 1980, **96,** 187–193.

Weil, W.B. Current controversies in childhood obesity. *Journal of Pediatrics,* 1977, **91,** 175–187.

Weiss, A.R. A behavioral approach to the treatment of adolescent obesity. *Behavior Therapy,* 1977, **8,** 720–726.

Wheeler, M.E., & Hess, K.W. Treatment of juvenile obesity by successive approximation control of eating. *Journal of Behavior Therapy and Experimental Psychiatry,* 1976, **7**, 235–241.

Williams, C.L., Carter, B.J., Arnold, C.B., & Wynder, E.L. Chronic disease risk factors among children: The "Know Your Body" study. *Journal of Chronic Diseases,* 1979, **32**, 505–513.

Wysocki, T., Hall, G., Iwata, B., & Riordan, M. Behavioral management of exercise: Contracting for aerobic points. *Journal of Applied Behavior Analysis,* 1979, **12**, 55–64.

Yager, J. Family issues in the pathogenesis of anorexia nervosa. *Psychosomatic Medicine,* 1982, **44**, 43–60.

Zack, P.M., Harlan, W.R., Leaverton, P.E., & Cornoni-Huntley, J. A longitudinal study of body fatness in childhood and adolescence. *Journal of Pediatrics,* 1979, **95**, 126–130.

# Part IV
## Pediatric Chronic Disorders

# Pediatric Chronic Disorders: Introductory Overview

As biomedical science has successfully developed treatment approaches to nutritional disorders and infectious diseases of childhood, there has been an increased emphasis on those children who now survive with marked physical impairment. As succinctly defined by Swezey (1978), "An *impairment* is a damaged, deteriorated, or injured organ or extremity, while a *handicap* is the disadvantage in function caused by the impairment. *Disability* is the inability to function effectively as a consequence of an excessive handicap resulting from an impairment [p. 1]." The goal of comprehensive management is to "minimize impairment and lessen the burden of the handicap so as to prevent disability [p. 2]." With the shift in disease epidemiology toward disorders in which chronic symptomatic management, rather than cure, represents a primary focus, coping, quality of life, and minimization of the limitations on the activities of daily living become key concerns (Cataldo, Russo, Bird, & Varni, 1980).

Although the total prevalence of children with chronic illnesses has been estimated at more than 10 percent (Pless, 1968; Pless & Douglas, 1971), many pediatric chronic disorders have a low incidence. However, the impact of these disorders is not accurately reflected in their incidence, since their chronicity imposes a disproportionately greater strain on the patients, their families, medical resources, and society (Meenan, Yelin, Nevitt, & Epstein, 1981; Zwaag, Mason, Joyner, & Runyan, 1980). In 1976 alone, 31 million school days were lost secondary to a chronic disease or disability (Department of Health, Education and Welfare, 1979).

Although biologically very diverse, pediatric chronic disorders have in common the features of significant duration (arbitrarily defined as longer than 3 months), and potential long-term, significant impact on the daily lives of the children and their families (Pless, 1980). The potential disruptions in school attendance, academic achievement, social relationships, lifestyle, and personal and financial costs, necessitate ongoing adaptation and long-term adjustment on the part of the child and his family. All these factors require a systematic comprehensive approach to the management of pediatric chronic disorders within the interdisciplinary health team model outlined in Chapter 1. Given the recognition that the difficulties of chronically ill and handicapped children and their families are similar regardless of the cause of the disability, interdisciplinary treatment strategies may be designed that can in many ways be generalized across different pediatric chronic conditions, for example, therapeutic adherence, parent training, and child self-management strategies. This approach holds forth the potential of providing coordinated longitudinal care which may significantly ameliorate the personal and financial costs of chronic disorders (see Stolov & Clowers, 1981, for review).

As previously suggested (Pless, 1980), pediatric chronic conditions represent a relatively homogeneous group, distinct in several fundamental aspects from the more common, episodical acute illnesses of childhood. These distinctive characteristics necessitate differences in the care of acutely ill and chronically ill or handicapped children (Battle, 1980). Pediatric chronic care requires multiple and comprehensive biobehavioral assessments over long periods of time, routine long-term follow-up, and ongoing family involvement. Whereas the acutely ill child can be treated and essentially "cured" within a relatively defined time by a primarily biomedical intervention, in the case of the child with a chronic disorder it is essential to consider the biobehavioral issues of active long-term self-management by the pediatric patient under the guidance of her parents and the health care team. With further advances in biomedical science and technology, it can be expected that there will be increasingly greater numbers of children who survive with chronic disorders, requiring ongoing biobehavioral comprehensive and interdisciplinary management.

In addition to the biomedical and biobehavioral considerations indigenous to the comprehensive care of children with chronic disorders, systematic attention must also be directed toward the behavioral and psychosocial adjustment of the child (Sumpter, 1980). This by no means implicates psychopathology, but means that children with life-threatening or chronic diseases are faced with acute and/or chronic stress situations that bring about major changes in daily living, requiring normal adaptive or coping mechanisms (Blum & Chang, 1981; Mattsson, 1972). A number of recent studies has demonstrated that for children with life-threatening or chronic diseases, the overall pattern is one of psychological normalcy rather than deviancy (Bedell, Giordani, Amour, Tavormina, & Boll, 1977; Kellerman, Zeltzer, Ellenberg, Dash, & Rigler, 1980; Tavormina, Kastner, Slater, & Watt, 1976; Zeltzer, Kellerman, Ellenberg, Dash, & Rigler, 1980).

Previous hypotheses in the older literature suggested that physically ill children demonstrate social maladjustment, low self-concept, increased anxiety and immaturity, and social isolation much more frequently than healthy children. However, most of these studies were based on assumptions, clinical impressions, subjective evaluations, or abbreviated projective techniques that may be considered of questionable reliability and validity. Tavormina et al. (1976) were the first investigators to utilize standardized, systematically reliable measurement instruments. In this initial investigation, 144 families who had a child with either diabetes, asthma, cystic fibrosis, or a hearing impairment were studied. The overall patterning of scores on the battery of standardized personality instruments utilized closely approximated scale norms for healthy children. The results further suggested a developmental progression for the children studied, aged 5 to 19 years, in which successful adaptation increased with age. Although exceptions were noted (and to be expected), the children's functional strengths and coping abilities noticeably outweighed their weaknesses.

In their study, Tavormina et al. (1976) employed the typical "snapshot" one-time evaluation of the children, which did not allow for a description of the children's functioning over time and especially during periods of acute exacerbations of the illness. In a subsequent study, Bedell et al. (1977) attempted to evaluate both life stress in general and life stress associated with these acute exacerbations and its relationship to the psychological functioning of chronically ill children. Forty-five children with a chronic illness, aged 6 to 15 years, were studied. The battery of test instruments included standardized life stress and anxiety inventories as well as the personality tests. After matching for age, a comparison of the life stress scores of the chronically ill children to the normative data indicated that 51 percent of the children had scored comparable to the average of the healthy group, and 49 percent had significantly higher scores. The type of chronic illness and the mean ages were evenly distributed in both the high and low stress groups, suggesting that the differences between the two groups reflected differences due to life stress and not other factors associated with the specific illness or their age. Further analysis of the data indicated that the low stress children experienced significantly fewer acute health problems than the high stress children. Additionally, the low stress children were found to have a more positive self-concept in general and rated themselves as being better behaved, more intelligent in school, more physically attractive, more socially popular, happier, and more satisfied with themselves than the high life stress children.

Bedell et al. (1977) interpreted their findings as suggesting that both social-environmental life stress and health-related factors were influential in determining the psychological well-being of the chronically ill children studied. Thus, these children's psychological status appeared to be a function of an interaction between acute illness episodes related to their chronic disorder and socioenvironmental stress factors, rather than merely a function of having a chronic illness *per se*.

Kellerman et al. (1980), in one of the better designed evaluation studies thus far, tested 349 healthy adolescents and 162 adolescents with various chronic or serious diseases on standardized measures of trait anxiety, self-esteem, and health locus of control (perception of self-control over health and illness). No differences in anxiety or self-esteem were found between the healthy or ill groups or between ill groups. Patients with oncologic, renal, cardiac, and rheumatologic disorders perceived significantly less control over their health than did healthy adolescents and patients with cystic fibrosis or diabetes mellitus. The stability of the disease prognosis was significantly related to low anxiety, as was the length of time since the initial diagnosis. Other variables including the course of the disease, visible signs of illness, severity, and number of hospitalizations did not significantly relate to the psychological variables. The authors interpreted the data as casting doubt upon previous assumptions that chronic or serious disease inevitably leads to psychopathology in adolescents. In contrast, the overall pattern found was one of psychological normalcy, with attitudes regarding control over health seen as reflecting realistic perceptions on the part of the patients. The authors further suggested the importance of looking at the effects of serious disease upon day-to-day functioning, rather than emphasizing inferred psychological deviance.

In the previous study by Bedell et al. (1977), it was noted that anxiety appeared to be related to life stress in healthy children but not in patients with chronic disease, suggesting that for healthy children stress is an anxiety provoking disruption in day-to-day normal functioning, whereas chronically ill children may learn to develop stress tolerance to the varying degrees of constant or frequent life disruptions. Thus, the chronically ill child may be seen to learn to live with his condition and to develop effective coping mechanisms. This perspective is supported by the Kellerman et al. (1980) findings that anxiety was negatively correlated with the time since initial diagnosis, suggesting the development of coping and adaptation over time.

The measure of anxiety used in the Kellerman et al. (1980) study was that of trait anxiety, a stable personality measure resistant to situational fluctuation. This does not mean that chronically ill adolescents do not experience situational (state) anxiety during acute illness exacerbations. Rather, it does indicate that chronically ill adolescents do not appear to be chronically anxious (trait anxiety). Further, Bedell et al. (1977) found that a comparison of the children's state and trait anxiety scores for the low and high stress groups indicated that there were no significant differences in their ratings. Again, these findings suggest the development of successful coping strategies by the children. It may be that successful coping with constant or frequent mild stress strengthens the adolescent's ability to cope with greater stress situations (Zeltzer et al., 1980). The prospect that successful coping can be further enhanced through the teaching of specific coping and self-management skills to the child appears to be a viable intervention strategy as will be illustrated in the subsequent chapters.

From a cognitive development perspective, chronically ill children's conceptualizations of their illness, the intent of the medical procedures, and the role of the treatment staff may further influence overall adjustment and adaptation. Brewster (1982) studied a group of 50 chronically ill hospitalized children, aged 5 to 12 years, testing them on five developmental tasks, scored in ascending order of cognitive maturation. The findings indicated a three-stage sequence of conceptual development in the children's understanding of the cause of illness: (1) In the first stage, generally ages less than 7 years, the children conceptualized disease as resulting entirely from human action, conceiving illness as the outcome of wrongdoing; (2) The second stage was characterized by the children's (typically ages 7 to 10 years) belief in singular physical causality, usually contending that illness is caused by germs; (3) The third stage was characterized by the children's acknowledgement that illness can have multiple causes, including the child's own actions, infection, and the body's lack of immunity. Stage 3 responses were not observed in any children younger than 9 years old.

In regards to the perceived intent of the medical procedures and the role of the treatment staff, a parallel three-stage sequence of understanding was found: (1) In the first stage, children under 7 years routinely stated that the medical procedures were done to punish them for being bad; (2) In the second stage (typically 7 to 10 year olds), the children accurately inferred the intention of the medical procedures and that treatment was intended to help them get well, but they believed that the staff's empathy was dependent on the child's expressing pain; (3) Stage 3 children (typically older than 9 years) could correctly infer both the intention of the medical procedures and the perceived empathy of the treatment staff.

A multivariate analysis of variance was performed on all five tasks for the four age groups studied, indicating a highly significant effect for age. That is, there was an ascending relationship between the age of the children and the children's scores on all five developmental tasks. Thus, the children processed the information about their illness and treatment through a predictable normal maturational cognitive sequence (see Chapter 2 for comparison to healthy children's similar processing). These findings further lend support to an overall normal psychological and cognitive developmental pattern in children with chronic illness.

Based on the recent literature and the author's experience, the perspective that will be followed in the subsequent chapters in regards to the behavioral and psychosocial adjustment of chronically ill or handicapped children is that they are not particularly "at risk" for psychopathology, but that they must face and cope with a number of life stress situations associated with episodical acute exacerbations of their chronic condition, as well as the potential long-term functional limitations in daily living which may also accompany their chronic disorder. As previously stated by Russo and Varni (1982), "Certainly, a number of children who develop chronic disease had adjustment difficulties before their illness and in a certain proportion of families marital difficulties, financial issues, and other factors existed which may work to subvert treatment. Nevertheless, it is our contention that in the main, children with chronic diseases are a psychologically normal population [p. 10]."

From this perspective, psychosocial maladjustment is not inevitable, but is another consideration in the overall comprehensive assessment of the pediatric patient and her family. Through a comprehensive biobehavioral management approach, stress may be managed through the active teaching of coping skills. This perspective is reflected in the following chapters on specific pediatric chronic disorders, where the emphasis is on comprehensive biobehavioral management through the teaching of self-management skills to the children and behavioral parenting skills to their parents in order to facilitate an overall successful adaptive coping process. Behavioral and psychosocial adjustment issues will be addressed separately in detail in Chapter 12.

# REFERENCES

Battle, C.U. The role of the primary care physician. In A.P. Scheiner & I.F. Abroms (Eds.), *The Practical Management of the Developmentally Disabled Child*. St. Louis: C.V. Mosby, 1980.
Bedell, J.R., Giordani, B., Amour, J.L., Tavormina, J., & Boll, T. Life stress and the psychological and medical adjustment of chronically ill children. *Journal of Psychosomatic Research*, 1977, **21**, 237–242.
Blum, R.W., & Chang, P.N. A group for adolescents facing chronic and terminal illness. *Journal of Child and Adolescent Medicine*, 1981, **3**, 7–12.
Brewster, A.B. Chronically ill hospitalized children's concepts of their illness. *Pediatrics*, 1982, **69**, 355–362.
Cataldo, M.F., Russo, D.C., Bird, B.L., & Varni, J.W. Assessment and management of chronic disorders. In J.M. Ferguson & C.B. Taylor (Eds.), *Comprehensive Handbook of Behavioral Medicine, Vol. 3: Extended Applications and Issues*. New York: Spectrum, 1980.
Department of Health, Education and Welfare, Public Health Service. *Public Policy and Chronic Disease* (NIH Publication No. 79-1896). Washington, D.C.: U.S. Government Printing Office, 1979.
Kellerman, J., Zeltzer, L., Ellenberg, L., Dash, J., & Rigler, D. Psychological effects of illness in adolescents. I. Anxiety, self-esteem, and perception of control. *Journal of Pediatrics*, 1980, **97**, 126–131.
Mattsson, A. Long-term physical illness in childhood: A challenge to psychosocial adaptation. *Pediatrics*, 1972, **50**, 801–811.
Meenan, R.F., Yelin, E.H., Nevitt, M., & Epstein, W.V. The impact of chronic disease: A sociomedical profile of rheumatoid arthritis. *Arthritis and Rheumatism*, 1981, **24**, 544–549.
Pless, I.B. Epidemiology of chronic disease. In M. Green & R.J. Haggerty (Eds.), *Ambulatory Pediatrics*. Philadelphia: W.B. Saunders, 1968.
Pless, I.B. Practical problems and their management. In A.P. Scheiner & I.F. Abroms (Eds.), *The Practical Management of the Developmentally Disabled Child*. St. Louis: C.V. Mosby, 1980.
Pless, I.B., & Douglas, J.W.B. Chronic illness in childhood: Part 1. Epidemiological and clinical characteristics. *Pediatrics*, 1971, **47**, 405–414.
Russo, D.C., & Varni, J.W. Behavioral pediatrics. In D.C. Russo & J.W. Varni (Eds.), *Behavioral Pediatrics: Research and Practice*. New York: Plenum Press, 1982.
Stolov, W.C., & Clowers, M.R. (Eds.) *Handbook of Severe Disability*. (Rehabilitation Services Administration). Washington, D.C.: U.S. Government Printing Office, 1981.

Sumpter, E.A. Behavioral aspects of pediatrics and chronic illness. In A.P. Scheiner &. I.F. Abroms (Eds.), *The Practical Management of the Developmentally Disabled Child.* St. Louis: C.V. Mosby, 1980.

Swezey, R.L. *Arthritis: Rational Therapy and Rehabilitation.* Philadelphia: W.B. Saunders, 1978.

Tavormina, J.B., Kastner, L.S., Slater, P.M., & Watt, S.L. Chronically ill children: A psychologically and emotionally deviant population? *Journal of Abnormal Child Psychology,* 1976, **4**, 99–110.

Zeltzer, L., Kellerman, J., Ellenberg, L., Dash, J., & Rigler, D. Psychological effects of illness in adolescents: II. Impact of illness in adolescents—crucial issues and coping styles. *Journal of Pediatrics,* 1980, **97**, 132–138.

Zwaag, R.V., Mason, W.B., Joyner, M.B., & Runyan, J.W. Cost of chronic disease care. *Journal of Chronic Diseases,* 1980, **33**, 713–720.

# 8
# Neurological/Neuromuscular Disorders: Myelomeningocele, Seizures, Tics, Cerebral Palsy

Pediatric neurological and neuromuscular disorders encompass a broad spectrum of conditions. Presently, the largest amount of biobehavioral empirical work has been conducted with children with myelomeningocele, seizures, tics, and cerebral palsy (see Bird, 1982, for review).

## MYELOMENINGOCELE

Myelomeningocele (spina bifida) is the most common congenital central nervous system defect, occurring with an incidence of one to three cases per 1,000 live births. This chronic disorder is characterized by myelodysplasia and cystic distension of the meninges, with associated neurogenic deficits (e.g., neurogenic incontinence) and lower extremity paralysis (Austin, Lindgren, & Dietrich, 1972; Shurtleff, 1980). The development of improved medical and surgical techniques has resulted in dramatically increased survival rates, with Dietrich (1979) reporting an 86 percent survival rate out of a total of 500 patients seen over a 16-year period. With such a high survival rate, opportunities now exist to focus on the habilitation and rehabilitation of associated chronic dysfunction in children with myelomeningocele (Akins, Davidson, & Hopkins, 1980; Manella, Jeffries, & Varni, 1983; Morrissy, 1978).

Biofeedback and nonbiofeedback biobehavioral techniques have thus far been applied to self-help skills, obesity, ambulation, and chronic urinary and fecal incontinence in children with myelomeningocele.

## Self-Help Skills

Marked developmental delays in self-help skills such as dressing, grooming, feeding, meal preparation, and hygiene have been found with children with

Table 8.1.    Format of Parent Training Program.

I. *First Session:* Skill Targeting and Baseline Procedures
   1. Overview of program stressing:
      a. data-keeping
      b. consistent attendance
   2. Operational definitions of target behaviors vs interpretations
      a. behavior-specific descriptions
   3. Self-help skill targeting
      a. selection of skills
      b. component steps of each skill
   4. Distribution of skill training manuals
   5. Explanation of data-keeping forms and baseline procedures
   6. Homework assignments
II. *Second Session:* Applications of Behavioral Principles to Skill Teaching
   1. Teaching concepts and procedures introduced
      a. task analysis
      b. get ready skills
      c. setting the stage
      d. shaping
      e. modeling
   2. Importance of data-keeping for teaching effectiveness evaluation
   3. Homework assignments
III. *Third Session:* Functional Analysis
   1. Antecedents ► Self-help Skills ► Consequences
   2. Antecedents as setting the stage for teaching and cueing performance
   3. Development of reinforcement menu
   4. Shaping and fading procedures
   5. Homework assignments
IV. *Fourth Session:* Troubleshooting for Teaching Problems
   1. Troubleshooting techniques
   2. Incidental teaching concept
   3. Homework assignments
V. *Fifth Session:* Videotaping and Critique of Teaching Sessions
   1. Videotaping of re-enactment of home teaching sessions
   2. Discussion and critique of videotaped sessions
   3. Distribution of behavior problems manuals
   4. Homework assignments
VI. *Sixth Session:* Definition, Targeting, and Measurement of Behavior Problems
   1. "A-B-C" (antecedents, behaviors, consequences) patterns
   2. Homework assignments
VII. *Seventh Session:* Identifying Alternative Consequences
   1. Extinction
   2. Response cost
   3. Differential reinforcement of other behaviors (DRO)
   4. Homework assignments
VIII. *Eighth Session:* Troubleshooting Behavior Problem Management and Play
   Activities as Skills
   1. Time-out as preferable to physical punishment
   2. Contingency contracting
   3. Homework assignments
IX. *Ninth Session:* Review
   1. Schedule follow-up sessions and follow-up data collection
   2. Overall evaluation of program

Source: Reprinted with permission from W.S. Feldman, K.J. Manella, L. Apodaca, and J.W. Varni. Behavioral group parent training in spina bifida. *Journal of Clinical Child Psychology*, 1982, **11**, 144–150.

myelomeningocele, resulting in much longer time periods for the achievement of functional independence (Sousa, Gordon, & Shurtleff, 1976). Feldman, Manella, Apodaca, and Varni (1982) described a behavioral group parent training program for the parents of four children with myelomeningocele. The training program was designed to teach the parents the behavioral techniques necessary in order for them to teach their children selected self-help skills. Table 8.1 contains an outline of the parent training program format.

At the beginning of the program, the parents were asked to select three self-help skills that they desired to teach their children. The parents were asked to use the following criteria in choosing the skills: (1) The child could already partially perform components of the overall skill; (2) It was important for her to learn; and (3) The parents would like to teach it. Following these criteria, a list of 12 self-help skills were generated (Table 8.2). Prior to the initiation of the

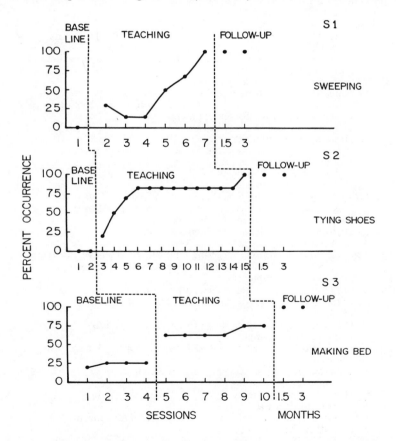

Fig. 8.1.   Percent occurrence of three self-help skills for three children with myelomeningocele during baseline and behavioral parent training phases.

Table 8.2.   A Comparison of Percent Mean
Self-Help Skill Proficiency Across the Four Children.

| Skill | Baseline | Teaching | Follow-Up |
|---|---|---|---|
| 1. Scraping/Stacking Dishes | 37.5 | 58.8 | 100.0 |
| 2. Sweeping | 0.0 | 45.8 | 100.0 |
| 3. Taking off Pants | 91.5 | 92.2 | 100.0 |
| 4. Putting on Pants | 57.0 | 90.1 | 100.0 |
| 5. Tying Shoes | 0.0 | 73.0 | 100.0 |
| 6. Changing Diaper | 30.0 | 74.5 | 100.0 |
| 7. Making a Bed | 23.8 | 76.0 | 100.0 |
| 8. Hanging up Pants | 33.0 | 87.5 | 100.0 |
| 9. Sweeping | 54.0 | 76.0 | 92.5 |
| 10. Brushing Hair | 60.0 | 95.8 | 100.0 |
| 11. Starting a Zipper | 66.7 | 75.0 | 90.0 |
| 12. Spreading with a knife | 54.3 | 95.0 | 100.0 |
| Mean Proficiency | 42.3 | 78.3 | 98.5 |

sessions, the parents and co-trainers signed a contingency contract, which specified the responsibilities of each participant. The behavioral parent training program (Table 8.1) resulted in a substantial increase in the mean proficiency level of all 12 skills for the four children (Table 8.2). Figure 8.1 illustrates the multiple-baseline design in sequentially teaching the self-help skills. This behavioral group parent training program has also been successfully extended to single parents with children with myelomeningocele (Feldman, Manella, & Varni, 1983) and to individual (nongroup) parent training (Feldman & Varni, 1983).

## Obesity

Obesity has been well recognized as a chronic problem in myelomeningocele (Hayes-Allen, 1972; Hayes-Allen & Tring, 1973). Factors that may place these children at high risk for becoming overweight include a reduced energy expenditure secondary to relative inactivity; some children are confined to wheelchairs, while others may walk only with bracing and/or crutches. These children may require a much lower caloric intake, perhaps even 50 percent of that of children without myelomeningocele (Llenado & Grogan, 1978). In one clinic population, over 90 percent of the teenagers with myelomeningocele were found to be overweight, as defined by a weight for height which exceeded the 75th percentile (Rickard, Brady, & Gresham, 1977). For the child with myelomeningocele, obesity may cause additional problems; for example, ambulation becomes increasingly harder, orthopedic surgeries are more difficult, and the potential for pressure sores is greater. The sum of these findings points to the importance of pediatric weight rehabilitation programs in myelomeningocele.

Killam, Apodaca, Manella, and Varni (1983) designed a weight control group program for five children (ages 7½ to 12 years) with myelomeningocele and their parents. At treatment initiation, the children averaged 52 percent overweight (range, 28 to 76 percent overweight). The children and their parents received instruction on selected aspects of diet, exercise, and specific behavioral techniques for altering eating and exercise habits (see Chapter 7 for a detailed description of the treatment program).

Table 8.3 contains a summary of the heights, weights, and percents overweight for the five children involved in the program, from the initial evaluation through the 6-month follow-up. Although there was wide variability in the change in percent overweight, four of the five children evidenced a therapeutic effect, averaging a 13 percent overweight loss. Table 8.4 reports both the objective therapeutic adherence data and the results of the adherence and social validity questionnaires (see Chapter 7). The measurements of therapeutic adherence also showed wide differences among the children, with greatest adherence tending to be positively related to the greatest percent overweight loss.

## Ambulation

Functional ambulation is strongly recommended for children with myelomeningocele because of the physiological complications (e.g., urinary stasis, bone atrophy, pressure sores) and psychological benefits of standing and walking in the child's development (Akins, Davidson, & Hopkins, 1980). Several studies of patients with myelomeningocele have demonstrated a corre-

Table 8.3.  Changes in Percent Overweight across Conditions.

| | Percent overweight | | | | |
|---|---|---|---|---|---|
| Children | Pretreatment assessment | 1st meeting | 4-month follow-up | 6-month follow-up | Net change (1st meeting to 6-month follow-up) |
| 1 | 25 | 28 | 6 | 4 | − 24 |
| 2 | 47 | 50 | 29 | 31 | − 19 |
| 3 | 54 | 56 | 54 | 49 | − 7 |
| 4 | 40 | 50 | 42 | 49 | − 1 |
| 5 | 71 | 76 | 86* | 97 | + 21 |

*6-week follow-up

Source: Reprinted with permission from P.E. Killam, L. Apodaca, K.J. Manella, & J.W. Varni. Behavioral pediatric weight rehabilitation for children with myelomeningocele. *MCN: American Journal of Maternal Child Nursing,* 1983, **8**, in press.

Table 8.4.    Relationship between Therapeutic Adherence Factors
and Percent Overweight Change.

| Measures | Children | | | | |
|---|---|---|---|---|---|
| | 1 | 2 | 3 | 4 | 5 |
| Percent Overweight Change (+ = gain, − = loss) | − 24 | − 19 | − 7 | − 1 | + 21 |
| Sessions Attended (Total possible = 13) | 13 | 8 | 13 | 7 | 6 |
| Children's use of Recording Tools (Total possible = 273) | 222 | 49* | 225* | 130 | 21* |
| Parents' use of Recording Tools (Total possible = 42) | 7 | 4 | 9 | 6 | 7 |
| Adherence Questionnaire Ratings | 2.2 | 2.0 | 1.5 | 2.1 | ** |
| Social Validity Ratings | 2.5 | 2.8 | 2.1 | 2.2 | 1.75 |

*Recorded by parents
**Did not compete

Source: Reprinted with permission from P.E. Killam, L. Apodaca, K.J. Manella, & J.W. Varni. Behavioral pediatric weight rehabilitation for children with myelomeningocele. *MCN: American Journal of Maternal Child Nursing,* 1983, **8**, in press.

lation between the spinal level of muscular paralysis and the likely ultimate level of ambulatory function (DeSouza & Carroll, 1976; Hoffer, Feiwell, Perry, Perry, & Bonnett, 1973; Huff & Ramsey, 1978). Those patients with sacral spinal cord lesions are far more likely to stand and walk, even without assistive devices such as bracing and crutches, than patients with lumbar or thoracic lesions. These patients may require considerable bracing just to stand and are less likely to achieve independent ambulation. However, regardless of lesion level, motivational factors may be instrumental in attaining functional ambulation in the young child with myelomeningocele.

Manella and Varni (1981) combined systematic therapist's reinforcement and behavioral parent training in teaching a 4½-year-old child with a repaired myelomeningocele at the third lumbar level (L₃) to stand and walk independently. Before the study began, the child had been attending a school for the orthopedically handicapped and was receiving physical therapy three times a week. Despite 6 months of physical therapy, the child demonstrated no independent walking, was confined to a stroller, and used crawling or scooting as her only modes of mobility. Reports from the school's physical therapist stated that the child had a short attention span and was not motivated to walk. She would frequently throw temper tantrums and refuse to walk during therapy sessions. This tantrum behavior also occurred at home when she was asked to walk. She would also frequently refuse to go to therapy sessions.

An initial evaluation revealed the presence of motor function through the third lumbar level ($L_3$). The iliopsoas muscles, hip adductor muscles, and quadriceps femoris muscles were graded 3 bilaterally on a scale of 0 to 5. Sensation was intact through the third lumbar dermatome. The orthotic prescription was polypropylene knee-ankle-foot orthoses with a thoracic band and gluteal sling.

The objectives of the behavioral physical therapy program were to attain functional independence in the following motor skills: (1) stands up, (2) stands erect, and (3) ambulates using a 4-point gait. Table 8.5 contains the functional components of these three motor skills. An assessment was made by the physical therapist to determine an appropriate reinforcement list for the child to motivate her adherence to the physical therapy regimen. Reinforcers identified included social praise and attention, encouragement, game playing, and physical contact. Initially, when the child complied with a request to stand up with her crutches, she was praised and allowed to play with stuffed animals for 5 minutes. Subsequently, this play activity and praise by the therapist were made contingent upon standing up and standing erect for 15 seconds (shaping procedure). Finally, in order to play with the stuffed animals and receive therapist approval, the child had to stand up, stand erect, and ambulate with a 4-point gait along a distance initially set at 20 feet and increased to 160 feet by the end of the program. In this way, the three motor skills were combined and led to functionally independent ambulation over increasingly longer distances. All inappropriate responses, such as refusing to move the crutches, temper tantrums, and deliberate loss of balance were ignored (extinction).

Table 8.5.    Functional Components of the Motor Skills:
Stands Up, Stands Erect, and Ambulates.

| Stands Up | Stands Erect | Ambulates |
|---|---|---|
| 1. rolls onto stomach | 1. stands with minimal lordosis | 1. moves one crutch forward |
| 2. places hands into leather loops of crutches | 2. stands with minimal hip flexion | 2. moves the opposite leg forward |
| 3. pushes up to quadruped position | 3. maintains erect position for 15 seconds | 3. moves other crutch forward |
| 4. positions one crutch and pushes up | | 4. moves other leg forward |
| 5. positions other crutch and pushes into standing | | |
| 6. re-positions crutches to secure balance | | |

Source: Reprinted with permission from K.J. Manella & J.W. Varni. Behavior therapy in a gait-training program for a child with myelomeningocele. *Physical Therapy*, 1981, **61**, 1284–1287.

The child's mother was trained in behavioral techniques after the child consistently exhibited appropriate walking behaviors in the clinic. After watching several clinic sessions, the mother practiced applying the behavioral techniques in the clinic under the supervision of the physical therapist. The program was then begun by the mother at home, with the mother recording the distance walked and the number of appropriate steps taken during each home

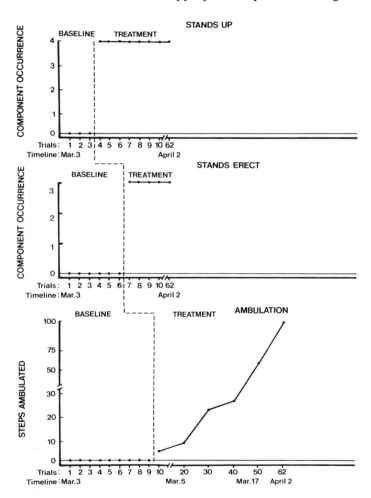

Fig. 8.2.   Occurrence of the motor skills stands up, stands erect, and ambulation during baseline and treatment sessions in the clinic.

Source: Reprinted with permission from K.J. Manella & J.W. Varni. Behavioral treatment of ambulatory function in a child with myelomeningocele. Manuscript submitted for publication, 1983.

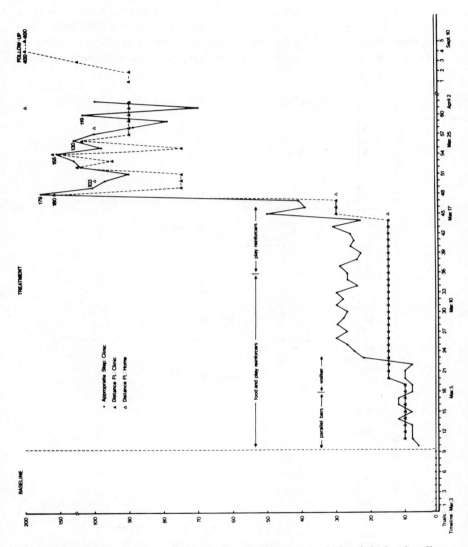

Fig. 8.3. Occurrence of appropriate steps and distance ambulated during baseline, treatment, and follow-up in the clinic and home settings.

Source: Reprinted with permission from K.J. Manella & J.W. Varni. Behavioral treatment of ambulatory function in a child with myelomeningocele. Manuscript submitted for publication, 1983.

session. With therapy progress, the child walked longer distances and developed enough muscle strength so as to require less bracing for independent ambulation.

Figures 8.2 and 8.3 contain similar data replicating the initial study with another young child with myelomeningocele (Manella & Varni, 1983). Within the multiple-baseline design across behaviors, it can be seen in Figure 8.2 that all components of the motor skills defined as stands up and stands erect were immediately exhibited upon initiation of the treatment program in the clinic. This result indicates that the child had been able to perform these skills completely and that the effect of the treatment program was to motivate her to perform them independently through contingent reinforcement. Figure 8.3 and the lower graph of Figure 8.2 illustrate a quite different kind of result for ambulation. At first, the child could not perform this skill. When reinforcement was contingent on ambulation, the number of steps taken and the distance walked began to increase gradually and steadily. These results illustrate a typical learning curve, indicating that the child was acquiring this motor skill within a shaping paradigm.

## Chronic Incontinence

Neurogenic urinary and fecal incontinence is prevalent in the vast majority of children with myelomeningocele because of the very low level of spinal cord innervation of bowel and bladder functions (Lorber, 1971). The myriad of physical and psychosocial difficulties associated with chronic incontinence in myelomeningocele can be quite profound (Hayden, Davenport, & Campbell, 1979; Shurtleff, Hayden, Chapman, Bnoy, & Hill, 1975). Particularly in wheelchair-bound patients, incontinence may contribute to excoriation of the perineal area which can progress to severe infection. Macerated, bacteria-laden skin is more prone to the development of pressure sores, with the moisture from chronic incontinence increasing the risk of pressure sore formation fivefold (Reuler & Cooney, 1981).

For children who are already hindered in social interactions with their peers by problems with ambulation and time-consuming physical care, incontinence may prove to be an almost insurmountable barrier. Evidence of incontinence (e.g., diapers and odor) evokes the most intense deprecation from peers (Chapman, Hill, & Shurtleff, 1979), hindering social interaction and the development of sexual identity (Shurtleff et al., 1975). Hunt (1981) identified chronic incontinence as causing greater distress than any of the other associated disabilities in myelomeningocele, being of primary significance in excluding the child from ordinary schooling. Thus, the psychosocial impact of incontinence, if untreated, may be quite profound.

The biobehavioral management of chronic incontinence is a relatively recent area of investigation in myelomeningocele (see Chapter 10 for a general review). Whitehead, Parker, Masek, Cataldo, and Freeman (1981) studied eight patients between 5 and 15 years old, all of whom had lifelong histories of severe fecal incontinence secondary to myelomeningocele. The biofeedback instrument consisted of a hollow cylinder to which two balloons were tied that were inserted into the anal canal (see Chapter 10). When inflated with air, these balloons abridged the anal canal, so that one balloon was surrounded by the internal anal sphincter, and a second was surrounded by the external anal sphincter. A third balloon was inserted through the cylinder into the rectum and was used to distend the rectum. Each balloon was connected to a pressure transducer. Transduced pressure changes were amplified and recorded on a polygraph.

Rectosphincteric biofeedback training initially involved teaching the patient to make an appropriate voluntary contraction of the external anal sphincter in the absence of rectal distension. The patients received feedback on sphincter responses by viewing the polygraph tracings. They were prompted verbally to contract the external anal sphincter and were praised for pen deflections in the appropriate direction (reflecting sphincter contractions). The next biofeedback training phase involved establishing contractions of the external anal sphincter following gradually greater rectal distensions and during reflex internal anal sphincter inhibition (relaxation). The final teaching phase consisted of establishing external anal sphincter contractive responses without feedback. The results showed that by the end of rectosphincteric biofeedback training, the patients could produce strong external anal sphincter contractions during rectal distension which were sustained for the duration of reflex internal anal sphincter inhibition. Following biofeedback training, six of the eight patients substantially reduced their incidents of fecal incontinence, with three of them becoming completely continent. Wald (1981), using a different rectosphincteric biofeedback training procedure, found that four of the eight patients who were treated with biofeedback had a good clinical response, with the disappearance of fecal soiling or a greater than 75 percent improvement in the frequency of soiling.

Since the studies by Whitehead et al. (1981) and Wald (1981) indicated that children with myelomeningocele could be taught to develop appropriate rectosphincteric responses, Jeffries, Killam, and Varni (1982) attempted a non-biofeedback biobehavioral intervention with the intent of motivating a 9-year-old child with a sacral level myelomeningocele to increase his attention to rectosphincteric responses. Prior to beginning fecal continence training, baseline data were obtained by recording the frequency of fecal incontinence. This was done by the parent and child for 3 weeks using a daily progress chart for recording the number of bowel movements, the time of their occurrence, and whether they occurred in the toilet, in his diapers, or in bed (Table 8.6). This

Table 8.6.    Daily Progress Chart for the
Biobehavioral Assessment of Urinary and Fecal Incontinence.

Child's Name: _____

| Date | | | | | | | |
|---|---|---|---|---|---|---|---|
| Day of Week | | | | | | | |
| Time | | | | | | | |
| 6:00 | | | | | | | |
| 7:00 | | | | | | | |
| 8:00 | | | | | | | |
| 9:00 | | | | | | | |
| 10:00 | | | | | | | |
| 11:00 | | | | | | | |
| 12:00 | | | | | | | |
| 1:00 | | | | | | | |
| 2:00 | | | | | | | |
| 3:00 | | | | | | | |
| 4:00 | | | | | | | |
| 5:00 | | | | | | | |
| 6:00 | | | | | | | |
| 7:00 | | | | | | | |
| 8:00 | | | | | | | |
| 9:00 | | | | | | | |

Code:  BMT = Bowel Movement in Toilet      UT = Urinates in Toilet
       BMP = Bowel Movement in Pants       UP = Urinates in Pants
       BMB = Bowel Movement in Bed         UB = Urinates in Bed
       DRY = No Bowel Movement or Urine

chart was used to collect data during baseline, treatment, and follow-up phases. During baseline, the mother was also instructed to identify positive reinforcers for her child that might motivate him to adhere to the management regimen. Positive reinforcers that were identified included daily earned television viewing time and weekly reinforcers such as a special late evening television program or a special trip. At the same time, behavior problems were identified and their frequency measured using a psychosocial assessment battery, which the mother completed prior to the intervention and again after treatment at follow-up.

The patient's mother was instructed in the use of the positive reinforcers and encouraged to socially reinforce the patient with praise and positive attention for each successful incident of fecal continence, in addition to the material reinforcers. This included reinforcement for both clean diapers and bowel movements in the toilet. Since the patient had repeatedly failed to attain bowel control with other methods, the procedure was divided into small steps to facilitate early success in the program and to encourage the child. When treatment was first started, the patient could earn his daily reinforcement if he had only one incident of fecal soiling a day. After one month of treatment, the patient demonstrated a consistent pattern of earning daily reinforcement. The criterion for reinforcement was increased over time and with success until complete fecal continence was required for reinforcement (shaping). There were also additional weekly reinforcers if the patient was clean initially 4 out of 7 days, then 5 out of 7 days, and finally 7 out of 7 days. Thus, both daily and weekly reinforcement were built into the program.

During the 3 weeks of baseline, the patient averaged 7.7 incidents of fecal soiling per week. With the initiation of the biobehavioral intervention, there was a steady decline in the frequency of fecal soiling so that the patient averaged 1.4 incidents of fecal soiling per week during treatment. During the 9 months of follow-up, the patient's weekly incidents of fecal incontinence averaged 0.16 per week, typically occurring only once a month. Additionally, the psychosocial assessments demonstrated a decline in most problem areas, complementing previous work with encopretic children (Levine, Marzonson, & Bakow, 1980). Thus, as the child achieved increased bowel control, he demonstrated fewer problems at school and with his peers and was reported to be more pleasant and cooperative at home.

Finally, it should be pointed out that the biobehavioral management of chronic urinary incontinence in myelomeningocele is just beginning to be investigated. Killam, Jeffries, and Varni (1983) have reported initial success using urodynamic biofeedback with children with myelomeningocele (see Chapter 10 for a detailed description of urodynamics). The potential of these techniques in decreasing chronic urinary incontinence by developing voluntary bladder and external urethral sphincter control is quite provocative and warrants considerable investigative attention.


# SEIZURES

Seizures are characterized by abnormal neural activity which disrupts normal brain functioning, resulting in transitory sensory, cognitive, and motor disturbances; epilepsy refers to chronically recurring seizures (Bird, 1982; Shin, 1977). Seizures have been categorized in terms of clinical, electroencephalographic, anatomical and etiological factors, and frequency (Ellison, Largent, & Bahr, 1981; Gastaut, 1970; Holmes, Sackellares, McKiernan, Ragland, & Dreifuss, 1980; Massey & Riley, 1980; Williams, Spiegel, & Mostofsky, 1978).

Advances in anticonvulsant drug therapy has resulted in some level of seizure control for 70 to 80 percent of children (Johnston & Freeman, 1981). The use of medications in the treatment of seizure disorders is primarily directed toward the prevention of seizures. Once a successful drug regimen has been established, it is prescribed as a routine part of the child's daily living pattern. However, little is known about the events that trigger or terminate a seizure, and little is known about the mechanism of the anticonvulsant action of the drugs (Johnston & Freeman, 1981). To further complicate the clinical management of childhood seizures, it has been found that noncompliance to the prescribed drug regimen is a considerable problem (Freiman & Buchanan, 1978). This finding is not surprising given that anticonvulsant therapy is a long-term prevention approach (i.e., when no symptoms are present), and the common drugs used may have a number of side effects (Gordon, 1982; Reynold, 1978). Although systematic research on enhancing adherence to the anticonvulsant drug regimen is generally lacking, clinical recommendations include monitoring anticonvulsant blood and saliva levels (Brett, 1977; Zysset, Rudeberg, Vassella, Kapfer, & Bircher, 1981), prescribing a once a day drug regimen rather than multiple doses per day (Johnston & Freeman, 1981), and when possible, reducing or completely withdrawing the drug regimen (Emerson, D'Souza, Vining, Holden, Mellits, & Freeman, 1981). Clearly, systematic investigations on biobehavioral techniques to assess and manage medication adherence in pediatric seizure disorders is needed and may result in further improvements in long-term seizure control and the reduction of toxic side effects.

In addition to enhancing medication adherence, biobehavioral management programs may be particularly instrumental by interfacing with the overall comprehensive care of the child with seizures, especially when anticonvulsant therapy has not obtained optimal seizure control. To date, biobehavioral interventions in seizure comprehensive care may be delineated into three major treatment categories: biofeedback, systematic desensitization, and contingency management (see Bird, 1982; Mostofsky & Balaschak, 1977, for reviews). The following studies exemplify these three areas.

## Biofeedback

Early neurophysiological studies on cats by Sterman and his colleagues led to the hypothesis that thalamic and cortical inhibitory responses are activated during the production of the sensorimotor rhythm (SMR). This rhythm is a 12 to 14 Hz sinusoidal waveform recorded from the scalp over the sensorimotor cortex. Sterman found that this rhythm appeared over the sensorimotor cortex during the suppression of motor activity. The observations on cats lead to research with human patients. Sterman and Friar (1972) reported that increasing SMR by EEG biofeedback conditioning reduced seizures in a patient not well-controlled by medication. Finley (1976) found similar positive effects with an adolescent patient.

Lubar and Bahler (1976) trained eight severely epileptic patients to increase 12–14 Hz EEG activity. The patients represented a cross section of several different types of epilepsy, including grand mal, myoclonic, akinetic, focal, and psychomotor types. Auditory and/or visual feedback was provided whenever one-half second of 12–14 Hz activity was detected in the EEG. The patients were provided with additional feedback keyed by the output of a 4–7 Hz filter which indicated the presence of epileptiform spike activity, slow waves, or motor movement. Feedback for SMR was inhibited whenever slow-wave activity spikes or movement were also present. During the treatment period, most of the patients showed varying degrees of improvement in seizure control, with the successful patients demonstrating an increase in the amount and amplitude of SMR during the training period. These findings supported the hypothesis that electroencephalographic feedback training reduced the incidence of seizures by presumably training the patient to modify EEG activity in a direction associated with an increased seizure threshold (Sterman & Friar, 1972).

Sterman and Macdonald (1978) compared the clinical effects of several central cortical EEG feedback training strategies in eight patients with poorly controlled seizures. Six of the eight patients reported significant and sustained seizure reduction following feedback for 12–15 Hz responses *or* 18–23 Hz responses in the absence of 6–9 Hz responses.

Kuhlman (1978) evaluated the clinical efficacy and mechanisms underlying EEG feedback training in five epileptic patients with poorly controlled seizures. When feedback was made contingent upon central 9–14 Hz activity, seizures declined by 60 percent in three patients. However, Kuhlman (1978) found that the clinical phenomenon of seizure reduction with EEG feedback training was obtained without enhancement of central 12–14 Hz activity (SMR). Kuhlman (1978) suggested that the positive results obtained in studies utilizing feedback for 12–14 Hz activity may have been due to reduction of abnormal epileptiform and slow wave activity or EEG desynchronization rather than to enhancement of a specific rhythm, particularly since the previous studies utilized multiple feedback contingencies that required patients to inhibit abnormal high amplitude-low frequency activity, which might result in a confounding of the proposed specific SMR effects.

Finally, Cott, Pavloski, and Black (1979) suggested that in the studies in which reduction in seizure frequency was reported following SMR training, the conditioning procedure included a clearly signaled time-out contingent on EEG slow waves, spike activity, or high-voltage scalp electromyographic activity. That is, SMR was not reinforced during epileptiform activity or gross motor movements, and the unavailability of reinforcement (time-out) was indicated to the patient by a signal, with the time-out contingency possibly suppressing EEG slow-wave and spike activity. Thus, the previous studies' findings that reduced seizure activity followed SMR training might be a result of the time-out procedure rather than SMR training itself. Cott et al. (1979) studied seven patients with epilepsy who had not responded well to medication, comparing time-out alone with SMR training plus time-out. Time-out was contingent on EEG slow waves, spike activity, or high-voltage scalp EMG activity, with a buzzer and a small lamp indicating time-out. For the patients who received SMR training, a SMR burst was reinforced when it occurred in the absence of EEG slow waves, spike activity, and high-voltage scalp EMG activity. The patients receiving just the time-out procedure were instructed to keep the time-out signals off as much as possible. The patients receiving the SMR training plus the time-out procedure were instructed to produce as many SMR feedback signals as possible, and told that SMR feedback would not be available whenever the time-out signals occurred. Cott et al. (1979) found that the time-out alone procedure was just as effective as the SMR training plus time-out procedure in reducing seizure rate. Thus, this study suggests that SMR conditioning does not appear to be the necessary component for a reduction in seizure rate, whereas time-out contingent on EEG slow waves, spike activity, and/or high-voltage scalp EMG activity may be a potentially effective component. Clearly, additional research is needed to clarify the mechanisms of EEG biofeedback effects on seizure rate.

## Systematic Desensitization

In *in vitro* systematic desensitization, the patient is initially taught relaxation techniques and then instructed to visualize or think of seizure-provoking scenes. Ince (1976) reported on a 12-year-old boy who exhibited both petit mal and grand mal seizures. The petit mal seizures were characterized by the child "blanking out," that is, staring into space and not responding from 45 seconds up to 2 minutes. Grand mal seizures were manifested by loss of speech, visual disturbances, falling, fainting, and convulsive movements of the trunk and extremities. The duration of the grand mal seizures was typically from 30 to 50 seconds, after which the patient fell asleep. None of the anticonvulsant drugs he was taking was effective in controlling his seizures. Several hierarchies of anxiety-provoking situations were constructed, including having seizures while in school and other public places, being ridiculed by other children, and receiving a new experimental anticonvulsant drug.

The child was initially taught relaxation techniques, and then systematic desensitization was begun. Each item on the hierarchies was paired with relaxation (as a counteranxious response), with progression from the least anxiety-provoking item on each hierarchy to the most anxiety-provoking item as the child was able to clearly visualize each scene without experiencing any anxiety. The child was also instructed to elicit his relaxation response whenever he felt the onset of a seizure approaching (he invariably had a preseizure aura). Prior to the *in vitro* systematic desensitization intervention, the child had between nine and ten grand mal seizures per week and from 25 to 26 petit mal seizures per week. During treatment, there was a substantial reduction in seizure rate, so that by a 6-month follow-up, neither grand mal nor petit mal seizures had occurred during that period.

## Contingency Management

Contingency management programs for seizure control may be divided into reinforcement for seizure-free periods (DRO schedule) and some form of punishment for seizure occurrence. Balaschak (1975) described a school-based intervention where the classroom teacher reinforced the seizure-free time periods of an 11-year-old girl with praise and treats. During the intervention, seizure rate decreased from 60 percent to 21 percent of the school days recorded.

Zlutnick, Mayville, and Moffat (1975) attempted to control seizures by applying consequences to the biobehaviors that reliably preceded the seizures. Zlutnick et al. (1975) hypothesized that if seizures are viewed as the terminal link in a chain of biobehaviors, they might be prevented by interrupting preseizure behaviors. The interruption procedure for preseizure behavior consisted of shouting "No!" loudly and grasping the child by the shoulders with both hands and shaking her vigorously once. Additionally, for one child, a differential reinforcement procedure was implemented contingent upon the preseizure behavior of arm raising. The child's hands were placed by her side, and she was reinforced after 5 seconds for "arms down." Some degree of seizure control was demonstrated for four of the five children studied.

Cataldo, Russo, and Freeman (1979) studied a 5-year-old girl with a mixed seizure disorder that included two types of seizures. The myoclonic seizures, which were brief episodes involving loss of neck tone, rapid random eye movements, and violent shaking of the upper body and arms for approximately one to ten seconds, occurred at variable rates of from 50 to 400 seizures per day. The grand mal seizures consisted of loss of balance, violent tonic-clonic convulsions lasting between 30 to 90 seconds, cyanosis, and urinary incontinence. The grand mal seizures occurred approximately one to six times per week, followed by sleep lasting as long as several hours. The use of most major antiepileptic drugs and a ketogenic diet were all unsuccessful in reducing the occurrence of seizures.

The intervention consisted of a time-out procedure. When the child's seizures reached a rate of 1.5 per minute for two consecutive 5-minute time periods, she was removed from the activity in which she was engaged, asked to sit in a chair in her room, close her eyes, and rest for 10 minutes. Thus, when the seizure rate was high, the child was removed from the hypothesized stimulating environment. This high-seizure-rate contingent time-out procedure resulted in a greatly reduced myoclonic seizure rate and a complete reduction of grand mal seizures. When the time-out contingency was removed, seizure rate returned to pretreatment frequency. These time-out procedures are comparable to the time-out contingency utilized by Cott et al. (1979) in their EEG biofeedback study and suggest the possible neurophysiological mechanisms for the effectiveness of time-out contingent on overt seizure behaviors.

## TICS

Although a number of attempts have been made to classify tics into various categories, the only clear-cut "tic-syndrome" is the Gilles de la Tourette's syndrome, which is characterized by compulsive jerking of the voluntary musculature, particularly the face, neck, and extremities (Yates, 1970). This syndrome is differentiated from other complex tics by the accompaniment of compulsive obscene utterances. Although tranquilizers and muscle relaxants have produced control over tics for some patients, these drugs may cause serious side effects (Shapiro, Shapiro, & Wayne, 1973).

Varni, Boyd, and Cataldo (1978) described in detail a treatment package for a 7-year-old child, which included self-monitoring, reinforcement for decreased tic frequency (DRL schedule), and tic contingent time-out. The child had a history of high rate multiple tic behaviors from the age of 2 years, accelerating to an even higher rate 6 months prior to the onset of the study. Four discrete tics were identified: facial grimaces, shoulder shrugging, rump protrusion, and the vocalization "huh." Facial grimaces were operationally defined as squinting both eyes, accompanied by mouth distortions. These two facial components occurred simultaneously. Shoulder shrugging was defined as a rapid up and down movement involving one or both shoulders. Rump protrusion was a rapid bending of both knees that resulted in the rump extending outward from the body angle. The vocalization "huh" was a rapid single syllable utterance. As treatment progressed, response definitions were extended to include topographically similar but less prominent tics, that is, less intense facial grimaces and less exaggerated shoulder shrugging and rump protrusion. The less intense facial grimaces included unilateral eye squinting, mouth twitching, and slight nose wrinkling. These facial behaviors often occurred singly.

Facial tics were initially selected for treatment in the clinic setting since they occurred at a higher frequency and greater intensity than the other tics. The initial phase of treatment was designed to make the child aware of the facial grimaces and to teach him to label and self-monitor these facial tics. First the child was asked to look in a mirror and verbalize what he was doing with his face. Facial grimaces were labeled as tics, and the child was prompted to indicate verbally each time a tic occurred. Consistent labeling with the use of the mirror was then faded to labeling without looking in the mirror and while engaging in other activities. After the child was reliably self-monitoring and labeling his facial tics (a matter of several minutes), the therapist explained to the child the contingencies for facial tics. Specifically, the therapist recorded

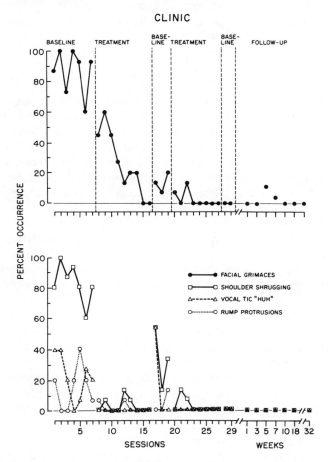

Fig. 8.4.    Percent occurrence of the tic behaviors across successive baseline and treatment reversals in the clinic. Only facial grimaces were directly treated.

Source: Reprinted with permission from J.W. Varni, E.F. Boyd, & M.F. Cataldo. Self-monitoring, external reinforcement, and time-out procedures in the control of high rate tic behaviors in a hyperactive child. *Journal of Behavior Therapy and Experimental Psychiatry*, 1978, **9**, 353–358.

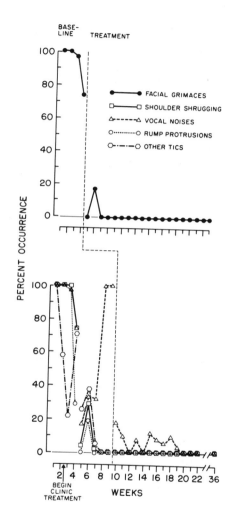

Fig. 8.5. Percent occurrence of the tic behaviors during baseline and treatment in the home. Facial grimaces were initially treated, then vocal noises. Shoulder shrugging, rump protrusions, and other tics were not directly treated.

Source: Reprinted with permission from J.W. Varni, E.F. Boyd, & M.F. Cataldo. Self-monitoring, external reinforcement, and time-out procedures in the control of high rate tic behaviors in a hyperactive child. *Journal of Behavior Therapy and Experimental Psychiatry,* 1978, **9**, 353–358.

each time the child reported a facial tic; if the child emitted fewer than ten facial tics in 5 minutes, he could go out into the corridor and play; however, if he did more than ten tics, he was placed in time-out (a chair in an empty room) for 5 minutes. The therapist positively reinforced the absence of facial tics with praise throughout the 5-minute treatment period.

During treatment, both response definitions and treatment contingencies were altered to shape zero rates of tic behavior (DRL schedule). As facial tics decreased in intensity, more subtle movements were identified as tics. Similarly, the contingencies on the number of facial tics for a free-play versus time-out consequence were systematically changed, requiring gradually fewer and fewer tics per 5-minute period (DRL schedule). As seen in Figure 8.4, the treatment package resulted in a gradually decreased frequency of facial tics in the clinic setting and generalized as well to the other tic behaviors that were not specifically treated.

In the home setting, the child's mother recorded the occurrence of tic behaviors as she went about her daily activities. Each half-hour she simply noted on a behavior checklist whether or not she had seen a tic occur during the previous half-hour period. Two weeks after treatment had begun in the clinic, the child's mother was instructed to implement treatment procedures for facial grimaces at home. When the child emitted a facial tic, he was told so by his mother, and then placed in time-out (a chair facing the corner of a room) for 5 minutes. If no tics were noted for one half-hour, the mother would praise the child and give him a gold star that could later be exchanged for preferred activities. On the tenth week of home treatment, similar contingencies were also placed on vocal tics. As initially seen in the clinic setting, the treatment package resulted in a complete cessation of tics in the home setting, maintained over an extended follow-up period (Figure 8.5).

# CEREBRAL PALSY

Cerebral palsy is a term that refers to a group of nonprogressive disorders of motor function caused by brain insult or injury in early development (Schain, 1977). The diagnosis of cerebral palsy may include some or all of the following symptoms: involuntary motor movement such as spasms, spinal cord abnormality, mental retardation, muscular weakness secondary to myopathy or neuropathy, and spastic paraplegia (Vining, Accardo, Rubenstein, Farrell, & Roizen, 1976). Children with spastic cerebral palsy may exhibit hemoplegia (muscular spasticity and/or paralysis involving two limbs on the same side), double hemoplegia (all four limbs with the upper extremities more affected), quadriplegia (all four limbs with the lower extremities slightly more involved), and diplegia (all four limbs with the lower extremities affected to a markedly greater degree than the uppers) (Vining et al., 1976). Children with cerebral palsy exhibit developmental delays in a number of physical and psychosocial functional abilities (Caputo & Biehl, 1973; Kaminer & Chinitz, 1982; Wright & Nicholson, 1973). Biobehavioral management strategies with children with cerebral palsy have generally included biofeedback and nonbiofeedback biobehavioral management procedures.

## Biofeedback

In the child with spastic cerebral palsy, the goal of physical habilitation is frequently the reduction of muscle tone so as to facilitate more normal motor patterns. EMG biofeedback has recently been investigated as a component of physical habilitation in normalizing muscle tone in children with spastic cerebral palsy (Cataldo, Bird, & Cunningham, 1978; Finley, Etherton, Dickman, Karimian, & Simpson, 1981; Finley, Niman, Standley, & Ender, 1976; Finley, Niman, Standley, & Wansley, 1977).

Finley et al. (1976) studied six patients selected on the basis of manifesting primarily athetoid cerebral palsy which was refractory to conventional forms of therapy. EMG biofeedback was targeted on the frontalis muscle, with surface electrodes placed in a bipolar configuration over this area. Visual feedback consisted of pen deflections on polygraph chart paper, with audio feedback provided by clicks. The intensity of both feedback modalities was proportional to the muscle activity recorded by the frontalis EMG. Each patient was instructed to strive to slow the clicks down until they stopped and to attempt to move the pen tracings on the polygraph chart paper to as near zero as possible. Biofeedback training resulted in a reduction in frontalis EMG for all patients. Additionally, improvements on speech and motor functions were also observed. Finley et al. (1976) suggested that frontalis EMG biofeedback may lead to general muscle relaxation over the entire body, consequently facilitating more normal motor movements from a point of muscle relaxation rather than spasticity.

Finley et al. (1977) extended their initial findings with frontalis EMG biofeedback to four younger children (6 to 10 years of age) with spastic cerebral palsy, adding a systematic motivational component. If the child's cumulative integrated frontalis EMG voltage fell below the designated cumulative voltage threshold during the biofeedback sessions, the child was immediately reinforced with a token, money, candy, or a toy. The children were not specifically told to relax, but were told that they should strive to slow the clicks (audio feedback) down until they stopped and to attempt to move the pen tracings on the polygraph chart paper (visual feedback) to as near zero as possible. In the early biofeedback sessions, the threshold for stopping the clicks was relatively high, so that a slight reduction in frontalis EMG would stop the clicks. As the biofeedback sessions progressed, the threshold for stopping the clicks was gradually made more difficult (shaping), thus requiring a greater degree of relaxation for reinforcement. The study results showed a decrease in frontalis muscle activity and some improvement in speech and motor skills. Additionally, a correspondence between frontalis EMG and forearm flexor EMG was noted under certain conditions, suggesting some generalization of relaxation training.

Cataldo, Bird, and Cunningham (1978) studied two young children and a young adult patient all with severe choreoathetoid cerebral palsy. The patients' inability to inhibit high levels of muscle tension and athetoid movements in their trunk area and upper extremities interfered with breath control, speech, and the acquisition of simple self-help skills. Depending on each patient's particular area of involvement, biofeedback training was selected to increase voluntary control over the biceps muscle of patient 1's right arm, the left and right pectoral muscles of patient 2, and the left biceps, left jaw muscle, and frontalis for patient 3. Clinical observations subsequent to biofeedback training suggested that reductions in EMG voltage levels were accompanied by an improvement in motor control in two patients.

Biofeedback training has also been applied to improve the gait of children with cerebral palsy (Conrad & Bleck, 1980; Seeger, Caudrey, & Scholes, 1981), and to correct head positioning (Wooldridge & Russell, 1976).

## Nonbiofeedback Biobehavioral Management

Riordan, Iwata, Wohl, and Finney (1980) worked with two children whose overall low level of food consumption placed them at risk for malnutrition. Both children exhibited self-feeding skills, however, they displayed a persistently low and highly selected food intake. The body weight and height of each child was below the fifth percentile for age. Neither child was diagnosed as having any significant oral motor or digestive difficulties that would account for the low food intake and body weight. Nutritional evaluations indicated that each child's diet was deficient in proteins, vitamins, and calories.

During meals, the number of bites of food and the sips of juice/milk were measured, in addition to inappropriate behaviors such as placing their hands in their mouth and removing food, tongue protrusions, leaving the table, and throwing food or utensils. Initially, a bite of a preferred food item and social praise were contingent upon the child feeding herself a bite of the food item targeted for ingestion. Over time, the number of bites required prior to the availability of the preferred food item was increased, while praise continued to be given for each bite. Finally, the child's preferred food was made available only if the child both consumed the required number of bites/sips of the target food and also showed the therapist that her mouth was empty of the target food. The new contingency was added because it was observed that both children would take a larger number of bites, hoard the food in their mouths, and later expel the entire quantity of food. During treatment, the number of

Neurological/Neuromuscular Disorders    189

bites/sips of the target foods increased substantially and inappropriate mealtime behaviors decreased for both children, resulting in a more well-balanced nutritional diet.

Thompson, Iwata, and Poynter (1979) treated the pathological tongue thrusts of a 10-year-old child with spastic cerebral palsy that interfered with feeding. The intervention consisted of differential reinforcement (presentation of food contingent upon tongue in) and punishment (gently pushing the tongue back into the mouth with a spoon). The results showed substantial decreases in pathological tongue thrusts and inappropriate food expulsion, and a large increase in appropriate chewing of food during meals.

Rapp (Rapp, 1980; Rapp & Bowers, 1979) treated chronic drooling in children with cerebral palsy by increasing the child's awareness of his drooling and by prompting swallowing. Rapp and Bowers (1979) developed an electronic device (the size of a cigarette pack) which was pinned to the child's clothing. Initially, the therapist worked with each child to shape an approximation to swallowing, as most of the children could not swallow effectively. A mirror was used during shaping as a visual aid for demonstration and feedback. Once the child's swallowing was learned and she was responding to verbal or gestural requests to swallow, prompting with the auditory cue (beeps) began. Initially, the device was switched on, emitting one beep simultaneously with the request to swallow. Eventually, the cues from the therapist were faded out and the auditory cues (beeps) solely served this prompting function. Beeps were emitted at predetermined set intervals so as to systematically prompt the child to swallow on a regular basis. Social praise was also contingent on dryness and swallowing. The rate of drooling was considerably reduced in every case, maintained over an extended follow-up period. Although the above biofeedback and nonbiofeedback biobehavioral interventions are encouraging, considerable empirical work remains to be conducted.

# REFERENCES

Akins, C., Davidson, R., & Hopkins, T. The child with myelodysplasia. In A.P. Scheiner & I.F. Abroms (Eds.), *The Practical Management of the Developmentally Disabled Child*. St. Louis: Mosby, 1980.

Austin, E.S., Lindgren, W.D., & Dietrich, S.L. Spina bifida and myelomeningocele. *American Family Physician*, 1972, **6**, 105–111.

Balaschak, B.A. Teacher-implemented behavior modification in a case of organically based epilepsy. *Journal of Consulting and Clinical Psychology*, 1976, **44**, 218–223.

Bird, B.L. Behavioral interventions in pediatric neurology. In D.C. Russo & J.W. Varni (Eds.), *Behavioral Pediatrics: Research and Practice*. New York: Plenum Press, 1982.

Brett, E. Implications of measuring anticonvulsant blood levels in epilepsy. *Developmental Medicine and Child Neurology*, 1977, **19**, 245–251.

Capute, A.J., & Biehl, R.F. Functional developmental evaluation: Prerequisite to habilitation. *Pediatric Clinics of North America*, 1973, **20**, 3–26.

Cataldo, M.F., Bird, B.L., & Cunningham, C.E. Experimental analysis of EMG feedback in treating cerebral palsy. *Journal of Behavioral Medicine*, 1978, **1**, 311–322.

Cataldo, M.F., Russo, D.C., & Freeman, J.M. A behavior analysis approach to high-rate myoclonic seizures. *Journal of Autism and Developmental Disorders*, 1979, **9**, 413–427.

Chapman, W.H., Hill, M.H., & Shurtleff, D.B. *Management of the Neurogenic Bowel and Bladder.* Oak Brook, Ill.: Eterna Press, 1979.

Conrad, L., & Bleck, E.E. Augmented auditory feedback in the treatment of equinus gait in children. *Developmental Medicine and Child Neurology*, 1980, **22**, 713–718.

Cott, A., Pavloski, R.P., & Black, A.H. Reducing epileptic seizures through operant conditioning of central nervous system activity: Procedural variables. *Science*, 1979, **103**, 73–75.

DeSouza, L.J., & Carroll, N. Ambulation of the braced myelomeningocele patient. *Journal of Bone and Joint Surgery*, 1976, **58**, 1112–1118.

Dietrich, S.L. Death and survival of spina bifida patients. Orthopaedic Hospital, unpublished manuscript, 1979.

Ellison, P.H., Largent, J.A., & Bahr, J.P. A scoring system to predict outcome following neonatal seizures. *Journal of Pediatrics*, 1981, **99**, 455–459.

Emerson, R., D'Souza, B.J., Vining, E.P., Holden, K.R., Mellits, E.D., & Freeman, J.M. Stopping medication in children with epilepsy. *New England Journal of Medicine*, 1981, **304**, 1125–1129.

Feldman, W.S., Manella, K.J., Apodaca, L., & Varni, J.W. Behavioral group parent training in spina bifida. *Journal of Clinical Child Psychology*, 1982, **11**, 144–150.

Feldman, W.S., Manella, K.J., & Varni, J.W. A behavioral parent training program for single mothers of physically handicapped children. *Child Care, Health and Development*, 1983, **9**, in press.

Feldman, W.S., & Varni, J.W. A parent training program for the child with spina bifida. *Spina Bifida Therapy*, 1983, **4**, in press.

Finley, W.W. Effects of sham feedback following successful SMR training in an epileptic: Follow-up study. *Biofeedback and Self-Regulation*, 1976, **1**, 227–235.

Finley, W.W., Etherton, M.D., Dickman, D., Karimian, D., & Simpson, R.W. A simple EMG-reward system for biofeedback training of children. *Biofeedback and Self-Regulation*, 1981, **6**, 169–180.

Finley, W.W., Niman, C.A., Standley, J., & Ender, P. Frontal EMG-biofeedback training of athetoid cerebral palsy patients: A report of six cases. *Biofeedback and Self-Regulation*, 1976, **1**, 169–182.

Finley, W.W., Niman, C.A., Standley, J., & Wansley, R.A. Electrophysiologic behavior modification of frontal EMG in cerebral-palsied children. *Biofeedback and Self-Regulation*, 1977, **2**, 59–79.

Freiman, J., & Buchanan, N. Drug compliance and therapeutic considerations in 75 black epileptic children. *Central African Journal of Medicine*, 1978, **24**, 136–140.

Gastaut, H. Clinical and electroencephalographical classification of epileptic seizures. *Epilepsia*, 1970, **11**, 102–113.

Gordon, N. Duration of treatment for childhood epilepsy. *Developmental Medicine and Child Neurology*, 1982, **24**, 84–88.

Hayden, P.W., Davenport, S.L., & Campbell, M.M. Adolescents with myelodysplasia: Impact of physical disability on emotional maturation. *Pediatrics*, 1979, **64**, 53–59.

Hayes-Allen, M.C. Obesity and short stature in children with myelomeningocele. *Developmental Medicine and Child Neurology*, 1972, **14**, 59–64.

Hayes-Allen, M.C., & Tring, F.C. Obesity: Another hazard for spina bifida children. *British Journal of Preventive and Social Medicine*, 1973, **27**, 192–196.

Hoffer, M.M., Feiwell, E., Perry, R., Perry, J., & Bonnett, C. Functional ambulation in patients with myelomeningocele. *Journal of Bone and Joint Surgery*, 1973, **55**, 137–148.

Holmes, G.L., Sackellares, J.C., McKiernan, J., Ragland, M., & Dreifuss, F.E. Evaluation of childhood pseudoseizures using EEG telemetry and video tape monitoring. *Journal of Pediatrics*, 1980, **97**, 554–558.

Huff, C.W., & Ramsey, P.L. Myelodysplasia: The influence of the quadriceps and hip abductor muscles on ambulatory function and stability of the hip. *Journal of Bone and Joint Surgery*, 1978, **60**, 432–443.

Hunt, G.M. Spina bifida: Implications for 100 children at school. *Developmental Medicine and Child Neurology*, 1981, **23**, 160–172.

Ince, L.P. The use of relaxation training and a conditioned stimulus in the elimination of epileptic seizures in a child: A case study. *Journal of Behavior Therapy and Experimental Psychiatry*, 1976, **7**, 39–42.

Jeffries, J.S., Killam, P.E., & Varni, J.W. Behavioral management of fecal incontinence in a child with myelomeningocele. *Pediatric Nursing*, 1982, **8**, 267–270.

Johnston, M.V., & Freeman, J.M. Pharmacologic advances in seizure control. *Pediatric Clinics of North America*, 1981, **28**, 179–194.

Kaminer, R.K., & Chinitz, S.P. Educational intervention with multiply handicapped preschool children. *Archives of Physical Medicine and Rehabilitation*, 1982, **63**, 82–86.

Killam, P.E., Apodaca, L., Manella, K.J., & Varni, J.W. Behavioral pediatric weight rehabilitation for children with myelomeningocele. *MCN: American Journal of Maternal Child Nursing*, 1983, **8**, in press.

Killam, P.E., Jeffries, J.S., & Varni, J.W. Urodynamic biofeedback treatment of urinary incontinence in children with myelomeningocele: Some initial observations. Paper presented at the Annual Meeting of the Society of Behavioral Medicine, Baltimore, March 1983.

Kuhlman, W.N. EEG feedback training of epileptic patients: Clinical and electroencephalographic analysis. *Electroencephalography and Clinical Neurophysiology*, 1978, **45**, 699–710.

Levine, M.D., Marzonson, P., & Bakow, H. Behavioral symptom substitution in children cured of encopresis. *American Journal of Diseases of Children*, 1980, **134**, 663–667.

Llenado, M., & Grogan, C. Myelomeningocele. In S. Palmer & S. Ekvall (Eds.), *Pediatric Nutrition in Developmental Disorders*. Springfield, Illinois: Charles C. Thomas, 1978.

Lorber, J. Results of treatment of myelomeningocele. *Developmental Medicine and Child Neurology*, 1971, **13**, 279–303.

Lubar, J.F., & Bahler, W.W. Behavioral management of epileptic seizures following EEG biofeedback training of the sensorimotor rhythm. *Biofeedback and Self-Regulation*, 1976, **1**, 77–104.

Manella, K.J., Jeffries, J.S., & Varni, J.W. Adherence to health care behaviors in the prevention of pressure sores by adolescents with spina bifida. Manuscript submitted for publication, 1983.

Manella, K.J., & Varni, J.W. Behavioral treatment of ambulatory function in a child with myelomeningocele. Manuscript submitted for publication, 1983.

Manella, K.J., & Varni, J.W. Behavior therapy in a gait-training program for a child with myelomeningocele. *Physical Therapy*, 1981, **61**, 1284–1287.

Massey, E.W., & Riley, T.L. Pseudoseizures: Recognition and treatment. *Psychosomatics*, 1980, **21**, 987–997.

Morrissy, R.T. Spina bifida: A new rehabilitation problem. *Orthopaedic Clinics of North America*, 1978, **9**, 379–389.

Mostofsky, D.I., & Balaschak, B.A. Psychobiological control of seizures. *Psychological Bulletin*, 1977, **84**, 723–750.

Rapp, D.L. Drool control: Long-term follow-up. *Developmental Medicine and Child Neurology*, 1980, **22**, 448–453.

Rapp, D.L., & Bowers, P.M. Meldreth dribble-control project. *Child Care, Health and Development*, 1979, **5**, 143–149.

Reuler, J.B., & Cooney, T.G. The pressure sore: Pathophysiology and principles of management. *Annals of Internal Medicine*, 1981, **94**, 661–666.

Reynold, E.H. Drug treatment of epilepsy. *Lancet*, 1978, **2**, 721–725.

Rickard, K., Brady, M.S., & Gresham, E.L. Nutritional management of the chronically ill child: Congenital heart disease and myelomeningocele. *Pediatric Clinics of North America*, 1977, **24**, 157–174.

Riordan, M.M., Iwata, B.A., Wohl, M.K., & Finney, J.W. Behavioral treatment of food refusal and selectivity in developmentally disabled children. *Applied Research in Mental Retardation*, 1980, **1**, 95–112.

Schain, R.J. *Neurology of Childhood Learning Disorders*. Baltimore: Williams and Wilkins, 1977.

Seeger, B.R., Caudrey, D.J., & Scholes, J.R. Biofeedback therapy to achieve symmetrical gait in hemiplegic cerebral palsied child. *Archives of Physical Medicine and Rehabilitation*, 1981, **62**, 364–368.

Shapiro, A.K., Shapiro, E., & Wayne, H. Treatment of Tourette's syndrome with haloperidol: Review of 34 cases. *Archives of General Psychiatry*, 1973, **24**, 92–97.

Shurtleff, D.B. Myelodysplasia: Management and treatment. *Current Problems in Pediatrics*, 1980, **10**, 7–41.

Shurtleff, D.B., Hayden, P.W., Chapman, W.H., Bnoy, A.B., & Hill, M.H. Myelodysplasia: Problems of long-term survival and social function. *Western Journal of Medicine*, 1975, **122**, 199–205.

Sousa, J.C., Gordon, L.H., & Shurtleff, D.B. Assessing developmental daily living skills in patients with spina bifida. *Developmental Medicine and Child Neurology*, 1976, **18**, 134–142.

Sterman, M.B., & Friar, L. Suppression of seizures in an epileptic following sensorimotor EEG feedback training. *Electroencephalography and Clinical Neurophysiology*, 1972, **33**, 89–95.

Sterman, M.B., & Macdonald, L.R. Effects of central cortical EEG feedback training on incidence of poorly controlled seizures. *Epilepsia*, 1978, **19**, 207–222.

Thompson, G.A., Iwata, B.A., & Poynter, H. Operant control of pathological tongue thrust in spastic cerebral palsy. *Journal of Applied Behavior Analysis*, 1979, **12**, 325–333.

Varni, J.W., Boyd, E.F., & Cataldo, M.F. Self-monitoring, external reinforcement, and time-out procedures in the control of high rate tic behaviors in a hyperactive child. *Journal of Behavior Therapy and Experimental Psychiatry*, 1978, **9**, 353–358.

Vining, E.P.G., Accardo, P.J., Rubenstein, J.E., Farrell, S.E., & Roizen, N.J. Cerebral palsy: A pediatric developmentalist's overview. *American Journal of Diseases of Children*, 1976, **130**, 643–349.

Wald, A. Use of biofeedback in treatment of fecal incontinence in patients with myelomeningocele. *Pediatrics*, 1981, **68**, 45–49.

Whitehead, W.E., Parker, L.H., Masek, B.J., Cataldo, M.F., & Freeman, J.M. Biofeedback treatment of fecal incontinence in patients with myelomeningocele. *Developmental Medicine and Child Neurology*, 1981, **23**, 313–322.

Williams, D.T., Spiegel, H., & Mostofsky, D.I. Neurogenic and hysterical seizures in children and adolescents: Differential diagnostic and therapeutic considerations. *American Journal of Psychiatry*, 1978, **135**, 82–86.

Wooldridge, C.P., & Russell, G. Head position training with the cerebral palsied child: An application of biofeedback techniques. *Archives of Physical Medicine and Rehabilitation*, 1976, **57**, 407–414.

Wright, T., & Nicholson, J. Physiotherapy for the spastic child: An evaluation. *Developmental Medicine and Child Neurology*, 1973, **15**, 146–163.

Yates, A.J. *Behavior Therapy*. New York: Wiley, 1970.

Zlutnick, S., Mayville, W.J., & Moffat, S. Modification of seizure disorders: The interruption of behavioral chains. *Journal of Applied Behavior Analysis*, 1975, **8**, 1–12.

Zysset, T., Rudeberg, A., Vassella, F., Kupfer, A., & Bircher, J. Phenytoin therapy for epileptic children: Evaluation of salivary and plasma concentrations and of methods of assessing compliance. *Developmental Medicine and Child Neurology*, 1981, **23**, 66–75.

## 9

# Hematology/Oncology: Childhood Cancer, Hemophilia

Pediatric hematology/oncology encompasses a wide variety of childhood disorders including cancer, hemophilia, sickle cell anemia, and thalassemia. Presently, the greatest amount of biobehavioral empirical work has been conducted with childhood cancer and hemophilia (see Kellerman & Varni, 1982a, for review).

## CHILDHOOD CANCER

Advances in medical treatment have led to a marked improvement in the survival rate for many forms of childhood cancer. This extended life expectancy has brought with it an increase in problems of adjustment and lifestyle changes encountered in other pediatric chronic disorders (see Kellerman & Varni, 1982a, 1982b, for reviews). Whereas most adult cancers are solid tumors of various body organs (e.g., lung, breast, ovaries, gastrointestinal system, cervix, and uterus), the modal pediatric cancers are the acute leukemias, comprising approximately 40 percent of all childhood malignancies. Tumors of the brain account for an additional 14 percent, with the remaining 46 percent made up of tumors of the kidney, lymphatic system, nervous system, bone, soft tissue, and eye (Siegel, 1980).

A number of biobehavioral factors have been conceived to influence the disease process in cancer. The role of life stress on cancer development through biochemical reactions transmitted by the neuroendocrine system and its effects on the immune system has been suggested (see Riley, 1981; Sklar & Anisman, 1981, for reviews). Such factors as dietary intake, smoking, and noncompliance to cancer treatment regimens are also suggested influences on the development and progression of cancer.

In childhood cancer, an increasing emphasis is being placed on the overall coping process given the improved prognosis for long-term survival (National

Cancer Institute, 1980). In addition to the assessment of psychological adjust-ment (Kellerman & Katz, 1977; Kellerman, Rigler, Siegel, & Katz, 1977; Koocher, O'Malley, Gogan, & Foster, 1980), neuropsychological performance (Goff, Anderson, & Cooper, 1980), and school reintegration (Katz, Kellerman, Rigler, Williams, & Siegel, 1977), the analysis of the coping process in child-hood cancer also requires the biobehavioral assessment and management of the potential iatrogenic effects of medical treatment.

In contrast to adult cancer, chronic, debilitating pain is comparatively uncommon in childhood cancer. The absence of long-term pain problems is primarily due to the differing nature of cancers in adults and children. For example, as opposed to the carcinomas seen in adults, childhood leukemias and lymphomas are not extremely painful diseases *per se,* although they may be accompanied by joint aches, headaches, fatigue, and fever during periods of active disease. Exceptions are the pain experienced by some children in the terminal stages of cancer, a period usually lasting no more than several weeks, and those with certain solid tumors.

A more common source of discomfort in childhood cancer lies in the acute distress, pain, nausea, emesis, anorexia, and taste aversions related to the diagnosis and treatment of cancer. The biobehavioral assessment and manage-ment of these iatrogenic effects of medical treatment will be the primary focus of this chapter section on childhood cancer.

## Nausea, Emesis, and Taste Aversions

Despite the advances in childhood cancer treatment (Smith, 1981), the com-monly utilized chemotherapy and radiotherapy modalities have many undesir-able side effects which may result in a high noncompliance rate and subsequently threaten the survival of the patient (Smith, Rosen, Trueworthy, & Lowman, 1979). Nausea, vomiting, and anorexia (loss of appetite) are an increasing problem as a result of more aggressive therapeutic modalities (Harris, 1978). These cancer treatment side effects are particularly distressing, since antiemetic drugs have a variable response and may produce additional side effects (Harris, 1978).

Nutritional problems resulting from treatment side effects are common in childhood cancer (National Cancer Institute, 1980). These side effects in-fluence a child's eating pattern, cause a loss of appetite, and a resulting loss of weight. The resulting loss of weight is of particular significance given the findings that weight loss has been found to be associated with a decreased median survival rate in cancer patients (Dewys, Begg, Lavin et al., 1980). These fluctuations in appetite and tolerance for food secondary to cancer treatment modalities may be conceived of within a learned taste aversion model and may be quite persistent when maintained through avoidance conditioning (e.g., Peck, 1978).

*Learned Taste Aversions*

Considerable data exist on the acquisition of taste aversions through conditioning paradigms in the animal literature (see Seligman & Hager, 1972). Learned food aversions in humans have also been found. Garb and Stunkard (1974) studied 696 healthy individuals ranging in age from early childhood to old age. Aversions were defined as the development of an intense dislike for a specific food as a result of becoming sick after eating the food item, whether or not the food item was responsible for the illness (i.e., the subsequent nausea and vomiting might be secondary to the flu and not the food itself). Thirty-eight percent of all subjects reported having had at least one aversion at some time in their lives. Gastrointestinal illness was associated with the acquisition of taste aversions in 87 percent of the subjects who developed food aversions. One pairing (one-trial learning) of food and illness was sufficient to produce aversions that lasted for many years. Acquisition of the aversion involved delays of as long as 6 hours between exposure to the food and the subsequent illness. The onset of the aversions was most common between the ages of 6 to 12 years, when the prevalence rate reached 30 percent.

Logue, Ophir, and Strauss (1981) interviewed 517 healthy university undergraduates regarding their acquisition of illness-induced aversions to foods and drinks, with 65 percent reporting at least one aversion. Eighty-three percent of the aversions were formed to the taste of the foods, rather than to the smell (51 percent), texture (32 percent), appearance (26 percent) or other aspects of the foods. Aversions occurred most frequently when food intake was subsequently followed by illness (average time delay was 2.5 hours), regardless of whether the illness was caused by the food. In 29 percent of the subjects, aversions generalized to similar foods. Extinction was more effective than forgetting in removing aversions; that is, in cases where the food was eaten again without resultant illness the aversion was lost to a much greater extent than when the food was never eaten again, even though the number of years since the aversion had first been acquired was essentially the same. This finding may have implications for the extinction of learned taste aversions in childhood cancer patients. Of further significance to cancer treatment-caused food aversions is the finding that only 57 percent of the subjects reported that the aversive food was the cause of their subsequent illness. Twenty-two percent reported that they did not know the cause of the illness, and 20 percent reported that they knew that the illness was not caused by a food. This finding suggests that learned taste aversions may occur on a noncognitive level, that is, that aversion conditioning resulted even when the subjects "knew" that the food item did not cause the subsequent illness. These data are consistent with traditional learning experiments on conditioning (see Seligman & Hager, 1972). Logue et al. (1981) also found that the more times the subjects were nauseated, the more aversions were subsequently conditioned. Finally, the reported aversions were formed to less familiar and less preferred foods, which is also significant for childhood cancer aversion conditioning given the specific food preferences of children. In sum, the findings by Logue et al. (1981) suggest that the taste aversions caused by cancer treatment-induced illness in childhood cancer patients are consistent with the laws of learning and may be amenable to learning-based treatment approaches.

Bernstein has empirically demonstrated that learned taste aversions occur in childhood cancer patients (Bernstein, 1978) and adult cancer patients (Bernstein & Webster, 1980) receiving cancer chemotherapy, as well as in animal cancer models (Bernstein & Sigmundi, 1980). In both the childhood and adult patients, aversion conditioning occurred with only one pairing between the specific food item and chemotherapy-induced gastrointestinal illness, even though the patients knew that the gastrointestinal illness was caused by the cancer treatment and not the food item. Bernstein suggests that these taste aversions may be one of the factors contributing to the anorexia and weight loss seen in patients with cancer. Deconditioning of these learned taste aversions through extinction and reinforcement techniques awaits systematic investigation (see Cairns & Altman, 1979, for a related case study).

## Biobehavioral Treatment of Nausea and Emesis

In addition to the nausea, emesis, and anorexia experienced as a physiological side effect of many chemotherapeutic agents and radiation therapy, anticipatory symptoms such as nausea, emesis, emotional withdrawal, and a general anxiety response may occur in reaction to the temporal and spatial stimuli associated with painful cancer treatment procedures (e.g., bone marrow aspirations, lumbar punctures, venipunctures, and chemotherapeutic injections). Additionally, Nesse, Carli, Curtis, and Kleinman (1980) have found that the odor of the clinic and similar odors elsewhere may elicit pretreatment or anticipatory nausea and emesis originally associated with chemotherapy-produced nausea and emesis. These anticipatory symptoms appear to be a conditioned response pattern in which the procedure is the unconditioned stimulus and various other stimuli such as the waiting room, procedure room, odor of the clinic, and sight of the white-coated nurse or doctor are conditioned to elicit specific biobehaviors (Kellerman & Varni, 1982a). For example, the child may learn to associate entering the hospital with receiving an unpleasant procedure and subsequently experience anticipatory psychophysiological changes such as palpatations, coldness in the extremities, tachycardia, pallor, nausea, and emesis (Kellerman & Varni, 1982b). A variety of methods that promote attention refocusing (distraction) and counteranxious responding through imagery techniques and relaxation training (e.g., hypnosis, guided imagery, progressive muscle relaxation, meditation, biofeedback) may decondition these conditioned anticipatory biobehaviors. A number of initial observations support this approach (Burish & Lyles, 1979; Burish, Shartner, & Lyles, 1981; Ellenberg, Kellerman, Dash, Higgins, & Zeltzer, 1980; LaBaw, Holton, Tewell, & Eccles, 1975; Olness, 1981; Redd, 1980a). Three recent studies with adult cancer patients will be discussed because of their empirical approaches and potential applicability to childhood cancer patients.

Burish and Lyles (1981) studied 16 adult cancer patients who were referred because they exhibited anticipatory anxiety, nausea, and/or vomiting to chemotherapy treatments in spite of the fact that they were receiving antiemetic drugs. The patients were randomly assigned to either a relaxation training or a no-relaxation training condition. Patients in the relaxation training condition received instruction on progressive muscle relaxation training and guided relaxation imagery prior to chemotherapy sessions. The patients were also instructed to practice the relaxation procedures at home daily and were given a brief set of written relaxation training instructions. The study's results showed that the patients in the relaxation training condition reported feeling significantly less anxious and nauseated during their chemotherapy than the patients not receiving relaxation training. The nurse who administered the chemotherapy also rated the patients in the relaxation training condition as displaying significantly less anxiety and nausea. Burish and Lyle (1981) suggest that a possible explanation for the observed effects of relaxation training was that it directly reduced the patients' distress by decreasing muscle tension and, in combination with the imagery instructions, by diverting the patients' attention away from the chemotherapy setting and its conditioned aversive stimuli (olfactory, visual, tactual, and other stimuli that had become associated before, during, and after chemotherapy treatment and elicited anxiety, nausea, and emesis). For example, some patients stated that they began to feel anxious and nauseated when they first saw the chemotherapy syringes and other treatment-related material. Attention refocusing on pleasant imagery may serve to provide an essential distraction from these provoking stimuli.

Lyles, Burish, Krozely, and Oldham (1982) extended their previously described techniques to a larger sample of adult cancer patients, studying 50 patients receiving chemotherapy, 25 by the push injection method and 25 by the drip infusion method. In comparison to a no-treatment control group and a therapist-attention control group, the progressive muscle relaxation training plus guided relaxation imagery treatment group reported feeling significantly less anxious and nauseated during chemotherapy, showed less physiological arousal, and reported less anxiety and depression immediately after chemotherapy and significantly less severe and protracted nausea at home following chemotherapy. The attending nurses' observations during chemotherapy confirmed the patient self-report data.

Redd, Andresen, and Minagawa (1982) studied six adult cancer patients who were selected because they consistently vomited before the actual chemotherapy injection. All of the patients had received various antiemetic drugs without any reduction in nausea and emesis. The study's hypnosis procedure was explained in social learning terms as a method of relaxation and distraction, utilizing deep muscle relaxation and relaxing, pleasant imagery. Assessment included the nurses' recorded observations of emesis while the patients waited for treatment and during the actual chemotherapy injection and the patients' ratings of nausea on a visual analogue scale. The scale consisted of a 10 cm line, with the severity of nausea rated by placing a mark along the line between "no nausea" labeled at the left end and "nausea as bad as it could be" labeled at the right end. For all six patients, hypnosis training resulted in a complete suppression of emesis and a substantial reduction in pre- and post-treatment nausea. Thus, these three studies suggest that a treatment approach combining guided imagery and progressive muscle relaxation techniques may provide a significant therapeutic effect for the management of nausea, emesis, and anxiety secondary to cancer chemotherapy. Morrow and Morrell (1982) have also found these techniques successful within a systematic desensitization format. A recent study by Zeltzer, Kellerman, Ellenberg, and Dash (1982) found statistically significant reductions in both the frequency and intensity of treatment-related emesis in nine adolescents with cancer subsequent to hypnosis training, further indicating the potential applicability of these techniques in the childhood population.

## Behavioral Distress Secondary to Medical Procedures

Conditioned anxiety in response to recurrent painful medical procedures such as bone marrow aspirations, lumbar punctures, and venipunctures occurs frequently in childhood cancer patients (Kellerman & Varni, 1982a, 1982b). Katz, Kellerman, and Siegel (1980) studied 115 children with cancer undergoing bone marrow aspirations in order to develop a reliable and valid measurement scale of behavioral distress. Given the difficulty in distinguishing between anxiety and pain since these terms refer to constructs (Shacham & Daut, 1981), behavioral distress has been defined as a general term encompassing the biobehaviors of negative affect, including anxiety, fear, and acute pain (Katz, Kellerman, & Siegel, 1981). Katz et al. (1980) found that behavioral distress (e.g., crying, clinging, screaming, verbal statements of pain or fear) in response to bone marrow aspirations was virtually ubiquitous and did not habituate in the children studied, clearly suggesting the need for clinical intervention. Jay, Ozolins, Elliott, and Caldwell (in press) found a relationship between parental anxiety and the children's distress, suggesting parent training as a necessary component.

Ellenberg et al. (1980) successfully taught hypnosis to an adolescent girl with leukemia who reacted with considerable behavioral distress to bone marrow aspirations. The patient was asked to record her subjective reactions following a bone marrow aspiration on a pain and anxiety rating scale from 1 (no symptoms) to 5 (severe symptoms) before, during, and after the procedure.

Following hypnosis training there was a clear decrease in self-reported pain and anxiety before, during, and after the bone marrow aspirations. Subsequent studies by Kellerman, Zeltzer, Ellenberg, and Dash (1982) and Zeltzer and LeBaron (1982) have extended this hypnotic approach to acute procedural distress to a larger group of children and adolescents with leukemia, demonstrating significant reductions in both self-reported anxiety and discomfort before, during, and after the procedure. Jay, Elliott, Ozolins, and Olson (1982) also reported the beneficial effects of a behavior therapy treatment consisting of breathing exercises, imagery, filmed modeling, behavioral rehearsal, and reinforcement for childhood cancer patients undergoing painful medical procedures.

## Biobehavioral Effects of Protected Environments

The growing trend in the use of chemotherapeutic agents that require careful inpatient monitoring of physiological parameters has resulted in more frequent and prolonged periods of hospitalization for children with cancer. The medical effectiveness of protected environments employing barrier isolation facilities, such as life islands and laminar flow rooms has been described in terms of reducing the rate of bacterial infections during periods of drug- and disease-induced granulocytopenia. The empirical findings concerning the biobehavioral effects of long-term hospitalization and treatment in protective isolation indicates the need for careful monitoring of the patients' biobehavioral responses in addition to the physiological parameters (Hollenbeck, Susman, Nannis, Strope, Hersh, Levine, & Pizzo, 1980; Kellerman, Rigler, & Siegel, 1977; Kellerman, Rigler, Siegel, McCue, Pospisil, & Uno, 1976).

Kellerman, Rigler, and Siegel (1979) conducted a behavioral observation study of 14 children with cancer treated in a laminar airflow protected environment unit. The daily rating scale included items on appetite, sleep pattern, physical discomfort, affect, perception, activity, management problems, and social-interpersonal parameters. The children received a comprehensive psychosocial support approach to prevent their stay in the protected environment from resembling a prolonged deprivation or sensory isolation experience (Hollenbeck et al., 1980). The approach included access to window views and clocks, the encouragement of a daily schedule, regular family entry into the units, providing the services of a play therapist and schoolteacher, family counseling and preparation, along with detailed biobehavioral monitoring by both the nursing and psychosocial staff. Within the context of this ongoing treatment approach, Kellerman et al. (1979) found no debilitating or long-term biobehavioral effects related to prolonged protected environment treatment. The treatment of acute biobehavioral effects has received some initial empirical attention with adult cancer patients in protected isolation (Redd, 1980b), but systematic application to childhood cancer patients needs to be conducted.

# HEMOPHILIA

Hemophilia is a congenital hereditary disorder of blood coagulation, transmitted as an X-linked recessive trait by a female carrier to her male child. True hemophilia in a female is extremely rare, with female carriers of the trait being protected by the production of sufficient clotting factor by cells under the control of the normal gene bearing X-chromosome. Because of its status as one of the most frequent spontaneous mutations known in medicine, about a third of all newly diagnosed patients evidence no known family history of hemophilia (Strauss, 1969). This life-long chronic disorder is characterized by recurrent, unpredictable internal hemorrhaging affecting any body part, especially the joints and the extremities. Although the severity of the disorder varies among individuals, the failure to produce one of the plasma proteins required to form a blood clot is the identifying characteristic. The process of blood coagulation involves a series of biochemical reactions, with each requiring one or more of the plasma clotting factors. Since one of the clotting factors is deficient in hemophiliacs, the time required for the formation of an effective blood clot is greatly prolonged. Consequently, bleeding from injured blood vessels continues for a much longer time and more blood is lost into the joint, muscle, or other site of injury.

Severe hemophiliacs have less than 1 percent of normal activity of the clotting factor; moderate hemophiliacs evidence about 1-5 percent of normal clotting factor activity; and mild hemophiliacs show 6-50 percent of normal clotting factor (Hilgartner, 1979). Small external cuts on the skin can usually be treated by pressure bandages; however, untreated internal bleeding (typically indicated by pain, loss of motion, and/or swelling) may be quite prolonged. Although internal bleeding episodes can occur as a result of obvious physical trauma, many bleeding episodes occur spontaneously, that is, without clear precipitating cause, but may be a result of unrecognized mild trauma (Arnold & Hilgartner, 1977). Spontaneous bleeding episodes are more common in severe hemophiliacs, whereas moderate to mild hemophiliacs may experience excessive internal bleeding only as a result of obvious physical injury. While severe hemophiliacs may hemorrhage internally as often as once or twice a week as children, moderate hemophiliacs may have as few as one or two bleeding episodes a year, and mild hemophiliacs may bleed excessively only during a surgical intervention.

A major breakthrough in the medical management of hemophilia came in the early 1960s with the discovery and separation of the essential clotting factors from the plasma of normal blood. Freeze-dried concentrates of the clotting factor proteins made from pooled plasma are now available and are reconstituted with sterile water. The intravenous infusion of the factor concentrate temporarily replaces the missing clotting factor and converts the clotting status to normal, allowing a functional blood clot to form. As a result of home-based administration and self-infusion of factor replacement (hemophilia home care program or supervised self-treatment), early treatment is now possible, consequently reducing the severity of bleeding episodes, facilitating patient psychosocial adjustment and increasing school and work attendance and other activities of daily living (Dietrich, 1976a; Kaufert, 1980; Lazerson, 1972; Levine & Britten, 1973; Sergis & Hilgartner, 1972; Smith, Keyes, & Forman, 1982).

Even though muscle and soft tissue hemorrhages (hematomas) may be quite serious, the most frequent problem and major cause of disability in severe hemophilia is repeated bleeding into the joint areas (hemarthroses) (Arnold & Hilgartner, 1977; Dietrich, 1976b; Dietrich, Luck, & Martinson, 1982). Hemarthroses of the knees, elbows, and ankles account for the majority of the more severe joint bleeds (Aronstam et al., 1979). With repeated hemarthroses, a pathophysiological condition similar to osteoarthritis develops, marked by articular cartilage destruction, pathological bone formation, and impaired function (Sokoloff, 1975). Although prophylactic administration of factor replacement to prevent hemarthrosis has been investigated, the expense of this form of treatment, the amount of factor replacement required, and the difficulties of multiple transfusions on an ongoing basis have made it unrealistic for most patients (Kisker, Perlman, & Benton, 1971). It is even questionable whether prophylaxis will totally prevent hemarthroses and the resultant degenerative arthropathy (Kasper, Dietrich, & Rapaport, 1970). Although untreated hemarthroses will most certainly result in severe degenerative arthropathy, even prompt treatment at the first sign of a bleed may not prevent some progressive joint changes (Guenthner, Hilgartner, Miller, & Vienne, 1980). An estimated 75 percent of hemophilic adolescents and adults are affected by degenerative hemophilic arthropathy, with chronic arthritic pain representing the most frequent problem in the care of adolescent and adult hemophiliacs (Dietrich, 1976b). Since pain represents such an outstanding characteristic of hemophilia, comprehensive pain management techniques have received increasing attention.

## Pain Management in Hemophilia

Whereas acute pain in the hemophiliac is associated with a specific bleeding episode, chronic arthritic pain represents a sustained condition over an extended period of time (Dietrich et al., 1982). Thus pain perception is complicated in the hemophiliac by the existence of both acute bleeding and chronic arthritic pain (Varni, 1981a). More specifically, the acute pain of hemorrhage provides a functional signal, indicating the necessity of intravenous infusion of factor replacement, allowing a functional blood clot to form. Arthritic pain, on the other hand, represents a potentially debilitating chronic condition which may result in impaired life functioning and analgesic dependence (Varni &

Gilbert, 1982). A substantial number of analgesics and anti-inflammatory medications are of limited usefulness, since they inhibit platelet aggregation and prolong the bleeding time in hemophiliacs (Arnold & Hilgartner, 1977). Consequently, the challenge has been to develop an effective intervention in the reduction of perceived chronic arthritic pain, while not interfering with the essential functional signal of acute bleeding pain.

Medical observations have suggested the possible therapeutic value of warming and heat application in the management of arthritic joints (Lehmann, Warren, & Scham, 1974). White (1973) reported data from a questionnaire administered to 30 osteoarthritic and rheumatoid arthritic patients, with 27 patients associating pain relief with past experiences of warmth and massage. In these patients, the application of a counterirritant (10 percent menthol and 15 percent methyl salicylate) produced active tissue hyperemia and a sensation of heat accompanied by decreased pain perception. Citing earlier findings by Wasserman, Oester, Oryshkevich, Montgomery, Poske, and Ruksha (1968) which demonstrated abnormal electromyographic readings in muscles adjacent to arthritic joints, White (1973) proposed that the counterirritant-produced hyperemia reduced the ischemia in the contracted muscles surrounding the arthritic joint. Swezey (1978) reviewed the evidence on the relative efficacy of superficial heating in articular disorders, suggesting that the threshold for pain may be raised by superficial heating, but cautioned that the increases in superficial circulation in relationship to pain relief and muscle relaxation needed to be experimentally determined. Hilgard's (1975) laboratory research on hypnosis-controlled experimental pain has indicated the role of distraction and refocusing of attention, anxiety reduction, suggestions of pain relief, and the imagination of past experiences that are incompatible with pain as potent cognitive variables in the reduction of pain perception.

Varni (1981a, 1981b) reported on the successful self-regulation of chronic arthritic pain perception by hemophiliacs involving a treatment strategy consisting of progressive muscle relaxation exercises, meditative breathing, and guided imagery techniques (see Chapter 4 for a detailed description of these techniques). In these studies, the patient was instructed to imagine himself actually in a scene previously identified or associated with past experiences of warmth and arthritic pain relief. The scene was initially evoked by a detailed multisensory description by the therapist, and further details of the scene were subsequently described out loud by the patient. Once the scene was clearly described and visualized by the patient, the therapist's suggestions included imagining the gentle flow of blood from the forehead down all the body parts to the targeted arthritic joint, images of warm colors such as red and orange, and the sensations of warm sand and sun on the joint in the context of a beach scene. Further suggestions consisted of statements indicating reduction of pain as the joint progressively felt warmer and more comfortable. Each patient had previously identified one joint as the site of greatest arthritic pain, and this joint was targeted for active warming during clinic and home practice sessions.

Table 9.1. Hemophilia Multidimensional Pain Assessment Instrument (HMPAI).

| DATE | TIME Start Stop | TYPE | INTENSITY SCALE | ANTECEDENTS | LOCATION | MEDICATION | PAIN REDUCTION | TENSION SCALE |
|------|------|------|------|------|------|------|------|------|
| | | | | | | | | |

CODE: TYPE = Arthritic Pain (A)
Bleeding Pain (B)
Other Pain (O)

LOCATION = e.g., left elbow, right knee

ANTECEDENT = e.g., physical trauma, interpersonal stress, unknown.

INTENSITY = 1 to 10
(mild) (severe)

MEDICATION = analgesic or concentrate; type and amount.

PAIN REDUCTION =
1   to   10
(not effective) (100% effective)

DAILY TENSION =
1   to   10
(relaxed) (stressed)

203

Table 9.2.    Comparative Assessment Inventory.

- *Comparative Pain:* How is your arthritic (bleeding) pain as compared to before you started using the self-regulation techniques? 3 = much better, 2 = moderately better, 1 = slightly better, 0 = the same, − 1 = slightly worse, − 2 = moderately worse, − 3 = much worse.
- *Comparative Mobility:* How is your ability to move, i.e., standing, walking, as compared to before you started using the self-regulation techniques? Same scale as above.
- *Comparative Sleep:* How is your ability to sleep during arthritic pain as compared to before you started using the self-regulation techniques? Same scale as above.
- *Overall Improvement:* How would you rate your overall level of general improvement as compared to before you started using the self-regulation techniques? 3 = complete or nearly complete improvement, 2 = moderate improvement, 1 = slight improvement, 0 = unchanged, − 1 = slightly worse, − 2 = moderately worse, − 3 = markedly worse.

In the initial investigation (Varni, 1981a), preliminary findings with two hemophiliacs suggested the potential utility of these self-regulation techniques in the reduction of chronic arthritic pain (described in detail in Chapter 4). The next investigation was designed to systematically extend these earlier findings to three additional hemophiliacs under improved methodological conditions, including longer baseline and follow-up assessments, and measurement of multiple subjective and medical parameters in relationship to chronic arthritic pain (Varni, 1981b). Each patient was instructed in the use of the daily self-monitoring Hemophilia Multidimensional Pain Assessment Instrument (Table 9.1 ). In addition, each patient's subjective evaluation of the overall impact of the intervention was determined by a comparative assessment inventory administered at the final follow-up session (Table 9.2). An analysis of each patient's medical chart and pharmacy records provided data on the number of analgesics ordered, factor replacement units required for the treatment of bleeding episodes, and the number of hemorrhages. These records were analyzed retrospectively at the completion of the investigation to represent the patient's status 6 months prior to the self-regulation intervention and during the follow-up period (averaged monthly for both pre- and postassessment). Finally, a thermal biofeedback unit served as a physiological assessment device rather than as a training technique, with the patient instructed to actively attempt to increase the temperature at the joint site during the self-regulation conditions without the benefit of moment-to-moment feedback.

An analysis of Figure 9.1 demonstrates that the self-regulation techniques were effective in significantly reducing the number of days of perceived chronic arthritic pain per week for all three patients, maintained over an extended follow-up assessment. Further analysis of the daily pain assessment instrument showed that on the 10-point scale (1 = mild pain, 10 = most severe pain), arthritic pain perception decreased from an average of 5.1 during baseline to

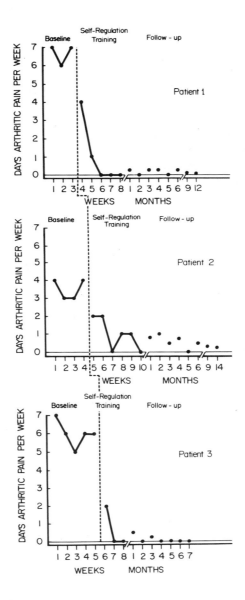

Fig. 9.1.   Days of total arthritic pain perception per week during baseline, self-regulation training, and follow-up for three hemophiliacs.

Source: Reprinted with permission from J.W. Varni. Self-regulation techniques in the management of chronic arthritic pain in hemophilia. *Behavior Therapy,* 1982, **12**, 185–194.

2.2 on those follow-up days in which arthritic pain occurred (Table 9.3). Average bleeding pain was essentially unchanged from baseline to follow-up conditions (6.9 to 6.8). Each patient's evaluation at the final follow-up session on the comparative assessment inventory indicated substantial positive changes in arthritic pain, mobility, sleep, and general overall functioning, with no reported changes in bleeding pain perception (Table 9.4). Assessment of the surface skin temperature over the targeted arthritic joint showed increased thermal readings from baseline to self-regulation conditions, averaging an increase of 4.1° F. These findings were consistent across patients and were maintained over the follow-up period (Table 9.5). The analysis of the medical charts and pharmacy records demonstrated that the units of factor replace-

Table 9.3.    Subjective Ratings on the 10-Point Scales.

| Patient | | Arthritic pain intensity | Bleeding pain intensity | Daily tension rating |
|---|---|---|---|---|
| 1 | Pre: | 5.3 | 6.8 | 5.6 |
|   | Post: | 1.8 | 6.9 | 4.9 |
| 2 | Pre: | 5.2 | 5.9 | 4.3 |
|   | Post: | 3.3 | 5.7 | 4.4 |
| 3 | Pre: | 4.8 | 7.9 | 3.6 |
|   | Post: | 1.4 | 7.7 | 2.9 |
| $\bar{x}$ | Pre: | 5.1 | 6.9 | 4.5 |
|   | Post: | 2.2 | 6.8 | 4.1 |

Source: Reprinted with permission from J.W. Varni. Self-regulation techniques in the management of chronic arthritic pain in hemophilia. *Behavior Therapy*, 1981, **12**, 185–194.

Table 9.4.    Subjective Evaluations of Improvement on the ± 3-Point Scales.

| Patient | Comparative arthritic pain | Comparative bleeding pain | Comparative mobility | Comparative sleep | Overall improvement |
|---|---|---|---|---|---|
| 1 | +3 | 0 | +3 | +3 | +3 |
| 2 | +2 | 0 | +2 | +2 | +2 |
| 3 | +3 | 0 | +2 | +2 | +3 |
| $\bar{x}$ | +2.7 | 0 | +2.3 | +2.3 | +2.7 |

Source: Reprinted with permission from J.W. Varni. Self-regulation techniques in the management of chronic arthritic pain in hemophilia. *Behavior Therapy*, 1981, **12**, 185–194.

Table 9.5.    Physiological and Medical Parameters.

| Patient | | Arthritic joint skin temperature (°F) | Analgesic tablets (#) | Factor replacement (units) | Bleeding frequency |
|---|---|---|---|---|---|
| 1 | Pre: | 84.4 | 4.3 | 10,667 | 5.1 |
|   | Post: | 87.9 | 0 | 9,893 | 4.8 |
| 2 | Pre: | 83.1 | 15.8 | 6,264 | 3.7 |
|   | Post: | 88.3 | 7.9 | 8,919 | 4.6 |
| 3 | Pre: | 85.8 | 2.7 | 1,166 | .33 |
|   | Post: | 89.3 | 0 | 858 | .29 |
| $\bar{x}$ | Pre: | 84.4 | 7.6 | 6,032 | 3.0 |
|   | Post: | 88.5 | 2.6 | 6,557 | 3.2 |

Source: Reprinted with permission from J.W. Varni. Self-regulation techniques in the management of chronic arthritic pain in hemophilia. *Behavior Therapy,* 1981, **12**, 185–194.

ment prescribed covaried with the number of bleeding episodes for all three patients, with the average number of bleeding episodes and units of factor replacement remaining essentially constant across pre- and postassessment periods. The number of analgesic tablets showed a consistent decrease across patients (Table 9.5).

These data on both the medical parameters of bleeding frequency and factor replacement units, as well as the subjective pain ratings, support the proposal that these self-regulation techniques did not affect acute bleeding pain perception. Substantial decreases in reported bleeding frequency and factor replacement units would have been expected had bleeding pain perception been affected. It is essential to emphasize that these techniques are not meant to supersede proper and correct medical care (i.e., factor replacement therapy). Nevertheless, in the case of hemophilic degenerative arthropathy, the chronic arthritic pain, in contrast to the acute bleeding pain, exceeds its functional intent, potentially resulting in limitations in normal activities, with the possibility of analgesic dependence always of concern (Varni & Gilbert, 1982). (These data are presented in Chapter 4.) Thus, within the context of a detailed consideration of each patient's physical and psychological status, these techniques represent a noninvasive and supportive therapeutic intervention that provide an additional treatment modality in the comprehensive management of hemophilia when applied within an interdisciplinary hemophilia comprehensive care center.

Pain management is also of concern for those hemophilic children who develop an inhibitor (antibody) to Factor VIII, subsequently presenting a serious problem in the management of each bleeding episode and the accompanying acute bleeding pain. Varni, Gilbert, and Dietrich (1981) reported on the successful biobehavioral management of pain and analgesic dependence in a 9-year-old hemophilic child with Factor VIII inhibitor. This study is described in detail in Chapter 4.

## Adherence to Proper Factor Replacement Techniques

The recognition of the advantages of prompt factor replacement therapy for each bleeding episode has served as a stimulus for the creation of the hemophilia home care program in an attempt to minimize or prevent the crippling effects of internal hemorrhaging (Dietrich, 1976a, 1976b). The home care program facilitates the prompt administration of factor replacement concentrate at home when a bleeding episode begins, potentially resulting in earlier recovery of joint function, greater self-sufficiency for the patient and his family, fewer absences from school or work, and a decrease in the cost of treatment (Lazerson, 1972; Kaufert, 1980; Sergis & Hilgartner, 1972; Smith et al., 1982). The home care program consists of teaching the hemophiliac, his parents, and other family members the techniques necessary for the administration of factor replacement products. Although the home care program (also called supervised self-treatment) has been adopted nationally through hemophilia comprehensive care centers, adherence to proper factor replacement procedures has only been recently investigated. If proper adherence to factor replacement procedures and sterile technique is not followed during the reconstitution and administration process, the following problems may result and adversely affect the patient: loss of potency in the factor concentrate, infection, damage to the veins, and spread of hepatitis to family members.

In pediatric chronic disorders, the adherence to long-term and complex treatment regimens such as the hemophilia home care program represents a serious and continuous problem (see Chapter 6). A review of the literature suggests that the instructional strategies employed by a clinician may influence adherence by improving the patient's comprehension and memory of the regimen (see Chapter 6). These instructional strategies include providing the information in incremental quantities over time, organizing the information into specific categories, and combining verbal and written instructions.

Sergis-Deavenport and Varni (1982, 1983) investigated the effectiveness of behavioral techniques and instructional strategies in the teaching of and the therapeutic adherence to proper factor replacement procedures for the hemophilia home care program. The instructional strategies included the techniques described above. The behavioral techniques consisted of the modeling of correct factor replacement procedures by the pediatric nurse practitioner, and the parent of the hemophilic child observing these modeled behaviors (observational learning). The parent's behavioral rehearsal of the observed techniques was recorded on a behavior checklist (Table 9.6), with the nurse providing corrective feedback and social reinforcement contingent on the parent's performance. The behavioral assessment instrument was designed to represent standard content for factor replacement therapy and consisted of the behaviors considered essential for the safe administration of concentrate to maintain aseptic technique and minimize the spread of hepatitis and damage to the veins.

Table 9.6.    Behavioral Assessment Instrument Sample Items
(Factor Replacement Therapy).

*Reconstitution Behaviors*
1. Wash hands
6. Double-ended needle—snap open
10. Insert needle end into sterile water bottle
14. Insert exposed needle into concentrate bottle
15. Add sterile water to concentrate
20. Sterile technique used throughout

*Syringe Preparation Behaviors*
2. Attach filter needle to syringe
7. Insert filter needle attached to syringe into concentrate bottle
9. Withdraw concentrate into syringe
11. Remove air bubbles
13. Twist filter needle off syringe
20. Sterile technique used throughout

*Infusion Behaviors*
4. Scalp vein needle—bend wing ends
6. Place tourniquet on hand or arm for venipuncture
7. Select venipuncture site
8. Swab skin surface with alcohol
12. Pierce needle through skin
13. Insert needle into vein
14. Secure needle in vein
15. Tape needle to skin
16. Release tourniquet
20. Attach scalp vein tubing to syringe
22. Inject concentrate slowly
27. Remove needle from skin
28. Apply pressure over venipuncture site
29. Place Band-Aid over venipuncture site
36. Sterile technique used throughout

Source: Reprinted with permission from E. Sergis-Deavenport, & J.W. Varni. Behavioral assessment and management of adherence to factor replacement therapy in hemophilia. *Journal of Pediatric Psychology,* 1983, **8,** in press.

Table 9.7.    Procedure Summary: Criteria Measures
for Teaching Factor Replacement Procedures.

| | Criteria Measures | Parents' Performance | Nursing Intervention |
|---|---|---|---|
| BASELINE PHASE | — | Demonstrate techniques thought to be appropriate for mixing and administering plasma concentrate | Without modeling F.R.P., obtain baseline data of level of skill across three classes of behavior in one session<br>1) baseline on reconstitution<br>2) baselines on syringe prep.<br>3) baselines on infusion |
| TREATMENT PHASE | | Observe modeled behaviors<br>Rehearse behaviors | Model reconstitution behaviors<br>a) double-ended needle technique<br>b) needle-syringe technique<br>Assess performance |
| | If score < 80% correct on reconstitution behaviors | Observe modeled behaviors<br>Rehearse behaviors<br>Trial #2 etc. | If score < 80% correct, model same behaviors again and reassess performance |
| | If score 80% correct or above | Reconstitution behaviors adequately learned | Advance parent to second classification of behaviors<br>Model syringe preparation<br>Assess performance |
| | | Observe modeled behaviors<br>Rehearse behaviors | |
| | If score < 80% correct on syringe prep. behaviors | Observe modeled behaviors<br>Rehearse behaviors<br>Trial #2 etc. | If score < 80% correct, model same behaviors again and reassess performance |
| | If score 80% correct or above | Syringe preparation behaviors adequately learned | Advance parent to third classification of behaviors<br>Model infusion behaviors on venipuncture and assess performance |

Table 9.7.   (cont'd)

| | Criteria Measures | Parents' Performance | Nursing Intervention |
|---|---|---|---|
| | | Observe modeled behaviors<br>Rehearse behaviors | |
| | If two consecutive scores < 85% correct on venipuncture model | Observe modeled behaviors<br>Rehearse behaviors Trial #2, etc. | If scores < 85% correct, model same behaviors again and reassess performance |
| | If two consecutive scores of 85% correct or above on venipuncture model | Infusion behaviors adequately learned on venipuncture model | Advance parent to practice venipuncture on adult volunteer |
| | | Rehearse behaviors on adult volunteer | Assess performance |
| | If two consecutive scores 85% correct on adult volunteer | Infusion behaviors adequately learned on adult volunteer | Advance parent to perform venipuncture on child |
| | | Rehearse behaviors on child | Assess performance |
| | Without modeling, if two separate scores 100% correct on child obtained during reconstitution, syringe preparation and infusion | Factor replacement procedures adequately learned without modeling | Advance parent for final testing |
| | Without modeling, if score 100% on all three classes of behaviors | Training completed in factor replacement procedures | Advance to home care program |
| FOLLOW-UP PHASE | | Demonstrate factor replacement procedures on model | Without modeling assess level of skill across three classes of behaviors |
| | If score < 100% correct | Rehearse behaviors on model | Model all three classes of behaviors |

Source: Reprinted with permission from E. Sergis-Deavenport, & J.W. Varni. Behavioral techniques in teaching hemophilia factor replacement procedures to families. *Pediatric Nursing,* 1982, **8**, 416–419.

Three classifications of factor replacement behaviors were delineated: (1) Reconstitution consisted of 20 behaviors; (2) Syringe preparation consisted of 20 behaviors; and (3) Infusion consisted of 36 behaviors. The parent's behavioral responses on each task performed were recorded on an occurrence/nonoccurrence basis on the checklist, with proper sequencing required for the correct responding of certain behaviors. Specific criteria were required before

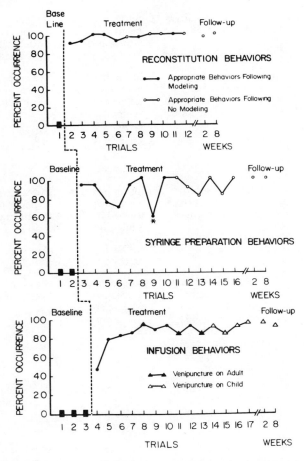

Fig. 9.2. A multiple-baseline model of percent occurrence of appropriate factor replacement behaviors across baseline, treatment, and follow-up phases on a parent of a hemophilic child. The asterisk in syringe preparation behaviors represents a 22-day delay in practicing syringe preparation behaviors.

Source: Reprinted with permission from E. Sergis-Deavenport, & J.W. Varni. Behavioral techniques in teaching hemophilia factor replacement procedures to families. *Pediatric Nursing,* 1982, **8**, 416–419.

learning each subsequent classification (Table 9.7). A representative multiple-baseline analysis of the training process for a parent is shown in Figure 9.2 (Sergis-Deavenport & Varni, 1982). In addition to a treatment group of five parents who received factor replacement training for the first time, a comparison group of seven parents who had been on the home care program for an average of 5 years was also tested on the behavior checklist (Sergis-Deavenport & Varni, 1983). The performance of the treatment group increased from 15 percent during baseline to 92 percent by the end of the treatment condition, maintained at 97 percent correct adherence over a long-term follow-up assessment. In contrast, the comparison group showed only 65 percent correct adherence when tested. These findings demonstrate the necessity and the potential of these techniques in improving long-term adherence to a complex treatment regimen for this chronic disorder, and have been recently successfully extended to the biobehavioral assessment and management of adherence to therapeutic exercise by children with hemophilia (Greenan, Powell, & Varni, 1983).

# REFERENCES

Aronstam, A., Rainsford, S.G., & Painter, M.J. Patterns of bleeding in adolescents with severe hemophilia A. *British Medical Journal,* 1979, **1**, 469–470.

Arnold, W.D., & Hilgartner, M.W. Hemophilic arthropathy: Current concepts of pathogenesis and management. *Journal of Bone and Joint Surgery,* 1977, **59**, 287–305.

Bernstein, I.L. Learned taste aversions in children receiving chemotherapy. *Science,* 1978, **200**, 1302–1303.

Bernstein, I.L., & Sigmundi, R.A. Tumor anorexia: A learned food aversion? *Science,* 1980, **209**, 416–418.

Bernstein, I.L., & Webster, M.M. Learned taste aversions in humans. *Physiology and Behavior,* 1980, **25**, 363–366.

Burish, T.G., & Lyles, J.N. Effectiveness of relaxation training in reducing adverse reactions to cancer chemotherapy. *Journal of Behavioral Medicine,* 1981, **4**, 65–78.

Burish, T.G., & Lyles, J.N. Effectiveness of relaxation training in reducing the aversiveness of chemotherapy in the treatment of cancer. *Journal of Behavior Therapy and Experimental Psychiatry,* 1979, **10**, 357–361.

Burish, T.G., Shartner, C.D., & Lyles, J.N. Effectiveness of multiple muscle-site EMG biofeedback and relaxation training in reducing the aversiveness of cancer chemotherapy. *Biofeedback and Self-Regulation,* 1981, **6**, 523–535.

Cairns, G.F., & Altman, K. Behavioral treatment of cancer-related anorexia. *Journal of Behavior Therapy and Experimental Psychiatry,* 1979, **10**, 353–356.

Dewys, W.D., Begg, C., Lavin, P.T. et al. Prognostic effect of weight loss prior to chemotherapy in cancer patients. *American Journal of Medicine,* 1980, **69**, 491–497.

Dietrich, S.L. Medical management of hemophilia. In D.C. Boone (Ed.), *Comprehensive Management of Hemophilia.* Philadelphia: Davis, 1976. (a)

Dietrich, S.L. Musculoskeletal problems. In M.W. Hilgartner (Ed.), *Hemophilia in Children.* Littleton, Mass.: Publishing Sciences Group, 1976. (b)

Dietrich, S.L., Luck, J.V., & Martinson, A.M. Musculoskeletal problems. In M.W. Hilgartner (Ed.), *Hemophilia in the Child and Adult.* New York: Masson Press, 1982.

Ellenberg, L., Kellerman, J., Dash, J., Higgins, G., & Zeltzer, L. Use of hypnosis for multiple symptoms in an adolescent girl with leukemia. *Journal of Adolescent Health Care,* 1980, **1,** 132–136.

Garb, J.L., & Stunkard, A.J. Taste aversions in man. *American Journal of Psychiatry,* 1974, **131,** 1204–1207.

Goff, J.R., Anderson, H.R., & Cooper, P.F. Distractibility and memory deficits in long-term survivors of acute lymphoblastic leukemia. *Journal of Developmental and Behavioral Pediatrics,* 1980, **1,** 158–163.

Greenan, E., Powell, C., & Varni, J.W. Adherence to therapeutic exercise by children with hemophilia. Manuscript submitted for publication, 1983.

Guenthner, E.E., Hilgartner, M.W., Miller, C.H., & Vienne, G. Hemophilic arthropathy: Effect of home care on treatment patterns and joint disease. *Journal of Pediatrics,* 1980, **97,** 378–382.

Harris, J.G. Nausea, vomiting and cancer treatment. *Cancer Journal for Clinicians,* 1978, **28,** 194–201.

Hilgard, E.R. The alleviation of pain by hypnosis. *Pain,* 1975, **1,** 213–231.

Hilgartner, M.W. *Comprehensive Care of Hemophilia.* Rockville, MD: Department of Health, Education and Welfare (DHEW Publication No. 79-5129), 1979.

Hollenbeck, A.R., Susman, E.J., Nannis, E.D., Strope, B.E., Hersh, S.P., Levine, A.S., & Pizzo, P.A. Children with serious illness: Behavioral correlates of separation and isolation. *Child Psychiatry and Human Development,* 1980, **11,** 3–11.

Jay, S.M., Elliott, C.H., Ozolins, M., & Olson, R.A. Behavioral management of children's distress during painful medical procedures. Paper presented at the Annual Meeting of the American Psychological Association, Washington, D.C., August 1982.

Jay, S.M., Ozolins, M., Elliott, C.H., & Caldwell, S. Assessment of children's distress during painful medical procedures. *Health Psychology,* in press.

Kasper, C.K., Dietrich, S.L., & Rapaport, S.I. Hemophilia prophylaxis with Factor VIII concentrate. *Archives of Internal Medicine,* 1970, **125,** 1004–1009.

Katz, E.R., Kellerman, J., Rigler, D., Williams, K.O., & Siegel, S.E. School intervention with pediatric cancer patients. *Journal of Pediatric Psychology,* 1977, **2,** 72–76.

Katz, E.R., Kellerman, J., & Siegel, S.E. Anxiety as an affective focus in the clinical study of acute behavioral distress: A reply to Shacham and Daut. *Journal of Consulting and Clinical Psychology,* 1981, **49,** 470–471.

Katz, E.R., Kellerman, J., & Siegel, S.E. Behavioral distress in children with cancer undergoing medical procedures: Developmental considerations. *Journal of Consulting and Clinical Psychology,* 1980, **48,** 356–365.

Kaufert, J.M. Social and psychological responses to home treatment of hemophilia. *Journal of Epidemiology and Community Health,* 1980, **34,** 194–200.

Kellerman, J., & Katz, E.R. The adolescent with cancer: Theoretical, clinical and research issues. *Journal of Pediatric Psychology,* 1977, **2,** 127–131.

Kellerman, J., Rigler, D., & Siegel, S.E. Psychological response of children to isolation in a protected environment. *Journal of Behavioral Medicine,* 1979, **3,** 263–274.

Kellerman, J., Rigler, D., & Siegel, S.E. The psychological effects of isolation in protected environments. *American Journal of Psychiatry,* 1977, **134,** 563–565.

Kellerman, J., Rigler, D., Siegel, S.E., & Katz, E.R. Disease-related communication and depression in pediatric cancer patients. *Journal of Pediatric Psychology,* 1977, **2,** 52–53.

Kellerman, J., Rigler, D., Siegel, S.E., McCue, K., Pospisil, J., & Uno, R. Psychological evaluation and management of pediatric oncology patients in protected environments. *Medical and Pediatric Oncology,* 1976, **2,** 353–360.

Kellerman, J., & Varni, J.W. Pediatric hematology/oncology. In D.C. Russo & J.W. Varni (Eds.), *Behavioral Pediatrics: Research and Practice.* New York: Plenum Press, 1982. (a)

Kellerman, J., & Varni, J.W. Psychosocial aspects of pediatric hematology-oncology. In M.L.N. Willoughby & S.E. Siegel (Eds.), *Modern Trends in Pediatrics.* London: Butterworth & Co., 1982. (b)

Kellerman, J., Zeltzer, L., Ellenberg, L., & Dash, J. Hypnotic reduction of distress associated with adolescent cancer and treatment: I. Acute pain and anxiety due to medical procedures. Manuscript submitted for publication, 1982.

Kisker, C.T., Perlman, A.W., & Benton, C. Arthritis in hemophilia. *Seminars in Arthritis,* 1971, **1**, 220–235.

Koocher, G.P., O'Malley, J.E., Gogan, J.L., & Foster, D.J. Psychological adjustment among pediatric cancer survivors. *Journal of Child Psychology and Psychiatry,* 1980, **21**, 163–173.

LaBaw, L., Holton, C., Tewell, K., & Eccles, D. The use of self-hypnosis by children with cancer. *American Journal of Clinical Hypnosis,* 1975, **17**, 233–238.

Lazerson, J. Hemophilia home transfusion program: Effect on school attendance. *Journal of Pediatrics,* 1972, **81**, 330–332.

Lehmann, J.F., Warren, C.G., & Scham, S.M. Therapeutic heat and cold. *Clinical Orthopedics and Related Research,* 1974, **99**, 207–245.

Levine, P.H., & Britten, F.H. Supervised patient-management of hemophilia: A study of 45 patients with hemophilia A and B. *Annals of Internal Medicine,* 1973, **78**, 195–201.

Logue, A.W., Ophir, I., & Strauss, K.E. The acquisition of taste aversions in humans. *Behaviour Research and Therapy,* 1981, **19**, 319–333.

Lyles, J.N., Burish, T.G., Krozely, M.G., & Oldham, R.K. Efficacy of relaxation training and guided imagery in reducing the aversiveness of cancer chemotherapy. *Journal of Consulting and Clinical Psychology,* 1982, **50**, 509–524.

Morrow, G.R., & Morrell, C. Behavioral treatment for the anticipatory nausea and vomiting induced by cancer chemotherapy. *New England Journal of Medicine,* 1982, **307**, 1476–1480.

National Cancer Institute. *Coping with Cancer.* Bethesda, MD: National Institutes of Health Publication No. 80-2080, 1980.

Nesse, R.M., Carli, T., Curtis, G.C., & Kleinman, P.D. Pretreatment nausea in cancer chemotherapy: A conditioned response? *Psychosomatic Medicine,* 1980, **42**, 33–36.

Olness, K. Imagery (self-hypnosis) as adjunct therapy in childhood cancer: Clinical experience with 25 patients. *American Journal of Pediatric Hematology/Oncology,* 1981, **3**, 313–321.

Peck, C.L. Modification of a learned vomiting ritual by change in stimulus conditions and self-controlled response prevention. *Journal of Behavior Therapy and Experimental Psychiatry,* 1978, **9**, 359–363.

Redd, W.H. In vivo desensitization in the treatment of chronic emesis following gastrointestinal surgery. *Behavior Therapy,* 1980, **11**, 421–427. (a)

Redd, W.H. Stimulus control and extinction of psychosomatic symptoms in cancer patients in protective isolation. *Journal of Consulting and Clinical Psychology,* 1980, **48**, 448–455. (b)

Redd, W.H., Andresen, G.V., & Minagawa, R.Y. Hypnotic control of anticipatory emesis in patients receiving cancer chemotherapy. *Journal of Consulting and Clinical Psychology,* 1982, **50**, 14–19.

Riley, V. Psychoneuroendocrine influences on immunocompetence and neoplasia. *Science,* 1981, **212**, 1100–1109.

Seligman, M.E.P., & Hager, J.L. (Eds.) *Biological Boundaries of Learning.* New York: Appleton-Century-Crofts, 1972.

Sergis, E., & Hilgartner, M.W. Hemophilia. *American Journal of Nursing,* 1972, **72**, 2011–2017.

Sergis-Deavenport, E., & Varni, J.W. Behavioral techniques in teaching hemophilia factor replacement procedures to families. *Pediatric Nursing,* 1982, **8**, 416–419.

Sergis-Deavenport, E., & Varni, J.W. Behavioral assessment and management of adherence to factor replacement therapy in hemophilia. *Journal of Pediatric Psychology,* 1983, **8**, in press.

Shacham, S., & Daut, R. Anxiety or pain: What does the scale measure? *Journal of Consulting and Clinical Psychology,* 1981, **49**, 468–469.

Siegel, S.E. The current outlook of childhood cancer: The medical background. In J. Kellerman (Ed.), *Psychological Aspects of Childhood Cancer.* Springfield, Ill.: Charles C. Thomas, 1980.

Sklar, L.S., & Anisman, H. Stress and cancer. *Psychological Bulletin,* 1981, **89**, 369–406.

Smith, P.S., Keyes, N.C., & Forman, E.N. Socioeconomic evaluation of a state-funded compre-

216     Clinical Behavioral Pediatrics

hensive hemophilia-care program. *New England Journal of Medicine,* 1982, **306**, 575–579.

Smith, S.D. Advances in the pharmacology of cancer chemotherapy. *Pediatric Clinics of North America,* 1981, **28**, 145–160.

Smith, S.D., Rosen, D., Trueworthy, R.C., & Lowman, J.T. A reliable method of evaluating drug compliance in children with cancer. *Cancer,* 1979, **43**, 169–173.

Sokoloff, L. Biochemical and physiological aspects of degenerative joint disease with special reference to hemophilic arthropathy. *Annals of New York Academy of Sciences,* 1975, **240**, 285–290.

Strauss, H.S. The perpetuation of hemophilia by mutation. *Pediatrics,* 1969, **39**, 186–193.

Swezey, R.L. *Arthritis: Rational Therapy and Rehabilitation.* Philadelphia: Saunders, 1978.

Varni, J.W. Behavioral medicine in hemophilia arthritic pain management: Two case studies. *Archives of Physical Medicine and Rehabilitation,* 1981, **62**, 183–187. (a)

Varni, J.W. Self-regulation techniques in the management of chronic arthritic pain in hemophilia. *Behavior Therapy,* 1981, **12**, 185–194. (b)

Varni, J.W., & Gilbert, A. Self-regulation of chronic arthritic pain and long-term analgesic dependence in a hemophiliac. *Rheumatology and Rehabilitation,* 1982, **21**, 171–174.

Varni, J.W., Gilbert, A., & Dietrich, S.L. Behavioral medicine in pain and analgesia management for the hemophilic child with Factor VIII inhibitor. *Pain,* 1981, **11**, 121–126.

Wasserman, R.R., Oester, Y.T., Oryshkevich, R.S., Montgomery, M.M., Poske, R.M., & Ruksha, A. Electromyographic, electrodiagnostic, and motor nerve conduction observations in patients with rheumatoid arthritis. *Archives of Physical Medicine and Rehabilitation,* 1968, **49**, 90–95.

White, J.R. Effects of a counterirritant on perceived pain and hand movement in patients with arthritis. *Physical Therapy,* 1973, **53**, 956–960.

Zeltzer, L., Kellerman, J., Ellenberg, L., & Dash, J. Hypnotic reduction of distress associated with adolescent cancer and treatment: II. Nausea and emesis. Manuscript submitted for publication, 1982.

Zeltzer, L., & LeBaron, S. Hypnosis and nonhypnotic techniques for reduction of pain and anxiety during painful procedures in children and adolescents with cancer. *Journal of Pediatrics,* 1982, **101**, 1032–1035.

# 10

# Urinary and Fecal Incontinence

## URINARY INCONTINENCE

Urinary incontinence may be classified into two broad categories: enuresis and neurogenic dysfunction. Neurogenic disorders are characterized by the presence of urological or neurological pathology. Enuresis, on the other hand, is considered a functional disorder with an absence of any underlying overt organic pathology. Most children with urinary incontinence are diagnosed as enuretic. Enuresis may be further delineated into diurnal (daytime) or nocturnal (nighttime) and primary or secondary. Primary enuresis refers to children who have never achieved continence, whereas secondary enuresis refers to children who have attained at least a 6-month period of continence before relapsing to incontinence. Most enuretic children evidence the primary-nocturnal pattern of enuresis (see Parker & Whitehead, 1982, for review).

Children with specific organic etiology for urinary incontinence include those with anatomical defects such as absent urethra, ectopic ureter, epispadias, exstrophy, and iatrogenic injury secondary to operations on the bladder or urethra, and those children with neuromuscular disorders such as myelomeningocele, sacral agenesis, spinal cord injury, and incontinence secondary to pelvic surgery or irradiation (Cook, Babcock, Swenson, & King, 1978). Although enuretic children do not traditionally evidence any of the above overt anatomical or neuromuscular pathology, urodynamic studies (described in a subsequent section) on children have demonstrated a neurogenic component to some enuretic children's incontinence (Blaivas, Labib, Bauer, & Retik, 1977a; Whiteside & Arnold, 1975). However, the issue of whether this neurogenic dysfunction causes or results from chronic incontinence has not been empirically resolved. Some authors describe this disorder as the pseudoneurogenic bladder (Hanna, Di Scipio, Suh, Kogan, Levitt, & Donner, 1981b), the non-neurogenic neurogenic bladder (Allen, 1977), or idiopathic bladder instability (Cardozo, Abrams, Stanton, & Feneley, 1978). This bladder instability is reflected by the findings of some investigators that enuretic children have a reduced functional bladder capacity. As discussed by Whiteside and Arnold (1975), this reduced functional capacity is due to the occurrence of uninhibited detrusor contractions, with the true bladder capacity under general anesthesia the same as for nonenuretic children. This detrusor instability with reduced functional bladder capacity may not only lead to diurnal and nocturnal enuresis in the child, but may also manifest itself in the adult as nocturia, daytime frequency, urgency, and urge incontinence.

Muellner (1960) has described five developmental steps in the attainment of voluntary control over micturition by the child: (1) sensory awareness that the bladder is full; (2) voluntary control over urination when the bladder is full or nearly full; (3) voluntary control over starting and stopping urine flow when the bladder is full; (4) voluntary control over starting urinary flow under any degree of bladder fullness; and (5) with voluntary control over bladder functioning, the next and final step is the voluntary control over functional bladder capacity. The physiological mechanisms of this micturitional control are discussed in a subsequent section.

The age of attaining voluntary micturitional control has been investigated a number of times, with Oppel, Harper, and Rider (1968) providing a relatively representative and comprehensive study of this area. In their 12-month prospective study of 859 children, Oppel et al. (1968) assessed both diurnal and nocturnal incontinence by three dimensions: (1) the cumulative percent of children who had attained continence for the first time, without regard for subsequent relapse; (2) the cumulative percent of children who attained continence without subsequent relapse to age 12; and (3) the percent of children who were continent at each specific age, irrespective of whether it was first or final continence. Table 10.1 contains a summary of the major findings of this study. As these data indicate, diurnal continence is attained prior to nocturnal continence at each age group.

Table 10.1.    Prevalence of Diurnal and Nocturnal Urinary Continence (Percent Occurrence).

| Age (yr) | Diurnal Continence | | | Nocturnal Continence | | |
|---|---|---|---|---|---|---|
| | First Continence | Final Continence | Age-specific Continence | First Continence | Final Continence | Age-specific Continence |
| 3 | 84 | 78 | 84 | 66 | 51 | 64 |
| 6 | 99 | 94 | 96 | 87 | 70 | 77 |
| 9 | 99 | 96 | 97 | 94 | 81 | 83 |
| 12 | 100 | 99 | 99 | 97 | 92 | 92 |

## Physiological Mechanisms

The main purpose of the urinary system is to clear the blood of waste products (Smith, 1978). The kidneys filter the blood, excreting excess water and the waste products of protein metabolism as urine. Urine flows from the tubules of the kidney and collects as the renal pelvis where it is subsequently transported down the ureter to the urinary bladder by peristalsis. The ureter enters the bladder wall at an oblique angle to form the ureterovesical junction that prevents reflux flow of urine back up the ureters.

The primary functions of the urinary bladder are the storage of urine and evacuation of intravesical content by a coordinated series of neuromuscular mechanisms (Bradley & Scott, 1978). The capacity for urine storage is a function of the distensibility of the epithelial, muscular, and connective tissue components of the urinary detrusor muscle (bladder wall). The average adult bladder has a reservoir capacity of 350-450 ml. Adaptation of the detrusor smooth muscle to increasing distention, provoked by further urine influx, is possible because of the elastic properties of smooth muscle and collagen intrinsic to the detrusor. The internal urethral sphincter, located approximately at the bladder neck, is not a true circular sphincter, but a thickening formed by interlaced and converging smooth muscle fibers of the detrusor as they pass distally to become the smooth musculature of the proximal, mid, and distal urethra. The external urethral sphincter and parts of the mid and distal urethra consist of striated muscle. The perineal muscles of the pelvic floor are also striated, act as an indirect sphincter, and contribute to sphincteric function.

Micturition (urination) is largely a function of a simple reflex reaction between the bladder and the sacral portion of the spinal cord, which in turn is under the control of higher midbrain and cortical centers (Bradley, Rockswold, Timm, & Scott, 1976). The spinal pathways involved in the innervation of the detrusor smooth muscle and the periurethral striated muscle include both motor and sensory pathways. However, the organization and distribution of the spinal pathways innervating the detrusor smooth muscle and periurethral striated muscle are considerably different (Bradley & Scott, 1978). Further, the detrusor and urethral smooth musculature are relatively unique—although innervated by the autonomic nervous system, they are under voluntary control (Lapides, Sweet, & Lewis, 1957). Lapides et al. (1957) observed that urinary continence could be maintained by either the smooth musculature of the internal sphincter or the striated musculature of the external sphincter. Micturition was found to be initiated and terminated voluntarily without the use of any striated muscle, but striated muscle was required for the sudden, rapid inhibition of urine flow.

Recent findings indicate that the striated muscle of the external urethral sphincter consists of specialized fibers (slow twitch type I) which are functionally capable of maintaining tone over long time periods without fatigue (Gosling, Dixon, Critchley, & Thompson, 1981). Unlike the external urethral sphincter, the levator ani additionally contains a population of fast twitch (type II) fibers functionally associated with rapid, forceful muscle contraction. In general, the periurethral striated muscle assists the external urethral sphincter in active urethral closure, not only to ensure continence but also to produce rapid, forceful occlusion of the urethra such as occurs during voluntary interruption of micturition. Thus, given the ability of the internal urethral sphincter to also maintain continence (Kleeman, 1970), both smooth and striated muscle may be viewed as functioning in a coordinated manner to preserve continence.

In the normal bladder, the gradual distension caused by urine influx results in little appreciable increase in intravesical pressure until a threshold volume (approximately 400 ml in the adult) is reached. At this point, sensations of fullness are transmitted to the sacral cord where, if voluntary (cerebral) control is lacking (as in infants and young children), neurochemical discharges through the motor side of the reflex arc cause powerful, sustained detrusor contraction and spontaneous involuntary voiding. With the development of the nervous system and toilet training by the parents, the young child gradually gains cerebral control over the sacral reflex and gradually develops social continence. At this point, micturition is completely under voluntary control so that the detrusor reflex contractile response to threshold volume can be inhibited, permitting the bladder to accommodate larger volumes of urine; conversely, detrusor contraction can be initiated whether at threshold volume or not. During detrusor reflex contraction, the contractile pull of this musculature widens and shortens the proximal urethra and opens the internal urethral sphincter. Normally, detrusor contraction is essentially simultaneously accompanied by reflex relaxation of the external urethral sphincter and pelvic floor musculature. In the absence of voluntary periurethral musculature contraction, unobstructed urinary flow is achieved and results in micturition.

The neurophysiological mechanisms of micturition represent an area of active research, with new data furthering the understanding of this complex process (see Bradley & Scott, 1978). Autonomic innervation of the smooth musculature of the urinary bladder may be differentiated into the parasympathetic and sympathetic nervous systems. The bladder is innervated throughout its entirety by the parasympathetic nervous system through the pelvic nerves which arise from the sacral spinal roots, $S_2$, $S_3$, and $S_4$. This innervation is cholinergic, and thus these bladder receptor sites are stimulated by the neurotransmitter acetylcholine. When stimulated, these sites cause a detrusor muscle contraction and are associated with bladder emptying. The sympathetic nervous system innervation is through the hypogastric nerve which arises through the spinal roots at $T_{11}$ to $L_2$. This innervation is adrenergic, and these bladder receptor sites are stimulated by the neurotransmitter norepinephrine.

When stimulated, these sites differentially relax the bladder wall and contract the bladder neck, resulting in urine storage (Raezer, Benson, Wein, & Duckett, 1977).

During the storage phase of bladder function, sensory impulses are elicited by stimulation of both tension receptors in the layers of collagen surrounding detrusor smooth muscle and stretch receptors located in the pelvic floor musculature. These sensory impulses converge in the spinal cord and travel cranially (ascend), activating many areas in the central nervous system, including the cerebellum, basal ganglia, and cerebral cortex. The detrusor motor area in the frontal lobes of the cerebral cortex receives sensory input from proprioceptive sensory endings in the detrusor smooth muscle. The cerebrocortical localization of the sensory pathways from the periurethral striated muscle is centered in the sensorimotor cortex. Through descending pathways synapsing on neurons in the gray matter of the spinal cord (primarily lumbar and sacral spinal cord), the areas of the cerebral cortex concerned with micturition provide for volitional control of contraction of the detrusor smooth muscle and the periurethral striated muscle.

Thus, the spinal pathways pertinent to the innervation of the detrusor smooth muscle and the periurethral striated muscle include both motor and sensory tracts. Ascending (afferent) proprioceptive sensory impulses originate from nerve endings in the detrusor muscle and muscle spindles and tendon organs in the pelvic floor musculature, as well as the anal sphincter. The descending (efferent) motor pathways innervate the detrusor, smooth muscle structures related to defecation and sexual function, and periurethral striated muscle. Both ascending and descending motor and sensory spinal pathways pass close to other ascending and descending pathways associated with postural mechanisms. Hence, bladder and bowel dysfunction may also be associated with other neuromuscular problems secondary to such spinal trauma as spinal cord injury or myelomeningocele. Since the organization and distribution of the spinal pathways innervating the detrusor smooth muscle and the periurethral striated muscle are considerably different, spinal cord lesions result in differential impairment of normal functioning. Relatively recent advances in urodynamic studies have greatly aided the understanding of the complex dynamics of micturition, both in normal functioning and in neurological impairment assessment.

## Urodynamic Assessment

Urodynamics is the field concerned with the identification and measurement of physiologic and pathologic factors involved in the storage, transportation, and evacuation of urine (Webster, 1982). Initially a research tool, urodynamic studies have increasingly become an essential diagnostic technique in clinical urology, specifically in the diagnosis of lower urinary tract dysfunction. With the development of sophisticated urodynamic equipment, greater accuracy in the assessment and treatment of voiding abnormalities in children are now possible (Firlit & Cook, 1977; Hanna, Di Scipio, Suh, Kogan, Levitt, & Donner, 1981a). The following urodynamic studies are the principal modes of current urodynamic assessment and provide a multifunction analysis of micturition mechanisms.

## Cystometry

Cystometry consists of the distention of the detrusor muscle with known volumes of catheter infused fluid or gas and concurrent recording of intravesical pressure. The most important clinical observation to be made during the analysis and interpretation of the cystometrogram (the graphic record of bladder pressure changes with progressive increases in bladder volume) is whether the patient develops a detrusor reflex and can suppress this reflex on command. Additional parameters studied through cystometry is the determination of the first sensation of bladder filling (normally at approximately 150ml to 250ml), the tonus limb (the accommodation of the detrusor to gradually increasing volumes of fluid), and the sensation of bladder fullness and urgency to void (normally 350ml to 550ml in the adult).

## Uroflowmetry

Uroflowmetry provides a measure of both flow rate and volume voided and is the only single test that evaluates the function of both the detrusor and the urethra. A normal flow rate in general indicates normal function in both of these structures. A normal adult flow rate is approximately 22ml per second.

## Urethral Pressure Profilometry

The urethral pressure profile is one of the most important measures of urethral function and provides a graphic recording of the pressure within the urethra at each point along its length. The urethral pressure profile graphic recording begins at the bladder. Through a mechanized constant withdrawal technique, resistance of the urethral walls to infused fluid is sequentially measured until the external meatus is reached. Normally, after a positive pressure deflection is recorded at the bladder neck, a progressive increase in urethral pressure is observed in the midportion of the urethra in the female and the membranous urethra in the male. Beyond this point, urethral pressure gradually decreases until the external meatus is reached.

*Sphincter Electromyography*

Electromyographic investigation of the external urethral sphincter provides a study of the bioelectric potentials generated by this striated musculature and as such is a method for determining functional integrity of innervation. In the relaxed state a low level of muscle activity is observed, with considerably greater electrical activity progressively evident under voluntary contraction in the normally innervated sphincter. In addition to testing for the presence or absence of voluntary sphincter control, sphincter electromyography also provides studies on the sphincter's response to bladder filling and sphincter response to attempts to void and interrupt voiding. In normal functioning, a minimum of electromyographic activity is present with an empty bladder, gradually increasing with bladder filling, and becoming quiescent during voiding.

The most common pediatric voiding problems are due to functional disturbances (Firlit & Cook, 1977). Organic causes are less frequently encountered but may result from myelomeningocele, sacral agenesis, structural abnormalities, infection, spinal cord injury, malignancy, or surgery. Multifunction urodynamic studies are particularly essential in the diagnosis of children with such organic-caused dysfunctional voiding patterns. For instance, many lesions thought to be complete spinal cord transections may spare certain pathways involved with micturition (Blaivas, Labib, Bauer, & Retik, 1977a, 1977b). Thus, one cannot predict bladder-sphincter dysfunction from the level of the spinal cord lesion; no correlation has been found between neurological spinal cord lesion level and the urodynamic pattern (Blaivas et al., 1977a, 1977b).

Although the value of urodynamic studies in the evaluation of enuresis is questionable, bladder dysfunction has been incriminated in the etiology of recurrent urinary infections, reflux, upper tract deterioration, and progressive renal damage. Thus, considerable clinical judgment is necessary to determine those children with dysfunctional voiding patterns in whom urodynamic studies are appropriate. Finally, urodynamic studies are quite useful in determining the effects of pharmacologic agents on bladder functioning.

## Pharmacologic Intervention

Pharmacologic intervention for neurogenic bladder dysfunction consists of drugs that mainly affect bladder function and drugs that chiefly affect the urethra (Raz & Bradley, 1979). The various effects of these different drugs are to increase intravesical pressure and facilitate emptying of the bladder, to decrease bladder contractions and increase bladder capacity, to increase urethral resistance, and to decrease urethral resistance. These drugs act specifically on the smooth muscle through the stimulation or inhibition of the parasympathetic or sympathetic nervous systems (Raezer et al., 1977). The neurophysiology of micturition determines the exact prescription of the drug that is required to attain the desired functional effect of either bladder emptying or urine storage. For instance, propantheline bromide is an anticholinergic agent which blocks the membrane receptor site activated by acetylcholine, which produces parasympathetically mediated contractions. Consequently, propantheline bromide would be prescribed to inhibit bladder contractions in an attempt to facilitate urine storage (see Raz & Bradley, 1979, and Raezer et al., 1977, for reviews).

## Urodynamic Biofeedback

Urodynamic biofeedback provides the patient with a learning situation where existing feedback from physiological functioning (e.g., proprioceptive cues) is augmented, or where physiological processes not usually in the patient's sensory awareness (or at least not systematically attended to) are presented on an immediate, moment-to-moment basis through biological feedback. Through urodynamic biofeedback, the patient is given the opportunity to learn to self-regulate (voluntarily control) physiological functions associated with micturition.

Initial studies on the treatment of urinary incontinence through biofeedback training using urodynamic equipment have recently appeared in the literature. Cardozo et al. (1978), in their two reports, studied a total of 33 adult female patients, ages 18 to 64 years, with symptoms of frequency, urgency, and urge incontinence due to idiopathic detrusor instability. Detrusor (bladder) pressure was measured by means of cystometry, with biological feedback provided through both auditory and visual modalities, thus making the patient aware of incremental changes in bladder pressure. A loudspeaker provided auditory feedback by increasing in pitch as the detrusor pressure rose and decreasing in pitch as the pressure fell. The detrusor pressure pen deflection recordings on the moving strip chart paper served as visual feedback. Under a condition of bladder filling (sterile water infusion) through a catheter inserted in the bladder, the patients were instructed to try to control the rise in pitch of the auditory signal by concentrating, deep breathing, fist clenching, general relaxation, or any other method that might be helpful for each individual patient. In this way, it was intended that by controlling the rise in pitch of the auditory signal, detrusor contractions, as measured by pressure recordings from the catheter in the bladder, would also be voluntarily controlled. Patients were considered to be subjectively cured if they no longer complained of frequency, urgency or urge incontinence, and objectively cured if they no longer exhibited uninhibited detrusor contractions, a pressure rise greater than 15cm of water, or leakage of urine at any time during cystometry. Of the 33 patients studied, 15 were considered objectively cured (14 subjectively) and five objectively improved (13 subjectively). Objective findings included increased functional bladder capacity, increased capacity before first sensation of bladder filling, reduction in uninhibited detrusor contractions, and reduction in pressure rise during bladder filling. Thus, through urodynamic biofeedback training, 20 of 33 patients were able to demonstrate self-regulation (voluntary control) of detrusor functioning.

Wear et al. (1979) studied four adult men and four adult women who demonstrated some degree of urinary incontinence or abnormal urinary retention. Periurethral electromyographic recordings were obtained via a catheter with surface electrodes located on either side of a ring on the catheter. An audio unit was set up so that a sound of proportional intensity and pitch would be produced at a significant elevation of electromyographic activity. Additionally, the strip chart recorder was placed in such a position so as to permit the patients to view the pen deflection recordings. The patients were instructed to initially relax and then contract their sphincters, using whatever techniques they found helpful, with constant auditory and visual feedback made available to guide their efforts. All patients were instructed to practice at home what they learned during the biofeedback training sessions. Since audio feedback appeared to be distracting, visual feedback proved to be most useful. Criteria for success included a marked reduction in the frequency and amount of incontinence, a reduction in residual urine, patient report of improvement, and cessation or marked reduction in the use of pharmacological agents and/or avoidance of surgical intervention. Based on these criteria, four of eight patients were successfully treated. Of interest, the following images appeared to facilitate the self-regulation of the external urethral sphincter:

1) Turn on the faucet and let the water come, 2) let go of the pucker string and let the urine fall out, 3) relax each muscle in sequence starting with your scalp and eyelids and work down your body, 4) think of a stream with water bubbling over the rocks and sparkling in the sunshine, 5) lean back and relax as if you were settling into a tub full of warm water, 6) squeeze the rectum as you would after a bowel movement, 7) shut off the urine as you would if someone suddenly opens the bathroom door while you are urinating, and 8) pinch off the waterhose so no water can get to the garden [p. 467].

Allen (1977) studied 21 children, ages 2½ to 12 years, with detrusor-sphincter dyssynergia, which is a discoordination between detrusor contraction and external urethral sphincter relaxation, resulting in abnormal voiding patterns, residual urine in the bladder, and potentially uninhibited detrusor contractions and other neurogeniclike dysfunction. Dyssynergia in these children was considered a functional or learned discoordination, not a result of an overt organic/neurological disorder. Nineteen of the 21 children studied demonstrated either diurnal or nocturnal incontinence. Voiding occurred in an intermittent or interrupted manner, without a sustained stream of good volume.

Allen suggested that in many cases this abnormal voiding pattern, caused by detrusor-external urethral sphincter discoordination, appeared to be a learned pattern. Consequently, Allen attempted a re-education or retraining program to teach detrusor-external urethral sphincter coordination through urodynamic biofeedback. By monitoring detrusor pressure, urine flow, and external urethral sphincter activity, the child was provided visual feedback of detrusor-sphincter functioning. The child was encouraged to relax the perineum and maintain a steady stream without straining, resulting in coordinated external urethral sphincter relaxation during detrusor contraction, producing a steady urine flow. However, Allen only provided a graphic display of the results on one 4-year-old boy. Although these urodynamic findings were quite clear, that is, the child was able to voluntarily reduce the electromyographic activity of the external urethral sphincter when a rise in bladder pressure occurred, resulting in a coordinated steady urine flow, no data were presented on the other children. Nevertheless, this single case presentation represents the first published report on urodynamic biofeedback in the pediatric population.

Maizels, King, and Firlit (1979) studied three girls, ages 9 to 14 years, with refractory detrusor-sphincter dyssynergia, resulting in abnormal voiding patterns, incomplete bladder emptying, incontinence, and a propensity for urinary infections. Two monopolar surface electrodes were applied to the perianal skin so as to monitor the electromyographic activity of the periurethral and pelvic floor musculature. The goal of biofeedback therapy was to retrain the external urethral sphincter to relax during voiding, using the visual feedback of the chart strip recordings of the sphincter electromyograms and urine flow rates. During the training trials, the children learned to relax the pelvic floor musculature during voiding, producing detrusor-sphincter synergia. Two of the children, both of whom demonstrated diurnal incontinence, became continent. The third child's condition was complicated by bilateral vesicoureteral reflux, progressive hydronephrosis and bilateral ureteral reimplants, and she was not able to attain synergia during the biofeedback sessions.

Hanna et al. (1981b) studied 83 children with self-sustained maladaptive voiding habits resulting in bladder dysfunction that mimicked obstructed and neuropathic disorders, yet on examination no overt neuropathology was evident. Most of the children had a prolonged history of urinary tract infections and urinary incontinence. Constipation and fecal soiling were also common (a finding supported by Allen [1977] on a similar pediatric population). Urodynamic testing revealed detrusor-sphincter dyssynergia as the most common underlying voiding pattern abnormality. Children who failed to respond to pharmacologic manipulation or surgery received biofeedback therapy. Twenty-four of the 35 patients who received biofeedback training in combination with pharmacologic intervention evidenced therapeutic gains, defined as free of symptoms for greater than 3 months and improved radiologically or significant urodynamic improvement as measured by flow rate and electromyography. Seven additional patients were rated as occasionally symptomatic and stable radiologically or moderate urodynamic improvement; only four of the 35 patients were judged as treatment failures. From an etiological perspective, Hanna et al. (1981b) speculated that the children studied had learned to contract their external urethral sphincters during increased bladder pressure, subsequently developing a maladaptive habit that became a self-sustained behavioral pattern over time. Additionally, they suggested that bladder ischemia during involuntary detrusor contractions and/or the high voiding pressure resulting from functional bladder outflow obstruction might result in a decreased blood flow to the bladder and increase its susceptibility to bacterial invasion. Finally, the authors estimated that biofeedback therapy "salvaged" 60 percent of their treatment failures originally treated through pharmacologic and/or surgical interventions.

The preceding studies were primarily conducted with children diagnosed as evidencing the "nonneurogenic neurogenic bladder" or the "pseudoneurogenic bladder" dysfunction, that is, bladder-sphincter dysfunction without overt neurological pathology. A case study by Schneider and Westendorf (1979) is unique in that it involved a 5-year-old girl, who as a result of an accidental fall 2 years prior to the study, was paralyzed below the waist. Subsequent to the spinal cord injury, the sensation of bladder distention was lost, urethral sphincter control was absent, and only some anal sphincter control was present. At the time of the study, the patient was wearing diapers and continually dribbled urine. In order to drain the bladder the child was catheterized three or four times a day. Urodynamic biofeedback involved inserting a flexible catheter into the bladder, which measured bladder pressure on a strip chart recorder. After the child consumed 475cc of fruit juice, the authors demonstrated various methods for increasing the pressure readings, such as raising her legs, tensing the diaphragm, and pressing the stomach manually. Reinforcement was provided for successfully effecting pressure changes on the chart paper. As the sessions progressed, gross bodily movements were restricted, and successive decrements in equipment sensitivity were made as a shaping technique, requiring greater and greater patient bladder control. Total spontaneous voiding, total volitional voiding, and total residual urine were measured for 12 days prior to biofeedback training, throughout the 8 days of biofeedback training, and for 16 days subsequent to the training sessions. With biofeedback training, the patient was able to completely reduce involuntary, spontaneous voiding, and no residual urine was found on catheterization. Instead, voluntary voiding was progressively achieved over the training trials. At an 18-month follow-up, these gains were found to be maintained, and the patient was continent. Although this study's findings are limited because of a number of methodological problems, they are nevertheless encouraging, since they represent the utilization of urodynamic biofeedback in the treatment of the child with overt neurological impairment.

As a clinical technique, urodynamic biofeedback holds considerable promise and hope for children with chronic urinary incontinence. However, additional research is needed to determine its utility for the treatment of children with overt neurological impairment. In this regard, Killam, Jeffries, and Varni (1983) have recently reported encouraging results utilizing urodynamic biofeedback in the treatment of chronic urinary incontinence in children with myelomeningocele. These initial data are quite provocative, in that these children with overt neurological (spinal) impairment were able to demonstrate voluntary control over bladder-sphincter functioning during the biofeedback training sessions, resulting in a decrease in urinary incontinence.

## Nonbiofeedback Biobehavioral Management

By far the greatest amount of clinical research effort on urinary incontinence has been directed toward the nonbiofeedback biobehavioral management of nocturnal incontinence.

### Nocturnal Incontinence

The literature on these clinical research efforts has emphasized three major treatment modalities: (1) the bell-and-pad (urine alarm) method, (2) urine retention training, and (3) dry-bed training.

**Bell-and-Pad Method.** The bell-and-pad or urine-alarm conditioning method was initially reported by Mowrer and Mowrer (1938). The typical apparatus consists of a sensing device in a pad that is placed on the bed and is activated by the passage of urine. The alarm may be in the form of a bell, buzzer, light, or even music, which should be of sufficient intensity to awaken the child. The child is then instructed to turn off the alarm, finish voiding in the bathroom, and then return to sleep. The theory behind the method reflects the Mowrers' belief that the ordinary method of parental arousing of children at night to urinate may condition the child to void when the bladder is only partly filled and consequently not at a sufficiently intense proprioceptive stimulus level to arouse the child. The Mowrers proposed that the urine-alarm method awakened the child only when the bladder capacity was at maximum level, requiring urination only with a full bladder, thus mimicking a normal pattern of responding. In a review of 25 studies published since 1938, Sloop (1977) reported an initial cure rate of more than 80 percent, with a relapse rate averaging approximately 25 percent. Considering the relapse rate, then only 55 percent of the children may be considered completely and permanently cured of nocturnal incontinence using the standard Mowrer procedure.

Modifications of the Mowrer bell-and-pad procedure have resulted in improved treatment and maintenance effects. Finley, Besserman, Bennett,

Clapp, and Finley (1973) programmed an intermittent scheduling of the urine alarm; only 70 percent of incontinence incidents were followed by the alarm. This schedule was proposed to be more resistant to extinction than the standard, continuous schedule. The rates of relapse (extinction of treatment gains) were substantially lower for the intermittent schedule group (13 percent) versus the continuous schedule group (44 percent). A second modification of the standard procedure was reported by Young and Morgan (1972), using what they termed an overlearning procedure. Overlearning requires the child to consume a large quantity of fluid, depending upon age and weight, prior to bedtime, after initially achieving nocturnal continence with the bell-and-pad method. The rationale for this increased fluid intake is that it provides a more rigorous test of prior conditioning, since the increased fluid intake should result in increased bladder fullness during the night. Young and Morgan (1972) reported a lower relapse rate (13 percent) for the patients receiving the overlearning/bell-and-pad method than the patients receiving the standard bell-and-pad method (35 percent).

Although the bell-and-pad method, particularly with modification, can be a highly effective treatment procedure for nocturnal incontinence, several practical factors may interfere with its successful utilization. In order to reach the generally accepted treatment criterion of 14 succesive dry nights, a treatment period of from 8 to 12 weeks can be expected. Often, the alarm not only awakens the child, but also all the other family members. Needless to say, a reasonably high dropout rate (noncompliance) may be expected given the length of time that the entire family must be subjected to midnight awakenings. This fact, in combination with "false alarms" (alarm activations in the absence of urination) may combine to limit the general acceptability of this treatment method.

*Urine Retention Training.* A functional bladder capacity of approximately 300ml to 350ml is typically required before a child can become nocturnally continent. Functional bladder capacity is defined as the amount of urine an individual will retain before voiding rather than the actual structural size of the bladder. Some investigators have compared the functional bladder capacity of nocturnally incontinent and continent children, finding a lower functional bladder capacity for incontinent children and a higher frequency of daytime urination in the nocturnally incontinent children. A small functional bladder capacity may suggest the need for "bladder stretching exercises" or urine retention training. Kimmel and Kimmel (1970) reported on a urine retention training method that was similar to the procedure originally proposed by Muellner (1960) for nocturnally incontinent children. The purpose of the regimen was to functionally increase bladder capacity by gradually increasing the period of time during the day in which bladder distension cues sensed by the child were sufficiently strong so as to provoke micturition, but micturition was intentionally voluntarily withheld. The child was instructed to inform the parent each time he felt the urge to void, and the parent subsequently instructed the child to "hold it" (for progressively longer time periods as the treatment progressed). Each time the child delayed urination, he received reinforcement. The original report by Kimmel and Kimmel (1970) was subsequently followed by two additional studies suggesting positive results (Paschalis, Kimmel, and Kimmel, 1971; Stedman, 1972). However, as more recently reviewed by Doleys (1980), subsequent studies have not supported this method when used alone as the treatment of choice for nocturnal incontinence. Although this method has resulted in an apparent increase in functional bladder capacity, a concomitant decrease in nocturnal incontinence has not been generally found in replication studies.

*Dry-Bed Training.* The dry-bed procedure (Azrin, Sneed, & Fox, 1974) was designed to involve one night of intensive training followed by the brief use of a urine-alarm apparatus. Major features of the procedure included: (1) increased fluid intake, (2) hourly awakenings, (3) teaching the child to awaken with progressively milder prompts, (4) practice in toileting, (5) reinforcement for appropriate urination in the toilet during the night, (6) use of the urine-alarm procedure, and (7) training in awareness of the dry versus wet condition of the bed. When bedwetting occurred, the child was required to change the bed sheets and practice arising from the bed and walking to the toilet. Azrin et al. (1974) termed these aspects of the procedure as cleanliness training and over-correction, respectively. Although the results of this study were highly significant, the authors sought to modify the procedures further.

The modified method included a daytime-training component (Azrin & Thienes, 1978). The principal change was to omit the urine-alarm apparatus. Another major change was to provide the one day of intensive training in the late afternoon and early evening rather than throughout the night so as to reduce inconvenience (and greater probability of noncompliance). A third major change was the addition of a "strain-and-hold" procedure whereby the child was instructed to initiate urination, but as soon as he felt about to urinate, to hold back. The purpose of this training component was to teach the child voluntary control over his urination and increase awareness of his bladder sensations. A fourth change was to train the child to inhibit urination until a large volume had collected (similar to the urine retention training method). A fifth change was to have the child behaviorally rehearse during the day the nighttime toileting actions, that is, getting out of bed and going to the toilet when a full bladder was sensed. Reinforcement was provided throughout the training procedure. All 50 children, aged 3 to 14 years, who used the procedure ceased evidencing nocturnal incontinence. A 20 percent relapse rate was rapidly reversed by a second training session. Subsequent studies designed to further make the techniques even more practical for widespread utilization have also reported substantial clinical effects (Azrin, Thienes-Hontos, & Besalel-Azrin, 1979; Besalel, Azrin, Thienes-Hontos, & McMorrow, 1980). In sum, the procedures of Azrin and his associates appear to be the treatment of choice for nocturnal incontinence at this time. A brief outline of the techniques described in Azrin and Thienes (1978) and Azrin et al., 1979 is contained in Table 10.2.

Table 10.2.    Intensive Training Procedure for Nocturnal Incontinence.

I.   *Late Afternoon*
   1. Child encouraged to drink large amounts of favorite beverages
   2. Child requested to attempt urination every one-half hour
       a. If child senses need to urinate, instruct to hold, for increasingly longer time periods
       b. If urination is absolutely necessary, engage in behavioral rehearsal, i.e., child lies in bed, gets up, and engages in appropriate toileting and is reinforced with favorite beverage and praise
   3. Progress chart of dry and wet nights posted
       a. Reinforcement list developed for dry nights
II.  *Evening: One hour prior to bedtime*
   1. Child rehearses cleanliness training
       a. Puts on pajamas
       b. Removes sheets and then puts them back on
   2. Child rehearses positive practice
       a. Lies in bed and counts to 50
       b. Gets up, goes to bathroom, attempts urination
       c. Returns to bed and repeats 20 more times
III. *Bedtime*
   1. Drinks favorite beverage
   2. Program re-explained by parents
IV.  *Periodic awakenings prior to parents' bedtime*
   1. Reinforce if dry and instruct to continue urinary control
   2. If needs to urinate, reinforce appropriate toileting and dry bed condition
   3. If wet, engage in cleanliness training and 20 trials of positive practice in appropriate toileting
V.   *Next Morning*
   1. Check one-half hour earlier than typical awakening time
   2. If dry, reinforce
   3. If wet, perform cleanliness training and 20 trials of positive practice

*Diurnal Incontinence*

Three major treatment approaches have been utilized for diurnal incontinence: (1) the pants-alarm method, (2) dry-pants training, and (3) bladder drill method.

***Pants-Alarm Method.*** The pants-alarm method was primarily designed for utilization with retarded children (Azrin, Bugle, & O'Brien, 1971). The apparatus is similar to the bell-and-pad apparatus, except that a portable instrument was designed to be worn by the child during the day. When combined with systematic reinforcement for appropriate toileting, the pants-alarm method was found to result in diurnal continence for the two profoundly retarded children reported on by Azrin et al. (1971). Mahoney, Van Wagenen and Meyerson (1971) used a similar portable urine-alarm appratus both with three normal children and five retarded children, again in combination with reinforcement for appropriate toileting. Seven of the eight children attained criterion continence. While these early studies are encouraging, the need for a portable urine-alarm apparatus limits their widespread utilization.

***Dry-Pants Training.*** Foxx and Azrin (1973) reported on the toilet training of normal, diurnally incontinent children, without the use of an urine-alarm apparatus. The essentials of the procedure consisted of the following steps: (1) Giving the child her favorite beverage at frequent intervals; (2) Reinforcing appropriate toileting, that is, walking to the commode, lowering pants, sitting or standing properly at the commode, urinating into the commode, and pulling up pants; and (3) Requiring cleanliness training and positive practice if wetting occurred. The specifics of the training regimen have been expanded into a training manual (Azrin & Foxx, 1974). Foxx and Azrin (1973) reported substantial clinical effects using this method by trained technicians. Its utilization by parents, in combination with three weekly instructional classes, resulted in 77 percent of the parents successfully toilet training their children (Butler, 1976). For young children, this method appears to be the current treatment of choice for diurnal incontinence.

***Bladder Drill Method.*** Although the bladder drill method has been used primarily with adult women with diurnal frequency, nocturnal frequency, urgency, urge incontinence, and stress incontinence, its similarity to the urine retention training method for nocturnal incontinence warrants discussion of its possible future use in pediatric diurnal voiding dysfunction. Jarvis and Miller (1980) studied 60 women, aged 27 to 79, with the above symptoms due to idiopathic detrusor instability as diagnosed by pressure-flow studies. Under general anesthesia, bladder capacity was 650ml or more for all patients. Each patient was then randomly assigned to either a bladder drill treatment group or a nontreatment control group. The control group was simply instructed to try and hold their urine for 4 hours. The treatment group received the bladder drill method, consisting of the following steps: (1) Patient instructed to pass urine at specific intervals during the day (usually every 1 ½ hours), and this interval was gradually increased by one-half hour intervals until a 4-hour interval schedule was attained, and (2) Patient instructed to maintain typical fluid intake throughout and to record fluid intake on a chart. After treatment, 27 of the 30 patients practicing the bladder drill method were continent and 25 were symptom free, whereas only 7 of the 30 controls were both continent and symptom free. At a 4-month follow-up, only one of the treatment subjects had relapsed. At this time, the bladder drill method may be the treatment of choice for detrusor instability in adult women. Its potential application to pediatric (e.g., DeLuca, Swenson, Fisher, & Loutfi, 1962) and neurogenic bladder dysfunction (e.g., Optiz, 1976) awaits further empirical investigation.

## FECAL INCONTINENCE

Fecal incontinence may be classified into two broad categories: encopresis and organic rectosphincteric dysfunction. Organic disorders are characterized by the presence of neurological or structural pathology, such as in myelomeningocele or Hirschsprung's disease. Encopresis, on the other hand, is considered a functional disorder with an absence of any underlying overt organic pathology. Most children with fecal incontinence are diagnosed as encopretic. Encopresis may be further delineated into primary or secondary categories. Primary encopresis refers to children who have never achieved continence, whereas secondary encopresis refers to children who have attained continence for at least several months, but have relapsed. In a descriptive analysis of 102 encopretic children, Levine (1975) found this sample to comprise approximately 3 percent of the total clinic population of a large children's hospital, a figure essentially consistent with the other incidence studies. The mean age of these children was 7 years, with a range of 4 to 13 years. The predominant pattern was one of secondary-diurnal incontinence. Thirty-two of the children also evidenced enuresis. Encopresis may also occur with constipation as the primary condition and overflow fecal incontinence as the secondary consequence (Schuster, 1977).

In the infant and young child, defecation is an uninhibited response initiated reflexively by meals that stimulate gastroileocolic motor activity (Schuster, 1977). Voluntary control of defecation through toilet training requires the child's gradual discrimination of subtle physiological cues indicating the need to evacuate, evoking appropriate toileting behaviors taught by the parents (Fleisher, 1976). The specific physiological mechanisms involved are discussed in the next section.

## Physiological Mechanisms

The major anatomical structures involved in defecation are the rectum, the internal anal sphincter, and the external anal sphincter. Fecal material is transported through peristalsis from the intestinal tract to the rectum, which has a capacity of approximately 12 to 15 cm. The awareness of the urge to defecate has both visceral sensory and somatic sensory components via the sacral spinal cord. The visceral sensory component involves afferent nerves within the autonomic plexi, which are excited by changes in mechanical tension within the rectal wall. Stretch receptors are located in the smooth muscle of the rectal wall. Tension is heightened by passive stretching or active contraction of the smooth muscle of the gut wall. Entrance of stool or gas distends the rectal lumen, causing an increase in the mechanical tension within the rectal wall, perceived as rectal fullness. The somatic sensory component involves afferent fibers that transmit sensory impulses from the anoderm to the central nervous system via the pudendal nerves. These impulses permit awareness of fecal material in the anal canal and awareness of the distinction between solid fecal material and gas.

Distension of the rectal wall causes a transient reflex relaxation of the smooth musculature of the internal anal sphincter and increases awareness of pending defecation. Internal anal sphincter tone is maintained via sympathetic innervation from the lumbar spinal cord ($L_4$, $L_5$); inhibition of internal anal sphincter tone is mediated through parasympathetic innervation from the sacral spinal cord ($S_1$, $S_2$, $S_3$). The striated musculature of the external anal sphincter, levator ani, and other muscles of the pelvic floor are somatically innervated through the sacral spinal cord ($S_2$, $S_3$, $S_4$) and are under voluntary control. Continence is normally maintained through voluntary contraction of the external anal sphincter and perianal musculature under conditions of reflexive relaxation of the internal anal sphincter secondary to rectal fullness. Defecation occurs with the voluntary relaxation of the striated musculature.

## Rectosphincteric Manometric Assessment

Schuster, Hookman, Hendrix, and Mendeloff (1965) first described the simultaneous manometric recording of internal and external anal sphincter responses under varying conditions of induced rectal fullness. The instrument for rectosphincteric manometry consists of two recording balloons on a hollow cylindrical core positioned in the anal canal. The outer balloon is situated so as to record external anal sphincter responses, and the inner balloon records internal anal sphincter responses. A third balloon is threaded through the cylinder and positioned in the rectum. Transient distension of this third balloon with air produces responses by both anal sphincters, which are recorded by transducers on a multichannel strip chart recording system similar to urodynamic instrumentation. Normally, rectal distension by air leads to reflex relaxation of the internal anal sphincter and simultaneous contraction of the external anal sphincter, proportional to the amount of rectal distension produced by the rectal balloon (Schuster et al., 1975; Schuster, 1973). Rectosphincteric manometry provides a sensitive measure of the function of both smooth and striated anal musculature and has served as a valuable diagnostic tool for the assessment of rectosphincteric responses in a number of neurological, structural, and idiopathic conditions such as myelomeningocele, Hirschsprung's disease, idiopathic constipation and incontinence, anal malformation, and anal imperforation (Alva, Mendeloff, & Schuster, 1967; Meunier, Mollard, & De Beaujeu, 1976; White, Suzuki, El Shafie, Kuman, Haller, & Schnaufer, 1972; Whitehead, Engel, & Schuster, 1980). Recently, rectosphincteric manometry has been extended to the biofeedback treatment of defecation dysfunction, as described in a subsequent section.

## Pharmacologic Intervention

Pharmacologic intervention is most widely utilized in the management of diarrhea, typically in infants and young children (see Angelides & Fitzgerald, 1981, for review). Three classes of antidiarrheal preparations are available: hydrophilic agents, absorbents, and antimotility agents. Medical interventions for fecal incontinence primarily include laxatives, enemas, and suppositories (see Parker & Whitehead, 1982, for review).

## Rectosphincteric Biofeedback

Engel, Nikoomanesh, and Schuster (1974) first reported on a series of five adult patients with chronic fecal incontinence secondary to laminectomy, proctectomy for tumor, idiopathic origin, hemorrhoidectomy, diabetes, and a 6-year-old child with myelomeningocele, utilizing rectosphincteric biofeedback as the training modality. The intervention consisted of three sequential phases. During phase 1, a diagnosis was made of the severity of impairment of rectosphincteric responses using the three-balloon manometry system developed by Schuster et al. (1965). After the diagnostic testing, each patient was instructed on normal rectosphincter responding and how their responding was different from normal responding (using the polygraph recordings on the strip chart). Phase 2, the beginning of the biofeedback training, provided the patient with the simultaneous visual feedback of the polygraph tracings of sphincteric responses under varying degrees of air-induced rectal fullness. Verbal reinforcement was provided by the therapist for gradually approximating normal responding. Phase 3 consisted of further refinement of rectosphincteric responding, with the patient now instructed to attempt to synchronize sphincteric responses so that the external anal sphincter contraction occurred simultaneously with internal anal sphincter relaxation. The final stage of phase 3 was to gradually require normal responding without the benefit of visual feedback, an attempt to reduce the patient's need for the instrument feedback, thus providing a further shaping step toward successful self-regulation of rectosphincteric responses.

The results of the study showed that all six patients completed the biofeedback training within four sessions or less. During phase 1, it was noted that for all six patients external anal sphincter responses were either diminished or absent, with internal anal sphincter responding varying from normal in some patients to completely absent for the child with myelomeningocele during various degrees of rectal fullness. All six patients demonstrated evidence of learned sphincteric control during the biofeedback training sessions. Follow-up assessments, ranging from 6 months to 5 years, found four of the patients completely continent since the biofeedback training, with substantially reduced incontinence in the other two patients.

As discussed by Engel et al. (1974), the biofeedback training is best viewed as affecting the rate of occurrence of existing responses, not the development of new associations. That is, all the patients must have had the capacity to produce sphincteric responses prior to the training, with biofeedback providing proprioceptive awareness through the subtle moment-to-moment feedback required for voluntary control (Schuster, 1977). Not only was biofeedback training successful in teaching voluntary control over the external anal sphincter striated musculature, but it was also effective in teaching voluntary control over the internal anal sphincter smooth musculature that is autonomically innervated (and previously presumed to be involuntary). This biofeedback conditioning of autonomically innervated smooth muscle is consistent with the previously reviewed findings on urodynamic biofeedback.

Cerulli, Nikoomanesh, and Schuster (1979) replicated these techniques with 50 patients (average age of 46 years, range of 6 to 97 years) with severe daily fecal incontinence for 1 to 38 years secondary to organic disease, generalized medical disorders, and postoperative complications of anorectal surgery. Thirty-six of the 50 patients successfully responded to biofeedback training as evidenced by the disappearance of fecal incontinence or a decrease in frequency of incontinence by 90 percent. Significantly, manometric improvement correlated with the clinical improvement and could be used to predict clinical improvement. Goldenberg, Hodges, Hersh, and Jinich (1980) replicated the rectosphincteric biofeedback training with 12 patients (ages 12 to 78 years) with fecal incontinence secondary to medical conditions or surgery. Follow-up assessments showed complete continence in six patients and a good response in four patients. Nine of these ten patients required only one biofeedback training session.

Olness, McParland, and Piper (1980) applied the rectosphincteric biofeedback procedures to 50 children (ages 4 to 18 years) with severe chronic fecal incontinence associated with either imperforate anus surgery in infancy or longstanding idiopathic constipation. Forty-seven of the children learned to have voluntary bowel movements, and 30 eliminated fecal soiling incidents completely during follow-up periods ranging from 6 months to 3 years. Significantly, 8 of the 10 patients with imperforate anus learned to defecate voluntarily with one to two biofeedback training sessions. An early case study by Kohlenberg (1973) also suggests the potential, as of yet unfulfilled, for biofeedback training in the management of fecal incontinence associated with Hirschsprung's disease.

Finally, fecal incontinence in children with myelomeningocele has also been selected for investigation. In their investigation of 50 patients, Cerulli et al. (1979) studied seven patients with myelomeningocele. Although the earlier Engel et al. (1974) study had reported the successful treatment of the one child with myelomeningocele, the Cerulli et al. (1979) study reported the successful treatment of only two of the seven patients with myelomeningocele. Wald (1981) used the three-balloon method with eight selected children, ages 5 to 17 years, with myelomeningocele, demonstrating a good clinical response in four of the children, defined as the disappearance of fecal soiling or a greater than 75 percent improvement in the frequency of soiling. Fortunately, another recent study (Whitehead, Parker, Masek, Cataldo, & Freeman, 1981), has reported greater success with a modified biofeedback procedure.

Whitehead et al. (1981) also utilized the three-balloon manometric system, but based on their diagnostic findings of the eight children with myelomeningocele studied (ages 5 to 15 years), they modified the rectosphincteric biofeedback teaching techniques used by the previous studies. Specifically, during the initial rectosphincteric manometric assessment, it was observed that these children's ability to sense rectal distension appeared to be normal, whereas the adult patients previously studied frequently reported a diminished ability to sense rectal distension. As suggested by Whitehead et al. (1981), the previous studies' biofeedback procedure may be conceptualized as sensory discrimination training, since it started with large volumes of air injected into the rectal balloon and then gradually required appropriate rectosphincteric responding with progressively smaller volumes. A further difference noted was that in the adult patients previously studied there was simply a weak or absent contraction of the external anal sphincter following rectal distension. In contrast, in seven of the eight children studied by Whitehead et al. (1981), the muscle tone of the external anal sphincter was actively inhibited following rectal distension, and this inhibition was directly proportional in magnitude to the volume of rectal distension, resulting in the children's inability to contract the external anal sphincter voluntarily.

These two observed differences, normal rectal sensation and reflexive inhibition of the external anal sphincter, led to a modified rectosphincteric biofeedback procedure based on response shaping rather than the previous stimulus discrimination training procedure. The biofeedback training consisted of four phases. Phase 1 consisted of the diagnosis of pretraining functioning through rectosphincteric manometry. Additionally, the subjective sensory threshold for rectal distension was determined by recording the smallest amount of rectal distension at which the child consistently reported sensation. Those children who were inconsistent in their reporting of initial sensation were given a forced-choice test, involving a presentation of 10 choice trials where they were required to identify which of two intervals air was injected into the rectal balloon. Air and no-air injections were randomized across the 10 trials. The child was considered to have subjective sensation at a particular distension level if able to correctly answer eight of the ten forced-choice trials.

Phase 2 began the response shaping biofeedback training procedure. The child was first taught to contract the external anal sphincter in the absence of rectal distension. Visual feedback was provided by viewing the polygraph chart strip tracings, and reinforcement was given for pen deflections in the appropriate direction (i.e., external anal sphincter contractions). Phase 3 involved the next step in the response shaping procedure, with the child now required to contract the external anal sphincter in response to gradually increasing amounts of air-produced rectal distension and associated reflexive internal anal sphincter relaxation. Rectal distension levels began at the previously determined subjective threshold and proceeded in increments of 5 to 10ml of injected air up to 60ml. Advancement to the next greater distension level was dependent on appropriate rectosphincteric responding at the previous level. During this phase the children were reinforced for synchronizing internal-external anal sphincteric responding. Finally, phase 4 was a continuation of phase 3 but without visual feedback, requiring the child to rely solely on subjective sensations. This provided the final shaping step toward the self-regulation of rectosphincteric responding. Following six biofeedback training sessions, five patients were fecally continent, and a sixth child evidenced an 80 percent reduction in the frequency of fecal incontinence. A clinically successful outcome was associated with the acquisition of a reliable contraction of the external anal sphincter subsequent to biofeedback training. At a 1 to 2 year follow-up, four children were having fecal soiling incidents once per month or less.

In sum, rectosphincteric biofeedback training provides a significant advancement in the treatment of chronic, severe fecal incontinence. Nonbiofeedback biobehavioral techniques may also prove valuable, as described next.

## Nonbiofeedback Biobehavioral Management

The largest amount of clinical research effort has been directed toward the nonbiofeedback biobehavioral management of encopresis, with fecal incontinence secondary to neurological impairment just beginning to be investigated from a nonbiofeedback biobehavioral management perspective (e.g., Epstein & McCoy, 1977; Jeffries, Killam, & Varni, 1982).

### Encopresis

The literature on the biobehavioral management of encopresis has emphasized two major treatment modalities: (1) utilization of reinforcement and punishment procedures to increase appropriate toileting behaviors and decrease the frequency of fecal soiling, and (2) an approach combining reinforcement/punishment procedures with evacuation aids (enemas, laxatives, suppositories) and/or gastroileocolic reflex conditioning.

*Reinforcement/Punishment Procedures.*  The recent studies utilizing reinforcement and punishment procedures have expanded on Foxx and Azrin's (1973) program of Full Cleanliness Training, which is a multicomponent training package (Crowley & Armstrong, 1977; Doleys, McWhorter, Williams, & Gentry, 1977). The three major components of this training package include:

1. *Periodic pants-checks and/or toileting.* The parents were instructed to check the child initially every hour for clean/soiled pants, followed by sitting on the toilet for a brief period.
2. *Full cleanliness training.* If the child's pants were soiled, he was required to correct this inappropriate toileting behavior by cleaning himself and his clothes, proposed as teaching responsibility for soiling and as further motivating appropriate toileting.
3. *Positive reinforcement for appropriate toileting behavior.* A reinforcement chart was placed in the bathroom. Each time the child defecated while sitting on the toilet he was given a token or point which could be exchanged from a previously developed reinforcement list.

Soiling was effectively eliminated in the three children studied by Doleys et al. (1977). Doleys et al. (1977) suggest that positive reinforcement for appropriate toileting behavior is an indispensable feature since it reduces the likelihood of a general suppression of defecation and instead increases a desirable toileting behavior pattern. Crowley and Armstrong (1977) have achieved similar results, that is, elimination of encopresis, using essentially an identical training package.

*Reinforcement/Punishment Procedures Combined with Evacuation Aids.* The goal of these procedures is to decrease fecal soiling by increasing the occurrence of regular and consistent bowel movements through the utilization of evacuation aids and/or the gastroileocolic reflex.

  Young (1973) described the physiological rationale behind gastroileocolic reflex training. Peristalsis in the colon usually occurs after a meal or fluid intake; this increase in colonic motor activity is called the gastrocolic reflex. Prior to the gastrocolic reflex the terminal ileum becomes hyperactive following food or fluid intake, termed the gastroileal reflex. The two processes together are termed the gastroileocolic reflex. During this reflex the entire small intestine demonstrates increased motility which is then transmitted to the large intestine. This colonic peristalsis is frequently followed by the urge to defecate. The training program developed by Young (1973) was designed to associate these reflexive responses with the toilet situation. Since the time interval from the ingestion of food or fluid to the occurrence of colonic sensation is approximately 20 to 30 minutes, and since another common time for the reflex to occur is during the first hour after arising in the morning, then these time periods were selected for the intervention. When the children went to bed at night they were given a mild laxative to assist the subsequent initiation of the reflex and to relieve colonic inertia. When the child awoke in the morning, a warm drink or food was given. Twenty to thirty minutes later the child was taken to the toilet. The child was reinforced for appropriate defecation or simply allowed to return to normal activities if defecation did not occur after sitting for 10 minutes. Additionally, the procedure was repeated during the day after meals. Young (1973) reported a successful outcome using this procedure with 19 of the 24 children so treated. Ashkenazi (1975) attained similar positive results with the insertion of a glycerine suppository as a stimulus for bowel movements immediately following meals, in combination with instructing the child to sit on the toilet within 15 to 20 minutes subsequent to meals/suppository insertion and reinforcement for appropriate toileting behaviors and no fecal soiling (DRO schedule).

A number of programs have utilized a combination of reinforcement/ punishment procedures, laxatives, enemas, and suppositories to achieve fecal continence (Christophersen & Rainey, 1976; Levine & Bakow, 1976; Wright & Walker, 1978). The essential components of these programs include the following: (1) The first active phase of treatment is vigorous bowel catharsis achieved by enemas and laxatives. (2) Once the initial bowel catharsis has been achieved, the child and parents are instructed to follow a program of the child going to the bathroom immediately upon awakening in the morning. If the child defecates, he is reinforced. (3) If defecation does not occur after sitting on the commode for 5 minutes, a glycerine suppository is inserted, and the child is then allowed to eat breakfast. (4) After breakfast the child is again instructed to go to the bathroom. (5) If defecation does not occur shortly prior to leaving for school, an enema is given (typically not necessary). (6) Throughout, the child is reinforced for regular, appropriate toileting behavior and no fecal soiling (DRO schedule). (7) After two consecutive weeks without fecal soiling, the program is gradually phased out and only reinstated if a relapse occurs. Wright and Walker (1978) report an 100 percent effectiveness for this program when carefully adhered to (see Chapter 8 for a description of the study by Jeffries et al. [1982] on the biobehavioral management of neurogenic fecal incontinence secondary to myelomeningocele).

# REFERENCES

Allen, T.D. The non-neurogenic neurogenic bladder. *Journal of Urology,* 1977, **117**, 232–238.
Alva, J., Mendeloff, A.I., & Schuster, M.M. Reflex and electromyographic abnormalities associated with fecal incontinence. *Gastroenterology,* 1976, **53**, 101–106.
Angelides, A., & Fitzgerald, J.F. Pharmacologic advances in the treatment of gastrointestinal diseases. *Pediatric Clinics of North America,* 1981, **28**, 95–112.

Ashkenazi, A. The treatment of encopresis using a discriminative stimulus and positive reinforcement. *Journal of Behavior Therapy and Experimental Psychiatry,* 1975, **6**, 155–157.

Azrin, N.H., Bugle, C., & O'Brien, F. Behavioral engineering: Two apparatuses for toilet training retarded children. *Journal of Applied Behavior Analysis,* 1971, **4**, 249–253.

Azrin, N.H., & Foxx, R.M. *Toilet Training in Less than a Day.* New York: Simon and Schuster, 1974.

Azrin, N.H., Sneed, T.J., & Foxx, R.M. Dry-bed Training: Rapid elimination of childhood enuresis. *Behaviour Research and Therapy,* 1974, **12**, 147–156.

Azrin, N.H., & Thienes, P.M. Rapid elimination of enuresis by intensive learning without a conditioning apparatus. *Behavior Therapy,* 1978, **9**, 342–354.

Azrin, N.H., Thienes-Hontos, P.T., & Besalel-Azrin, V. Elimination of enuresis without a conditioning apparatus: An extension by office instruction of the child and parents. *Behavior Therapy,* 1979, **10**, 14–19.

Besalel, V.A., Azrin, N.H., Thienes-Hontos, P., & McMorrow, M. Evaluation of a parent's manual for training enuretic children. *Behaviour Research and Therapy,* 1980, **18**, 358–360.

Blaivas, J.G., Labib, K.L., Bauer, S.B., & Retik, A.B. Changing concepts in the urodynamic evaluation of children. *Journal of Urology,* 1977, **117**, 778–781. (a)

Blaivas, J.G., Labib, K.L., Bauer, S.B., & Retik, A.B. New approach to electromyography of the external urethral sphincter. *Journal of Urology,* 1977, **117**, 773–777. (b)

Bradley, W.E., Rockswold, G.L., Timm, G.W., & Scott, F.B. Neurology of micturition. *Journal of Urology,* 1976, **115**, 481–486.

Bradley, W.E., & Scott, F.B. Physiology of the urinary bladder. In J.H. Harrison, R.F. Gittes, A.D. Perlmutter, T.A. Stamey, & P.L. Walsh (Eds.), *Campbell's Urology.* Vol. 1. Philadelphia: W.B. Saunders, 1978.

Butler, J.F. The toilet training success of parents after reading *Toilet Training in Less Than a Day. Behavior Therapy,* 1976, **7**, 185–191.

Cardozo, L.D., Abrams, P.D., Stanton, S.L., & Feneley, R.C.L. Idiopathic bladder instability treated by biofeedback. *British Journal of Urology,* 1978, **50**, 521–523.

Cardozo, L., Stanton, S.L., Hafner, J., & Allan, V. Biofeedback in the treatment of detrusor instability. *British Journal of Urology,* 1978, **50**, 250–254.

Cerulli, M.A., Nikoomanesh, P., & Schuster, M.M. Progress in biofeedback conditioning for fecal incontinence. *Gastroenterology,* 1979, **76**, 742–746.

Christophersen, E.R., & Rainey, S.K. Management of encopresis through a pediatric outpatient clinic. *Journal of Pediatric Psychology,* 1976, **4**, 38–41.

Cook, W.A., Babcock, J.R., Swenson, O.S., & King, L.R. Incontinence in children. *Urologic Clinics of North America,* 1978, **5**, 353–374.

Crowley, L.P., & Armstrong, P.M. Positive practice, overcorrection and behavioral rehearsal in the treatment of three cases of encopresis. *Journal of Behavior Therapy and Experimental Psychiatry,* 1977, **8**, 411–416.

DeLuca, F.G., Swenson, O., Fisher, J.H., & Loutfi, A.H. The dysfunctional "lazy" bladder syndrome in children. *Archives of Disease in Childhood,* 1962, **34**, 117–121.

Doleys, D.M. Enuresis. In J.M. Ferguson & C.B. Taylor (Eds.), *Comprehensive Handbook of Behavioral Medicine. Vol. 1: Systems Intervention.* Jamaica, NY: Spectrum, 1980.

Doleys, D.M., McWhorter, A.Q., Williams, S.C., & Gentry, W.R. Encopresis: Its treatment and relation to nocturnal enuresis. *Behavior Therapy,* 1977, **8**, 77–82.

Engel, B.T., Nikoomanesh, P., & Schuster, M.M. Operant conditioning of rectosphincteric responses in the treatment of fecal incontinence. *New England Journal of Medicine,* 1974, **290**, 646–649.

Epstein, L.H., & McCoy, J.F. Bladder and bowel control in Hirschsprung's disease. *Journal of Behavior Therapy and Experimental Psychiatry,* 1977, **8**, 97–99.

Finley, W.W., Besserman, R.L., Bennett, F.L., Clapp, R.K., & Finley, P.K. The effect of continuous, intermittent, and "placebo" reinforcement on the effectiveness of the conditioning treatment of enuresis nocturna. *Behaviour Research and Therapy,* 1973, **11**, 289–297.

242    Clinical Behavioral Pediatrics

Firlit, C.F., & Cook, W.A. Voiding pattern abnormalities in children. *Urology,* 1977, **10**, 25–29.
Fleisher, D.R. Diagnosis and treatment of disorders of defecation in children. *Pediatric Annals,* 1976, **5**, 71–101.
Foxx, R.M., & Azrin, N.H. Dry pants: A rapid method of toilet training children. *Behaviour Research and Therapy,* 1973, **11**, 435–442.
Foxx, R.M., & Azrin, N.H. *Toilet Training the Retarded.* Champaign, Illinois: Research Press, 1973.
Goldenberg, D.A., Hodges, K., Hersh, T., & Jinich, H. Biofeedback therapy for fecal incontinence. *American Journal of Gastroenterology,* 1980, **74**, 342–345.
Gosling, J.A., Dixon, J.S., Critchley, H.O.D., & Thompson, S.A. A comparative study of the human external sphincter and periurethral levator ani muscles. *British Journal of Urology,* 1981, **53**, 35–41.
Hanna, M.K., Di Scipio, W., Suh, K.K., Kogan, S.J., Levitt, S.B., & Donner, K. Urodynamics in children: Part I. Methodology. *Journal of Urology,* 1981, **125**, 530–533. (a)
Hanna, M.K., Di Scipio, W., Suh, K.K., Kogan, S.J., Levitt, S.B., & Donner, K. Urodynamics in children: Part II. The pseudoneurogenic bladder. *Journal of Urology,* 1981, **125**, 534–537. (b)
Jarvis, G.J., & Millar, D.R. Controlled trial of bladder drill for detrusor instability. *British Medical Journal,* 1980, **281**, 1322–1323.
Jeffries, J.S., Killam, P.E., & Varni, J.W. Behavioral management of fecal incontinence in a child with myelomeningocele. *Pediatric Nursing,* 1982, **8**, 267–270.
Killam, P.E., Jeffries, J.S., & Varni, J.W. Urodynamic biofeedback treatment of urinary incontinence in children with myelomeningocele: Some initial observations. Paper presented at the Annual Meeting of the Society of Behavioral Medicine, Baltimore, March 1983.
Kimmel, H.D., & Kimmel, E. An instrumental conditioning method for the treatment of enuresis. *Journal of Behavior Therapy and Experimental Psychiatry,* 1970, **1**, 121–123.
Kohlenberg, R.J. Operant conditioning of human anal sphincter pressure. *Journal of Applied Behavior Analysis,* 1973, **6**, 201–208.
Kleeman, F.J. The physiology of the internal urinary sphincter. *Journal of Urology,* 1970, **104**, 549–554.
Lapides, J., Sweet, R.B., & Lewis, L.W. Role of striated muscle in urination. *Journal of Urology,* 1957, **77**, 247–250.
Levine, M.D. Children with encopresis: A descriptive analysis. *Pediatrics,* 1975, **56**, 412–416.
Levine, M.D., & Bakow, H. Children with encopresis: A study of treatment outcome. *Pediatrics,* 1976, **58**, 845–852.
Mahoney, K., Van Wagenen, R.K., & Meyerson, L. Toilet training of normal and retarded children. *Journal of Applied Behavior Analysis,* 1971, **4**, 173–181.
Maizels, M., King, L.R., & Firlit, C.F. Urodynamic biofeedback: A new approach to treat vesical sphincter dyssynergia. *Journal of Urology,* 1979, **122**, 205–209.
Muellner, S.R. Development of urinary control in children: A new concept in cause, prevention and treatment of primary enuresis. *Journal of Urology,* 1960, **84**, 714–716.
Meunier, P., Mollard, P., & DeBeaujeu, M.J. Manometric studies of anorectal disorders in infancy and childhood: An investigation of the physiopathology of continence and defecation. *British Journal of Surgery,* 1976, **63**, 402–407.
Mowrer, O.H., & Mowrer, W.A. Enuresis: A method for its study and treatment. *American Journal of Orthopsychiatry,* 1938, **8**, 436–447.
Olness, K., McParland, F.A., & Piper, J. Biofeedback: A new modality in the management of children with fecal soiling. *Journal of Pediatrics,* 1980, **96**, 505–509.
Opitz, J.L. Bladder retraining: An organized program. *Mayo Clinic Proceedings,* 1976, **51**, 367–372.
Oppel, W.C., Harper, P.A., & Rider, R.V. The age of attaining bladder control. *Pediatrics,* 1968, **42**, 614–626.

Parker, L., & Whitehead, W.E. Treatment of urinary and fecal incontinence in children. In D.C. Russo & J.W. Varni (Eds.), *Behavioral Pediatrics: Research and Practice.* New York: Plenum Press, 1982.

Paschalis, A., Kimmel, H.D., & Kimmel, E. Further study of diurnal instrumental conditioning in the treatment of enuresis nocturna. *Journal of Behavior Therapy and Experimental Psychiatry,* 1972, **3**, 253–256.

Raezer, D.M., Benson, G.S., Wein, A.J., & Duckett, J.W. The functional approach to the management of the pediatric neuropathic bladder: A clinical study. *Journal of Urology,* 1977, **117**, 649–654.

Raz, S., & Bradley, W.E. Neuromuscular dysfunction of the lower urinary tract. In J.H. Harrison, R.F. Gittes, A.D. Perlmutter, T.A. Stamey, & P.C. Walsh (Eds.), *Campbell's Urology.* Vol. 2. Philadelphia: W.B. Saunders, 1979.

Schneider, R.D., & Westendorf, K. Adjuvant bladder-pressure biofeedback in treating neurogenic bladder dysfunction: A case study. *Behavior Therapist,* 1979, **2**, 29–31.

Schuster, M.M. Diagnostic value of anal sphincter pressure measurements. *Hospital Practice,* 1973, April, 114–122.

Schuster, M.M. Constipation and anorectal disorders. *Clinics in Gastroenterology,* 1977, **6**, 643–658.

Schuster, M.M. Biofeedback treatment of gastrointestinal disorders. *Medical Clinics of North America,* 1977, **61**, 907–912.

Schuster, M.M., Hookman, P., Hendrix, T.R., & Mendeloff, A.I. Simultaneous manometric recording of internal and external anal sphincteric reflexes. *Bulletin Johns Hopkins Hospital,* 1965, **79**, 79–88.

Sloop, E.W. Urinary disorders. In R.B. Williams & W.D. Gentry (Eds.), *Behavioral Approaches to Medical Treatment.* Cambridge, Mass.: Ballinger, 1977.

Smith, D.R. *General Urology.* Los Altos, Calif.: Lange, 1978.

Stedman, J.M. An extension of the Kimmel treatment for enuresis to an adolescent: A case report. *Journal of Behavior Therapy and Experimental Psychiatry,* 1972, **3**, 307–309.

Wald, A. Use of biofeedback in treatment of fecal incontinence in patients with meningomyelocele. *Pediatrics,* 1981, **68**, 45–49.

Wear, J.B., Wear, R.B., & Cleeland, C. Biofeedback in urology using urodynamics: Preliminary observations. *Journal of Urology,* 1979, **121**, 464–468.

Webster, G.D. Urodynamic studies. In M.I. Resnick & R.A. Older (Eds.), *Diagnosis of Diseases of the Genitourinary System.* New York: Thieme-Stratton, 1982.

White J.J., Suzuki, H., El Shafie, M., Kumar, A.P.M., Haller, J.A., & Schnaufer, L. A physiologic rationale for the management of neurologic rectal incontinence in children. *Pediatrics,* 1972, **49**, 888–893.

Whitehead, W.E., Engel, B.T., & Schuster, M.M. Irritable bowel syndrome: Physiological and psychological differences between diarrhea-predominant and constipation-predominant patients. *Digestive Diseases and Sciences,* 1980, **25**, 404–413.

Whitehead, W.E., Parker, L.H., Masek, B.J., Cataldo, M.F., & Freeman, J.M. Biofeedback treatment of fecal incontinence in patients with myelomeningocele. *Developmental Medicine and Child Neurology,* 1981, **23**, 313–322.

Whiteside, C.G., & Arnold, E.P. Persistent primary enuresis: A urodynamic assessment. *British Medical Journal,* 1975, **1**, 364–367.

Wright, L., & Walker, C.E. A simple behavioral treatment program for psychogenic encopresis. *Behaviour Research and Therapy,* 1978, **16**, 209–212.

Young, G.C. The treatment of childhood encopresis by conditioned gastro-ileal reflex training. *Behaviour Research and Therapy,* 1973, **11**, 499–503.

Young, G.C., & Morgan, R.T. Overlearning in the conditioning treatment of enuresis. *Behaviour Research and Therapy,* 1972, **10**, 147–151.

# 11

# Bronchial Asthma, Insulin-Dependent Juvenile Diabetes Mellitus, End-Stage Renal Disease

The pediatric chronic disorders, bronchial asthma, insulin-dependent juvenile diabetes mellitus, and end-stage renal disease have been grouped together because a substantial body of biobehavioral clinical research does not yet exist that would warrant independent chapter status. However, it is anticipated that future editions of the text will reflect empirical development in these areas, subsequently resulting in three separate chapters.

## BRONCHIAL ASTHMA

Asthma is a respiratory disorder that results in a recurrent, intermittent, and variable pattern of reversible airway obstruction, ranging in intensity from a sensation of tightness in the chest accompanied by a slight wheeze to status asthmaticus (see Creer, Renne, & Chai, 1982, for review). The more severe the disease, the less complete the airway obstruction reversibility. There are a variety of stimuli that may provoke airway obstruction in asthmatic patients, including allergens, aspirin and related substances, infections, emotional factors, exercise and irritants (Creer et al., 1982). Creer et al. (1982) further provide the physiological basis for these precipitants of asthmatic attacks. Generally, asthma attacks are a function of one of three physiological responses: bronchoconstriction due to contraction or spasms in the smooth muscle surrounding the airways, mucus or mucus plugs that clog the airways, or edema of the epithelial lining of the bronchial tubes. Estimates of the incidence of asthma vary from between 5 to 15 percent of all children under 12 years of age, with a more frequent occurrence among boys.

The long-term prognosis is dependent on the age of onset and the severity of disease. In a prospective study, Martin, McLennan, Landau, and Phelan (1980) randomly selected 331 children who had started to wheeze in childhood and followed them from age 7 to 21 years of age. Approximately half the children who started wheezing before age 7 were wheeze-free in early adulthood, with the frequency of wheezing decreasing for those more severely affected children. Early onset and an infrequent rate of wheezing were found to be favorable prognostic signs.

Although asthma-related mortality is low, its impact in terms of activity restriction and cost are high. Emergency room visits and hospitalizations result in a pattern of missed school days and can be a costly and time consuming burden for the family. In an attempt to reduce unnecessary hospitalization and relapse after discharge, Fischl, Pitchenik, and Gardner (1981) developed a predictive index using a combination of seven presenting factors: pulse rate greater than or equal to 120 per minute, respiratory rate greater than or equal to 30 per minute, pulses paradoxus greater than or equal to 18 mm Hg, peak expiratory flow rate less than or equal to 120 liters per minute, moderate to severe dyspnea, accessory-muscle use, and wheezing. The index ranged from 0 to 7, increasing with the severity of the symptoms. The authors found that an index score of 4 or higher was 96 percent accurate in predicting the need for hospitalization and 95 percent accurate in predicting the risk of relapse for patients with severe bronchial asthma. This multifactorial assessment approach may eventually lead to a reduction in the long hours that patients evidencing an acute bronchial asthma episode have to spend in the emergency room before a decision to hospitalize or discharge is made.

## Medication Adherence

A widely prescribed and efficacious treatment for asthma has been the bronchodilator drug theophylline. The value of this drug is that it is slowly absorbed and therefore ideal for continuous therapy. In inpatient studies where adherence is not a variable under patient control, it has been clearly demonstrated that there is a significant correlation between serum theophylline levels and improvement in pulmonary function. However, the clinical usefulness of this pharmacologic agent may be distorted in the outpatient treatment of asthma by a lack of adherence to the medication regimen.

Eney and Goldstein (1976) studied a group of 43 ambulatory asthmatic children, measuring serum and/or salivary theophylline levels. Only 11 percent of the children studied had theophylline levels in the therapeutic range; 65 percent had values below the accepted therapeutic level; and 23 percent had no detectable level of theophylline. In a second group of 47 asthmatic children, Eney and Goldstein (1976) informed the patients that they would be monitoring theophylline levels. This simple intervention resulted in 42 percent of the children studied showing theophylline levels in the therapeutic range; 51 percent had levels below the therapeutic level; and 6.3 percent had zero levels of theophylline. Thus, while improved, medication noncompliance continued to be a major problem.

In a subsequent study, Sublett, Pollard, Kadlec, and Karibo (1979) found subtherapeutic levels in 49 (98 percent) of the 50 ambulatory asthmatic children studied. In a further analysis of the data, however, it was discovered that physician error was the reason for the subtherapeutic theophylline levels in 24.5 percent of the patients; these patients had been treated with inappropriate medications such as antihistamines, decongestants, including over-the-counter preparations, or had been prescribed inadequate doses of bronchodilators. This physician error rather than patient noncompliance contributed to continued symptomatology in this subgroup of patients. Nevertheless, of the appropriately treated group, 75.5 percent had subtherapeutic theophylline levels. Sublett et al. (1979) suggest that inadequate patient (parent) instruction regarding the nature of the illness and the need to take all medications prescribed significantly contributed to the noncompliance rate. Becker, Radius, Rosenstock, Drachman, Schuberth, and Teets (1978) have further indicated the significance of material health beliefs, attitudes, and motivation as contributing factors in the adherence to the theophylline regimen. However, these studies are mainly descriptive; biobehavioral treatment interventions to improve theophylline adherence remain to be empirically demonstrated.

## Biofeedback and Relaxation Therapy

Assessment of pulmonary functioning through the spirometer and peak flow meter is a mandatory evaluation component of any treatment program for asthmatic children. The spirometer measures forced vital capacity (FVC), forced expiratory volume in 1 second ($FEV_1$), and maximum midexpiratory flow rate (MMFR). The FVC refers to the maximum amount of air that can be expired following a maximum inspiration; the $FEV_1$ is the volume of air that is expired during the first second of a forced expiration following an inspiration of maximum capacity. The peak flow meter measures the peak expiratory flow rate (PEFR), which refers to the amount of expiratory air blown in the initial 0.1 second following a maximum inspiration. It is essential to note that symptomatic data on the frequency, duration, and severity of asthma attacks may correlate only marginally with pulmonary functioning (Creer et al., 1982). Therefore, it is mandatory to include pulmonary functioning measures in any evaluation of biofeedback and relaxation therapy effects.

Biofeedback and relaxation training have not proven effective when the criterion of producing *clinically* significant (rather than only *statistically* significant) changes in pulmonary functioning is the measure (see King, 1980, for review). Alexander, Cropp, and Chai (1979), in a well-designed investigation that attempted to correct the methodological problems of previous research in this area, studied the potential effects of relaxation training in the treatment of 14 chronic severely asthmatic children. Each child received 11 sessions, divided into three experimental phases. Phase 1 involved three sessions of simple resting (quiet reading of comic books), in which the effects on pulmonary function of inactivity or resting quietly were assessed as a baseline measure. Phase 2 consisted of five sessions of relaxation training. Phase 3 assessed the effects of relaxation techniques on pulmonary function in comparison with the simple resting in Phase 1. Each pulmonary function assessment consisted of measurement of lung volumes and airway resistance in a whole body plethysmograph, followed by a slow vital capacity and two satisfactory forced vital capacity efforts into a spirometer. Additional measures included a "wheezing score," frontalis electromyographic activity, heart rate, respiratory rate, skin conductance, and digital skin temperature. As stated by Alexander et al. (1979) in the discussion of their findings, "The effects of relaxation on pulmonary mechanics obtained in these severely asthmatic youngsters were consistently unremarkable [p. 32]." Further, "Neither the clinical judgment scores nor the daily asthma data indicated any significant changes supportive of the usefulness of relaxation therapy [p. 33]."

As suggested by Alexander et al. (1979) and Creer et al. (1982), relaxation therapy may be best utilized as a component of systematic desensitization therapy where the reduction of maladaptive anxiety/fear responses secondary to asthma are targeted for intervention rather than the alteration of lung function. This is supported by the findings of Miklich, Renne, Creer, Alexander, Chai, Davis, Hoffman, and Danker-Brown (1977), who taught 19 asthmatic children to associate relaxation with imagined anxiety-provoking situations (i.e., *in vitro* systematic desensitization). The desensitization hierarchies included a list of imaginable scenes that aroused anxiety in the patient, such as: sensations experienced during an asthma attack, situations where the child experienced emotional arousal in relation to having or thinking about asthma, the parents' or child's reported emotional precipitants of symptoms, and nonemotional precipitants such as allergen exposure. The mean amount of improvement in pulmonary functions was statistically significant, but was considered as clinically insignificant. The authors also concluded that since systematic desensitization has been proven successful in the treatment of anxiety disorders (see Wolpe, 1973), its value is for those asthmatics who experience fear and panic at the thought or occurrence of asthma-related symptoms. Well-designed studies targeting *in vivo* anxiety measurement and anxiety reduction *per se* in asthmatics have yet to be conducted.

The research emphasis on the therapeutic modification of pulmonary functions through biofeedback and relaxation therapy has resulted in a lack of systematic attention directed toward what might be the most parsimonious biobehavioral interventions. Three areas of investigation that might be more profitably applicable to asthma comprehensive care are described below.

## Utilization of Inhalation Therapy Equipment

The incorrect utilization of inhalation therapy equipment reduces the maximum benefit derived from the medication it provides. Inhaled medication is often prescribed for use in the initial stage of treatment since the nebulized substances quickly reach the bronchial area and promote rapid bronchodilation. Even with repeated instructions, it is not uncommon for patients to not know how to use the equipment properly. Renne and Creer (1976) sought to improve the teaching method for the utilization of the intermittent positive pressure equipment. This equipment converts liquid bronchodilator medication into inhalable form and delivers it under positive pressure to the patient's airways. Improper care of the equipment impedes the treatment process since the medication fails to reach the site of lung obstruction, resulting in the potential worsening of the asthma attack and the need for additional medications and treatment.

Renne and Creer (1976) delineated three classes of behaviors that needed to occur concurrently for proper use of the equipment: eye fixation, facial posturing, and diaphragmatic breathing. The authors provided a detailed operational definition of each behavioral sequence, sequentially shaping the correct responses in each child. Reinforcement was provided for each sequential correct responding pattern. The intervention was not only highly successful in teaching the asthmatic children correct technique, but it was also found that the children required less symptomatic medication to alleviate their asthma attack after they had been taught to correctly use the equipment. After demonstration of this method of instruction, the authors report that the procedures were utilized by the nursing staff as part of their standard procedure for teaching inhalation equipment techniques to other asthmatic children.

## Behavior Problem Management

Creer (Creer, 1970; Creer, Weinberg, & Molk, 1974) has studied asthmatic children who appear to seek hospital admission and who make an effort to remain hospitalized even with remission of their illness. These children appear to attempt to exaggerate their symptoms in order to be hospitalized and prolong their stay once there, by making complaints that vaguely indicate an asthma attack or other illness. The rationale for the use of a time-out procedure by Creer was that aspects of the hospital environment were reinforcing this inappropriate behavior pattern. By systematically reinforcing the children for socially appropriate behaviors and reducing the reinforcement for inappropriate behaviors, the frequency and duration of unnecessary hospitalizations were dramatically reduced. Similar positive effects on the reduction of inappropriate symptom reporting have been found on both inpatient (Hochstadt, Shepard, & Lulla, 1980) and outpatient (Neisworth & Moore, 1972) studies of asthmatic children, as well as increases in school attendance and academic performance (Creer & Yoches, 1971).

## Self-Management Skills Training

Much of the emphasis of asthma treatment reflects an acute care, emergency intervention approach. As pointed out by Creer et al. (1982), a more parsimonious approach would be to teach the children the skills necessary to prevent the occurrence of asthma attacks and live in a manner that promotes continued good health. In this regard, self-management skills training may make a significant contribution to asthma comprehensive care.

In the self-management skills model, Creer (Creer, 1980; Creer et al., 1982) has delineated several major components: (1) *Self-observation,* which consists of the selected observation of a specific asthma-related biobehavioral pattern and the systematic monitoring of this biobehavioral pattern, such as recording on an asthma diary form the frequency of asthma attacks or the exact amounts and timing of asthma medication ingested. (2) *Self-instructions,* which are the verbal statements the child makes to prompt, direct, or maintain healthy biobehavioral patterns and guide behavior during asthma attacks. (3) *Decision-making skills,* which further guide the decision-making process during asthma attacks, directing the generation of proper biomedical solutions to asthma attack amelioration and treatment sources. Additionally, the children are taught what their limits are regarding physical activity and how to deal with peer pressure to smoke as part of the decision-making process. (4) *Self-induced stimulus or response change* which teaches the child to alter the conditions (stimuli) within his/her environment that may precipitate an attack (e.g., pets or smoke-filled rooms) and to alter their own responses so as to avoid either an asthma attack or a worsening of the episode.

Two studies on self-management skills training for asthmatic children highlight various aspects of Creer's proposed comprehensive program. Taplin and Creer (1978) taught two young children with chronic asthma to use a Wright Peak Flow mini-meter to obtain two daily measurements of peak expiratory flow rate and to record their data on an asthma diary form, along with the occurrence of all asthma attacks. The results of this exploratory investigation demonstrated that patient knowledge of the critical peak expiratory flow rate score lead to a slightly greater than three-fold increase in the predictability of asthma attacks in both children. As suggested by Taplin and Creer (1978), this self-monitoring procedure may be extremely useful as an early indication of an impending asthma attack. This information may lead to early treatment which may reduce the severity of the subsequent attack and consequently reduce unnecessary hospitalization.

Fireman, Friday, Gira, Vierthaler, and Michaels (1981) have conducted the most comprehensive self-management study to date for asthmatic children. This study will be discussed in detail, since it provides a valuable model for future research and clinical practice for many pediatric chronic disorders. The purpose of the study was to determine whether teaching self-management skills to asthmatic children and their parents in an ambulatory setting by a nurse-educator would alter the course of their disease. The specific aims of the study were to reduce the number and severity of asthma attacks, to reduce school absenteeism due to asthma, to reduce emergency room visits and hospitalizations due to asthma, and to develop positive family attitudes toward the management of asthma.

The 26 patients in the study ranged in age from 2 to 14 years, and each had a history of six or more asthmatic episodes. Following an initial evaluation by the pediatric allergist, a management plan was developed for each patient. The plan included avoidance of etiologic factors (stimuli that provoke asthmatic symptoms), appropriate bronchodilator and other drug therapy, and immunotherapy with inhalant allergens for those patients with a documented specific allergic etiology for their asthma and/or allergic rhinitis. The patients were then sequentially assigned to either the study or the comparison group (13 children per group), matched for age. All patients and families, whether in the study or comparison group, were given the same general instructions concerning asthma by the pediatric allergist.

The education curriculum provided by the nurse-educator to the study patients and families included a description of the anatomy of the lung, review of elementary pulmonary physiology and pathophysiology, and an explanation of the factors that can provoke asthma (i.e., allergens, infections, exercise, irritant inhalants, and emotions). The pharmacologic action of the drugs prescribed were explained. The importance of the avoidance and control of provocative stimuli in the patient's environment such as exposure to allergens and other pathogenetic inhalants was stressed, along with potential psychosocial factors that may be detrimental.

The self-management skills taught the children included the following components:

1. observation—being able to observe situations that might lead to an asthma attack;
2. discrimination—being able to discriminate those changes that would indicate an impending or actual asthma attack;
3. decision making—being able to make decisions, to take action themselves, or to get help to prevent or stop an asthma attack;
4. communication—being able to tell parents, doctors, or others what is happening just before and during an asthma attack;
5. self-reliance—having a strong positive attitude about being able to do things that help with asthma self-management.

Parental behavior considered to promote self-management by their children included:

1. positive reinforcement of their child when exhibiting self-management;
2. removal of reinforcement contingent on unnecessary dependent behavior;
3. creating opportunities for the child to initiate and practice self-management behavior.

The assessment of the patient's asthma consisted of the utilization of a symptom and medication diary, review of school attendance records, and tabulation of medical visits to the emergency room and hospitalizations. There was telephone monitoring by the nurse-educator every 2 to 3 months to ensure that the symptoms and medication diary was kept up-to-date and completed. Costs of care were estimated from the use of the emergency room and hospital facilities based on third party reimbursement rates. Family attitudes and knowledge were assessed through a telephone survey conducted at the completion of the investigation (average study duration of 12 months).

The findings of the study are as follows: (1) The study group experienced 1.5 asthma attacks per patient, which was four times less than the average six attacks per patient experienced by the comparison group. An asthma attack was operationally defined as sufficient wheezing to interfere with or alter the patient's daily routine. (2) The study group experienced 3.1 wheezing days per patient per month, which was not statistically significantly less than the 4.6 wheezing days per patient per month noted by the comparision group. (3) The study group was absent an average of 0.5 school days per patient due to asthma, whereas the comparison group was absent an average of 4.6 school days per patient due to asthma. (4) During the investigation the study group had no hospitalizations as contrasted to four hospitalizations (total of 10 hospital days) for the comparison group, at a cost of $2,500 versus zero dollars expended for the study group. (5) The study group required only one emergency room visit, while the comparison group required 13, representing a cost of $35 versus $455, respectively. For each of three age groups (2 to 6 years, 6 to 11 years, and 11 to 14 years), the outcomes were similar to the total group findings, that is, the study patients had fewer asthma attacks, fewer wheezing days, fewer school absences due to asthma, and fewer hospitalizations. Only in the 6-to-11-year-old children were emergency room visits the same in both groups.

Prior to the investigation, all of the children in both groups received frequent bronchodilator therapy, including oral theophylline and oral sympathomimetics. During the investigation, the study group used almost twice as much theophylline and sympathomimetic oral bronchodilators as the comparison group. Since the control of asthmatic symptoms is dependent in large part upon the patient's and family's adherence to an appropriate medication regimen and is an essential component of asthma self-management, Fireman et al. (1981) suggest that the study patients demonstrated greater medication adherence given their greater utilization of the oral bronchodilators. Fireman et al.

(1981) further suggest that the study patients might have initiated drug therapy sooner, since they demonstrated significantly fewer asthmatic attacks even though both groups had almost the same number of wheezing days. Whether enhanced medication adherence may have additionally contributed to less school absenteeism due to asthma and fewer emergency room visits and hospitalizations for asthma in the study group is difficult to document from the investigation's design and awaits further research. Finally, the cost of the additional medication used and the cost of the time spent by the nurse-educator in patient instruction and telephone counseling was 50 percent less than the $2,955 in direct costs related to the comparison group's emergency room visits and hospitalizations. In the study, it was the authors' intent to utilize a nonphysician educator, since previous studies have suggested that a potential reason for patient noncompliance is that the physician's office routine makes it difficult for patients to ask questions of the physician and to receive didactic instructions. The amount of time spent by the nurse-educator on patient instruction was not only cost efficient when contrasted to the comparison group, but may have enhanced patient adherence. As in all well-conducted clinical research, this study suggests a number of areas where future research may lead to further refinement of clinical methods, not only for asthmatic children, but for the management of pediatric chronic disorders in general.

## INSULIN-DEPENDENT JUVENILE DIABETES MELLITUS

Diabetes mellitus is a chronic disorder of carboyhdrate, lipid, and protein metabolism resulting from the inadequate production or utilization of insulin. Insulin, produced by the pancreas, acts primarily at the cell membrane, facilitating the transport of the sugar glucose into the cells. The principal symptoms associated with diabetes mellitus are elevated blood sugar (hyperglycemia), sugar in the urine (glycosuria), excessive urine production (polyuria), excessive thirst (polydipsia), and increase in food intake (polyphagia). The potential long-term consequences of diabetes mellitus include kidney failure, nerve damage, blindness, and a variety of cardiovascular and circulatory problems (Chase & Glasgow, 1976; Kannel & McGee, 1979; Kolata, 1979; White, Waltman, Krupin, & Santiago, 1981). The two main clinical forms of diabetes are insulin-dependent diabetes mellitus and noninsulin-dependent diabetes mellitus. Insulin-dependent diabetes mellitus generally begins during one of two childhood growth spurts: ages 5 to 6 or 10 to 12 (Fleegler, Roger, Drash, Rosenbloom, Travis, & Court, 1979). The insulin-dependent diabetic patient produces little or no endogenous insulin and requires insulin injections on a once or twice daily regimen (Langdon, James, & Sperling, 1981), with close monitoring of plasma insulin essential for potentiating overall health maintenance (Malone & Root, 1981).

## Stress Factors

The results of a number of studies have not shown emotional stress to be of etiologic significance in the onset of diabetes, nor have controlled studies supported the notion that there are psychiatric differences between diabetics and nondiabetics (see Greydanus & Hofmann, 1979; Hauser & Pollets, 1979, for reviews). Sullivan (1979a, 1979b) tested 105 adolescent girls with juvenile diabetes, finding this group to be relatively well adjusted. Stress factors may not be of particular biobehavioral interest in psychosocial issues *per se*, but rather in the physiological effects of stress on diabetes regulation (see Johnson, 1980, for review).

In the nondiabetic individual, stress results in the production of pituitary hormones and catecholamines, which result in a decrease in insulin production and an increase in free fatty acids and blood glucose. With the termination of stress, an increase in insulin production results in a return to normal homeostasis. However, in the diabetic, insulin injection is required to counteract the stress effects. Baker, Barcai, Kaye, and Haque (1969) found that a stress situation produced marked elevations in blood glucose and plasma free fatty acids concentrations in two diabetic children studied. This was interpreted to indicate that endogenous catecholamines play a key role in the mediation of the diabetic condition given their finding that beta adrenergic blockers of epinephrine can attenuate the metabolic consequences of a stress situation. Chase and Jackson (1981) studied 84 children and adolescents with insulin-dependent diabetes mellitus and found a relationship between common stress factors and both long-term and short-term sugar control as measured by glycosylated hemoglobin and fasting serum glucose concentrations, respectively. The authors interpreted their findings to indicate that stressful events, in addition to insulin dosage, exercise, and diet, are significant in diabetes regulation. Thus, the factors that are commonly used to measure diabetes control (i.e., ketones, glucose, free fatty acids) appear to be influenced by life stresses and stress-specific situations (see Tarnow & Silverman, 1981, for review). This would suggest that stress reduction techniques, such as relaxation therapy (e.g., Fowler, Budzynski, & VandenBergh, 1976) may be a useful adjunctive therapeutic modality. Empirical evidence must now be gathered to support this view and to identify potential contraindications (e.g., Seeburg & DeBoer, 1980).

## Therapeutic Adherence

The successful management of insulin-dependent juvenile diabetes mellitus requires strict adherence by the pediatric patient and her parents to a long-term and complex regimen consisting of insulin injections, collection of urine and/or serum specimens, specific diet behaviors, exercise, and hygiene behaviors.

The dosage and frequency that insulin is given depends on the individual patient and the physician prescribing it. It is important that urine specimens be accurately collected and labeled. Blood specimens may also be collected. A well-balanced diet adequate in all the basic essentials is required, that is, carbohydrates, proteins, fats, vitamins, minerals, and fluids. The age, weight, and physical activity of the patient is important in planning an appropriate diet. Because of poor circulation, the feet require special care and need to be kept clean and dry and regularly inspected for cuts or sores.

As reviewed by Simonds (1979), studies of children's and adolescents' adherence to the diabetes regimen indicate that noncompliance is a pervasive and serious problem. The complexity of the regimen provides many occasions for noncompliance, including noncompliant behaviors related to:

1. Insulin injections—omitting injections, giving injections at wrong or irregular time intervals, injecting the incorrect dosage, failing to alternate injection sites;
2. Diet—skipping meals or prescribed snack intervals, eating too much, eating sweets;
3. Urine testing—not testing at all, testing at incorrect times, reporting false results;
4. Exercise—not adjusting insulin dose and diet to changes in activity level;
5. Hygiene—not cleaning and checking feet, teeth, and skin on a regular basis.

In older children and adolescents, a self-management training approach may be the most appropriate orientation for enhancing therapeutic adherence, whereas in younger children, the parents must be intimately involved since they are primarily responsible for administering the program in the home. In all cases, therapeutic adherence must be considered within the context of the family and its facilitative or nonfacilitative effect on patient adherence (Wishner & O'Brien, 1978).

*Patient Education*

Given the complexity of the diabetes daily regimen, pediatric patient and parent education is a necessary first step toward optimizing therapeutic adherence. Lane and Evans (1979) have described a comprehensive patient education program for diabetes management incorporating instructions on the following elements: (1) Physiological measurements, i.e., blood sugar levels, urine glucose levels, urine acetone levels, weight, severe complications (insulin shock and diabetic acidosis), insulin complications, uncontrolled episodes, and symptoms associated with hyperglycemia; (2) Adherence factors, i.e., insulin administration, oral hypoglycemics, urine testing, diet, hygiene, and exercise; (3) Diabetes knowledge, i.e., basic pathophysiology of diabetes, relationship between insulin, diet, and exercise for proper self-management on a daily basis; (4) Utilization of health services, i.e., proper use of clinic appointments, hospitalization, and telephone "hotline"; (5) Psychosocial adaptation, i.e., attitudes, emotions, interpersonal relationships, and coping with the problems of living with diabetes. Although such a comprehensive patient education program serves an essential first step (see Table 6.1), optimizing therapeutic adherence requires further intervention beyond basic education. Initial programs which have attempted to enhance patient performance are described below.

### Self-Injection Regimen

Before a child can be expected to adhere to a daily regimen of self-injection of insulin, he must first be instructed on proper technique and how to control any anxiety that may be related to sticking himself with a needle. Such an instructional program has been described in a preliminary study by Gilbert, Johnson, Spillar, McCallum, Silverstein, and Rosenbloom (1982). The study was designed to investigate the effects of a peer-modeling film on anxiety reduction and skill acquisition of insulin-dependent diabetic children, aged 6 to 9 years, learning to self-inject insulin. The 28 children studied had insulin-dependent diabetes for an average of 2.9 years. The peer-modeling film displayed two children aged 6 to 8 years undergoing self-injection training, culminating in successful self-injection. The film dialogue consisted of information giving, self-descriptions of feelings, appropriate coping statements, self-instructions, and self-praise statements by the children. The primary dependent measures included a state anxiety inventory, a behavior checklist of anxiety-related behaviors, a palmer sweat index (intended as a physiological measure of anxiety), and a 27-item behavior checklist of proper self-injection techniques. Although several methodological problems limit the clinical significance of this preliminary study, it does suggest an approach that may be successfully implemented with further systematic empirical investigation, particularly its use of a behavioral skills test for the objective assessment of proper self-injection techniques.

### Hygiene, Diet, and Urine Testing Regimens

Lowe and Lutzker (1979) described a therapeutic adherence program incorporating parental home monitoring and contingency management procedures with a 9-year-old child with juvenile diabetes. Three behaviors were selected for intervention: adherence to foot care, diet, and urine testing. Although the patient and her mother had previously been given detailed verbal and written instructions on diet, insulin injections, urine testing, and skin care, the patient neglected to test her urine or engage in foot care on a regular basis, as well as neglecting to eat at scheduled times or eat all of the food on her plate.

The specific behavioral components required included: (1) *Urine testing* before breakfast, lunch, dinner, and at bedtime; (2) *Diet*, eating all food on her plate, eating at scheduled times that coincided with insulin injections, and decreasing intake of snacks with a high sugar content; (3) *Foot care*, putting on clean, color-fast socks each day, washing her feet with mild soap, patting them dry, and inspecting them for cuts and bruises every evening. Therapeutic adherence was operationally defined as the completion of a task at the pre-scribed time or within 15 minutes before or after that time. If the child did not complete the task within the time allotted, a "no" was scored for adherence on a daily chart by her mother. For noncompliance, the patient's mother was instructed to prompt her to complete the task.

The intervention consisted of two conditions: (1) A memo condition in which the instructions for completion of the three tasks were written in a memo or pamphlet form in easy-to-understand, step-by-step instructions and given to the child; (2) A token exchange point system in which the child could earn points for adhering to the regimen, which could later be exchanged for daily and weekly reinforcers. Importantly, a pretest was administered in the clinic setting prior to the implementation of the memo and token points conditions in the home to assess whether the child could in fact perform the required behaviors. In fact, there were several skill deficits that needed to be remediated prior to the application of the memo and contingency program. For instance, the child could correctly perform the urine tests for glucose, but not for acetone. She inspected and washed her feet correctly, but vigorously rubbed her feet rather than patting them dry. She understood which foods were needed for her health maintenance, but did not understand the food exchange system or the seriousness of delaying or skipping a meal. Subsequently, the child was taught the correct urine acetone testing procedure and proper feet patting through modeling and behavioral rehearsal. She was instructed on the specifics of proper diet management and then required to explain the food system and safety rules for dieting and to practice selecting sample meals from the food exchange lists utilizing her prescribed diet. After all these skills were achieved, the parent was then given the data sheets (daily chart) and instructed to take baseline data for 1 week on all three behavioral categories.

A multiple-baseline design across foot care behaviors, diet behaviors, and urine testing behaviors was implemented to evaluate the effectiveness of the intervention program. Following baseline, the memos were sequentially given to the child, and she was required to read them aloud. They were then posted in the bathroom or kitchen areas of the home. Adherence was calculated by dividing the number of times the child performed the required behaviors by the total number of prescribed behaviors required to be completed for the day. The results showed that the memo condition was sufficient to promote adherence to the diet regimen, but was ineffective in increasing adherence to the foot care and urine testing regimens. The token exchange point system was highly effective in enhancing adherence to these two regimens. At follow-up assessment, all three regimens were being adhered to at an 100 percent correct performance level.

## Self-Monitoring of Urine Glucose Levels

Patient self-monitoring of urine glucose and/or blood glucose concentrations is an essential component of an overall diabetes self-management regimen (Tattersall & Gale, 1981). Typically, the process involves the regulation of blood glucose levels (assessed in the clinic setting) by the self-monitoring of urine glucose levels (assessed in the home setting), and the adjustment of diet, exercise and/or insulin dose to maintain low blood glucose levels. However, improper or inaccurate testing of urine glucose reduces the potential for the proper adjustment of those factors that influence serum glucose levels. Although urine glucose testing has a relatively poor correlation with blood glucose levels and is a relatively poor prior warning system of potential hypoglycemia (Tattersall & Gale, 1981), the technical difficulties currently associated with home self-monitoring of blood glucose levels need to be resolved before this method of assessment can practically replace urine glucose testing. Given this precaution, the following studies are instructive as initial methods for improving the accuracy of and the adherence to the self-monitoring of glucose levels by the juvenile diabetic.

In a preliminary study, Epstein, Coburn, Becker, Drash, and Siminerio (1980) developed a standardized procedure for the measurement of urine glucose accuracy. The measurement procedure involved providing seven test tubes containing glucose concentrations corresponding to determinations available using the Clinitest method. The Clinitest method consists of mixing urine and water in specified proportions, applying a reagent, and comparing the color of the solution after a designated time interval to a standard color chart for the determination of urine glucose level. For the 81 diabetic children tested, Epstein et al. (1980) found a correct testing score of only 48 percent, with the majority of the errors associated with underestimates of glucose levels. Epstein, Figueroa, Farkas, and Beck (1981) attempted to improve the accuracy of urine glucose testing in the clinic setting in a subsequent study with diabetic children, ages 6 to 16 years, by simply providing systematic feedback for correct or incorrect test findings. This simple training procedure increased testing accuracy from 36 percent to 72 percent. This method may be considered a teaching component in the initial phase of self-management training.

A more comprehensive management approach has recently been described by Epstein, Beck, Figueroa, Farkas, Kazdin, Daneman, and Becker (1981). The study was designed as an initial evaluation of a biobehavioral program to decrease the amount of urine glucose in insulin-dependent diabetic children by regulating eating and exercise behaviors and adjusting insulin dosage through a combination of self-management training for the children and behavioral parent training.

Epstein et al. (1981) assessed a number of self-report and biochemical indices of metabolic control during the course of their study, including: (1) *Daily urine glucose testing using the Clinitest procedure*. The major dependent measure derived from the daily urine testing was percentage of negative tests (i.e., no presence of any glucose in the urine), since the presence of any glucose in the urine suggests that greater than normal glucose concentrations are present in the blood and that the renal threshold has been exceeded. (2) *A marked item technique* was used to measure adherence. The technique involved making placebo Clinitest tablets similar in appearance to the regular Clinitest tablets, but were inert when added to the urine/water test solution. Predetermined quantities of placebo tablets were bottled with a greater number of active Clinitest tablets than would be used and were given to the children. The children had previously received the Epstein et al. (1981) urine testing training. The parents were given a code that identified the correct number of placebos distributed for the week. At the end of each week, the parents tested the tablets remaining in each bottle and added the number of identified placebo tablets to the number of placebo tablets found by the children's testing. Comparison of the number of placebo tablets found by the parents and the children to the actual number of placebos distributed for the week provided a measure of the children's adherence to the urine glucose testing regimen on a weekly basis. (3) *Insulin dosage*, the amount and type of insulin taken by the child was assessed at least on a weekly basis. (4) *Glycoslated hemoglobin measurement* was used as a long-term estimate of blood glucose control. (5) *Fasting plasma glucose*. (6) *Fasting serum cholesterol* and *triglycerides*.

A multiple-baseline across groups design provided the evaluation of the intervention for the 20 families assigned to one of three treatment groups, which differed according to when the treatment was implemented (i.e., after 2, 4, or 6 weeks of baseline data collection). The intervention began with instruction on insulin adjustment and was followed sequentially by training in the regulation of diet and exercise behaviors. All information was provided in modular format for each topic area. Every child was tested on his knowledge of each area subsequent to the teaching session. In order to advance to the next module, the child had to score at least 80 percent on the test. The parents were further instructed in the development of a token exchange point system to reinforce their children's correct self-management behaviors.

During baseline, the children could earn points for the correct measurement of urine glucose, identifying the correct number of placebo tablets, and successfully matching the urine glucose values found by their parents during periodic parental reliability checks on the Clinitest procedure. Once the treatment phase began, the children could also earn points for diabetes control, initially defined as two or more urine glucose tests per day which measured less than 1 percent on the Clinitest 7-step color chart. After 2 weeks on this contingency, the children were required to demonstrate three tests a day of 1 percent or less urine glucose levels before earning token exchange points.

The results of the study indicated a significant increase in the percentage of negative urine glucose tests found sequentially across the three treatment groups within the multiple-baseline design. Additionally, the percent agreement between the number of placebo tablets identified by the children and the number provided was 76 percent. The percent agreement on the Clinitest findings between the parents and their children was 73 percent. However, the findings on the parameters of metabolic control were equivocal. Thus, while the goal of measuring and increasing adherence to the urine testing regimen was successful, there were no clinically significant improvements in the biochemical measures of control, particularly glycoslated hemoglobin, and only a statistically significant reduction in triglyceride levels was found. However, given the relatively short study follow-up period (2.5 months) and the long-term estimate of blood glucose indigenous to glycoslated hemoglobin, subsequent studies must include a substantially longer follow-up period before a definitive statement of concomitant metabolic regulation can be made.

Since the insulin dose did not change across the groups, the authors suggest that a reduction of simple sugars and/or an increase in exercise may have improved the short-term utilization of insulin given the substantial increase in the number of reported negative urine glucose tests. It should be noted that previous work has shown that standardized exercise invariably reduces serum glucose values (Langdon et al., 1981), may affect tissue sensitivity to insulin (Soman, Koivisto, Deibert, Felig, & DeFronzo, 1979) and may in general be instrumental in preventing or retarding certain cardiovascular complications in the diabetic patient (Chase & Glasgow, 1976; Richter, Ruderman, & Schneider, 1981). However, an exercise regimen must be conducted within a comprehensive management program in order to prevent a marked decrease in serum glucose that may lead to symptomatic hypoglycemia and because the metabolic and hormonal response to exercise in insulin-dependent diabetics varies with the degree of metabolic control at the onset of exercise and, more specifically, with the ambient level of insulin (Richter et al., 1981). Thus, in any program that attempts to regulate eating and exercise behaviors, the biobehavioral complexities of comprehensive diabetes management necessitate systematic assessment of both behavioral and biochemical/physiological parameters. In this regard, the Epstein et al. (1981) study represents a step in the correct direction for children, and a recent study by Schafer et al. (1982) provides a similar approach for diabetic adolescents. Further advances in the evaluation of comprehensive care programs for insulin-dependent juvenile diabetes will depend on further advances in behavioral-medical assessment techniques.

# END-STAGE RENAL DISEASE

Renal dysfunction may be divided into two broad categories that are clinically useful: renal insufficiency and renal failure (Merrill, 1978). Renal insufficiency is defined by the inability of the kidney to perform tests of normal functioning, such as the excretion of inulin and paraaminohippurate, as well as the inability to concentrate and dilute filtrate. Renal failure is defined by the inability of the kidney to excrete metabolite at normal plasma levels under conditions of normal intake, or conversely, to retain electrolyte under conditions of normal intake. In essence, renal failure has occurred when the plasma values for urea, creatinine, and phosphate rise significantly, even with a normal intake of precursors for these substances. Plasma values of these substances rise as the ability of the kidney to filter and excrete these substances per unit time decreases (Merrill, 1978).

Various causes of progressive renal dysfunction lead eventually to end-stage or terminal renal failure (Reimold, 1981). A variety of disorders are associated with end-stage renal disease. Either a primary renal process (e.g., glomerulonephritis, pyelonephritis, congenital hypoplasis) or a secondary one (e.g., a kidney affected by a systemic process such a diabetes mellitus or lupus erythematosus) may be at fault. Minor physiological alterations secondary to dehydration, infection, or hypertension may put a borderline patient into uncompensated, clinical uremia (Amend & Vincenti, 1978). Symptoms such as pruritus, generalized malaise, lassitude, forgetfulness, loss of libido, nausea, and altered behavior patterns are subtle complaints in this chronic disorder. Growth failure is a primary complaint in preadolescent patients.

Conservative management is offered until it becomes impossible for patients to continue their typical lifestyle. Conservative management includes dietary, protein, and potassium restriction as well as close attention to sodium balance in the diet so that patients do not retain sodium or become sodium depleted (Merrill, 1979). However, a steady decline in renal function is observed in children with chronic progressive renal failure, terminating in end-stage renal disease (Reimold, 1981). Long-term hemodialysis using semipermeable dialysis membranes is now widely used in the treatment of end-stage renal disease. Treatment is intermittent, usually 5 to 8 hours three times weekly, either in the medical setting or home. With the development of immunosuppression techniques and genetic matching, renal transplantation has become an acceptable alternative to maintenance hemodialysis (Salvatierra & Feduska, 1978). Transplantation reestablishes nearly normal constant body physiology and chemistry without intermittent dialysis and somewhat normalizes the diet. The disadvantages of transplantation include bone marrow suppression, susceptibility to infection, cushingoid body habitus, and the uncertainty of the success of the transplant. Nevertheless, the results of renal transplantation in children are generally good (Martin, 1979).

The advances in medical treatment have resulted in children with end-stage renal disease now being maintained for years on hemodialysis, and some children may now also receive multiple kidney transplantations. These improvements in medical management are reflected in an 89 percent survival rate 5 years after the initial diagnosis (Avner, Harmon, Grupe, Ingelfinger, Eraklis, & Levey, 1981). Given the increased survival rate of these children, then the frequent medical procedures and the prescribed drug and dietary regimens which are associated with hemodialysis and renal transplantation result in long-term lifestyle modifications as would be expected in a chronic disorder (Russo, Bennett, Harmon, & Brown, 1981). With this chronicity, physical and vocational rehabilitation, psychosocial adjustment, and therapeutic adherence to the prescribed long-term and complex medical regimens become salient components of the patient's overall maintenance of health and survival (Gutman, Stead, & Robinson, 1981; Kutner & Cardenas, 1981). From a biobehavioral perspective, therapeutic adherence has received the most systematic attention thus far in the literature.

## Therapeutic Adherence

Noncompliance to the prescribed dietary regimen associated with hemodialysis therapy results in elevated levels of toxic waste products, which produce symptoms of fatigue, dizziness, headache, nausea, and the need for ultrafiltration. Noncompliance to immunosuppressive treatment following renal transplantation may lead to impaired renal function or complete allograft failure. Korsch, Fine, and Negrete (1978) found that of 80 children studied, 17.5 percent (14 patients) were not adhering to immunosuppressive treatment as suspected by diminution in cushingoid features, sudden unexplained weight loss, or unexplained change in the patients' renal function on routine follow-up observations. Of these 14 patients, eight (57 percent) lost their allograft, and six (43 percent) evidenced decreased allograft function. The possibility of improving adherence by working with the family in specific areas of family functioning has been suggested as a potential method in need of investigation (Steidl, Finkelstein, Wexler, Feigenbaum, Kitsen, Kliger, & Quinland, 1980).

### Hemodialysis Regimen

Given that the instructional strategies utilized by a clinician may facilitate therapeutic adherence (see Chapter 6), the study by Lira and Mlott (1976) provides a methodology that may enhance adherence to the hemodialysis regimen. Lira and Mlott (1976) developed a home dialysis training program designed to increase the active participation of the patient in his hemodialysis treatment. Ten patients were assigned either to the experimental training group or a traditional training control group. Control group patients received a customary method of dialysis training outlined by typewritten procedures for the Drake Willock hemodialysis #4019 machine. Each of the procedures was divided into a number of steps that could be concisely defined and easily scored as 1 (indicating successfully mastered) or 0 (indicating that further training was needed). Patients in the experimental group were provided with a Hemodialysis Training Progress Chart, which was a behavior checklist of 65 specific steps required for proper hemodialysis. The patient was required to achieve mastery of all preceding steps before progressing to the next training step.

During each training session, the nurse-instructor explained those steps to be learned. The patient was instructed to perform all the procedural steps previously rehearsed, and the nurse scored each step on the chart in the presence of the patient. Each step was designed to be small enough to be learned readily and operationally defined, so as to be easily scored for mastery. Social reinforcement and corrective feedback regarding progress was provided on an ongoing basis. The number of training sessions required was determined by the amount of training necessary to master each of the steps comprising the entire procedure. Mastery was defined as a perfect score (100 percent correct responding) on the Hemodialysis Training Progress Chart. When mastery was achieved, the patients conducted the hemodialysis regimen in their home. One week after the completion of training, the patients were again tested on the behavior checklist. Failure on any step necessitated a review of the procedure. A number of failures necessitated reconsidering the patient's readiness to administer hemodialysis therapy at home (see Chapter 9 for a similar approach to hemophilia factor replacement therapy training).

As reported by Lira and Mlott (1976), the nursing staff noted a number of distinct advantages to the behavioral training method: (1) The clearly defined step-by-step procedure provided a readily observable account of the progress of the patient, identifying both weak areas and mastered steps. (2) The training sequence was provided in easily manageable learning increments so that the patients were not overwhelmed by the entire procedure. (3) The ongoing documented feedback regarding task mastery provided the staff with a systematic and immediate assessment of the effectiveness of their teaching efforts. (4) The behavioral training methodology facilitated the learning process so that the experimental group demonstrated an average training time of 36 days while the traditional training group required 47 days. Finally, the patients who received the behavioral training reported assuming greater participation in and responsibility for the home-based hemodialysis program. They also felt more confident in their ability to successfully perform the hemodialysis regimen because of the step-by-step approach where learning increments were readily integrated into the complete regimen based on successive success at each step.

*Dietary Regimen*

The prescribed diet for the child on maintenance hemodialysis is both a complex and long-term regimen, requiring modification of dietary protein, sodium, fluid, potassium, and phosphorus. The goals for the nutritional management of the child on maintenance hemodialysis include the following: (1) to ingest sufficient protein for positive nitrogen balance without causing uremic toxicity; (2) to eat enough nonprotein calories to meet energy needs and promote protein sparing; (3) to prevent excessive shifts in fluid status; and (4) to maintain electrolyte balance (Cadwallader, 1981). One of the major problems for children on hemodialysis is the provision of adequate nutrients and calories to maintain normal growth. The required restrictions on dietary potassium, protein, and fluid intake are calculated on the basis of body weight, so that the dietary regimen for those children who are small in size is even more restrictive than for adults. Children who are noncompliant to their prescribed dietary regimen are at increased risk for congestive heart failure, hypertension, bone disease, fluid overload uremia, and excessive serum potassium. While several studies with adult patients on dietary regimen adherence have been conducted (e.g., Barnes, 1976; Cummings, Becker, Kirscht, & Levin, 1981; Hart, 1979; Hartman & Becker, 1978), the following study with children exemplifies the current status in pediatric dietary adherence.

Magrab and Papadopoulou (1977) designed a token economy management program to promote adherence to the prescribed dietary regimen for four children, aged 11 to 18 years, on maintenance hemodialysis. All the children received dialysis two to three times per week. Adherence to dietary restriction was a serious and continuous problem for three of the four children, even though they had received numerous previous attempts at promoting therapeutic adherence (e.g., dietary instructions, parent counseling, medical consultation, increased staff attention).

Three dependent measures were targeted for assessment: weight, blood urea nitrogen (BUN), and serum potassium. Weight was measured pre- and post-dialysis on the same scale, at the same time of day, and with the same amount of clothing worn. Weight gain between dialysis sessions was considered to be a primary measure of fluid intake. An acceptable weight gain between dialysis sessions was defined as two pounds, representing the amount of fluid that could safely be dialyzed for each subject. BUN and potassium serum levels were also routinely obtained through the dialysis lines, without requiring further venipuncture of the child. A BUN level of 100 and a potassium level of 6 were defined as acceptable. Each child was informed of the new dietary program by the head nurse, and an individualized reinforcement list was developed for each child (e.g., toys, games, trips, craft projects, television time at the hospital, puzzles, comic books, model car and airplane kits). Eighteen points were designated equivalent to approximately $2.00 of conversion value for purchasing items from the reinforcement list.

Before beginning the program, each child was instructed by the dietician on the requirements for their special diet. Each child received a designated number of points for maintaining acceptable levels of weight (2 to 3 points), potassium (2 to 3 points), and BUN (2 to 3 points), depending on the number of days per week he received dialysis, up to a maximum of 18 points per week. Thus, children on dialysis twice a week received 3 points for each dependent measure, while children on dialysis three times per week received 2 points per dependent measure. A reinforcement chart was posted in the hemodialysis unit to further encourage adherence through social reinforcement by peers and staff. At the end of a week, each child reviewed the number of points earned as recorded on the reinforcement chart and then exchanged these points for the items on the reinforcement list (points could also be saved and exchanged after several weeks for more expensive items).

Baseline measures showed an average weight gain between dialysis for all four children of 2.18 pounds, with a range of 1.13 to 3.91 pounds. During the token economy program, average weight gain was 0.97 pounds, with a range of 0.55 to 1.26 pounds. BUN and potassium levels remained at acceptable levels for those children whose baseline levels initially were acceptable and were regulated to within acceptable levels for those children whose initial levels were not appropriate. These initial findings need to be replicated with larger populations of children with end-stage renal disease.

# REFERENCES

Alexander, A.B., Cropp, G.J.A., & Chai, H. Effects of relaxation training on pulmonary mechanics in children with asthma. *Journal of Applied Behavior Analysis*, 1979, **12**, 27–35.

Amend, W.J.C., & Vincenti, F. Chronic renal failure and dialysis. In D.R. Smith (Ed.), *General Urology*. Los Altos, CA: Lange, 1978.

Avner, E.D., Harmon, W.E., Grupe, W.E., Ingelfinger, J.R., Eraklis, A.J., & Levey, R.H. Mortality of chronic hemodialysis and renal transplantation in pediatric end-stage renal disease. *Pediatrics*, 1981, **67**, 412–416.

Baker, L., Barcai, A., Kaye, R., & Haque, N. Beta adrenergic blockage and juvenile diabetes: Acute studies and long-term therapeutic trial: Evidence for the role of catecholamines in mediating diabetic decompensation following emotional arousal. *Journal of Pediatrics*, 1969, **75**, 19–29.

Barnes, M.R. Token economy control of fluid overload in a patient receiving hemodialysis. *Journal of Behavior Therapy and Experimental Psychiatry*, 1976, **7**, 305–306.

Becker, M.H., Radius, S.M., Rosenstock, I.M., Drachman, R.H., Schuberth, K.C., & Teets, K.C. Compliance with a medical regimen for asthma: A test of the Health Belief Model. *Public Health Reports*, 1978, **93**, 268–277.

Cadwallader, A. Dietary therapy for the individual on hemodialysis. *Behavioral Medicine Update*, 1981, **3**, 12–14.

Chase, H.P., & Glasgow, A.M. Juvenile diabetes mellitus and serum lipids and lipoprotein levels. *American Journal of Diseases of Children*, 1976, **130**, 1113–1117.

Chase, H.P., & Jackson, G.G. Stress and sugar control in children with insulin-dependent diabetes mellitus. *Journal of Pediatrics*, 1981, **98**, 1011–1013.

Creer, T.L. The use of a time-out from positive reinforcement procedure with asthmatic children. *Journal of Psychosomatic Research*, 1970, **14**, 117–120.

Creer, T.L. Self-management behavioral strategies for asthmatics. *Behavioral Medicine*, 1980, **7**, 14–24.

Creer, T.L., Renne, C.M., & Chai, H. The application of behavioral techniques to childhood asthma. In D.C. Russo & J.W. Varni (Eds.), *Behavioral Pediatrics: Research and Practice*. New York: Plenum Press, 1982.

Creer, T.L., Weinberg, E., & Molk, L. Managing a hospital behavior problem: Malingering. *Journal of Behavior Therapy and Experimental Psychiatry*, 1974, **5**, 259–262.

Creer, T.L., & Yoches, C. The modification of an inappropriate behavioral pattern in asthmatic children. *Journal of Chronic Diseases*, 1971, **24**, 507–513.

Cummings, K.M., Becker, M.H., Kirscht, J.P., & Levin, N.W. Intervention strategies to improve compliance with medical regimens by ambulatory hemodialysis patients. *Journal of Behavioral Medicine*, 1981, **4**, 111–127.

Eney, R.D., & Goldstein, E.D. Compliance of chronic asthmatics with oral administration of theophylline as measured by serum and salivary levels. *Pediatrics*, 1976, **57**, 513–517.

Epstein, L.H., Beck, S., Figueroa, J., Farkas, G., Kazdin, A.E., Daneman, D., & Becker, D. The effects of targeting improvements in urine glucose on metabolic control in children with insulin dependent diabetes. *Journal of Applied Behavior Analysis*, 1981, **14**, 365–375.

Epstein, L.H., Coburn, P.L., Becker, D., Drash, A., & Siminerio, L. Measurement and modification of the accuracy of determinations of glucose concentrations. *Diabetes Care*, 1980, **3**, 535–536.

Epstein, L.H., Figueroa, J., Farkas, G.M., & Beck, S. The short-term effects of feedback on accuracy of urine glucose determinations in insulin-dependent diabetic children. *Behavior Therapy*, 1981, **12**, 560–564.

Fireman, P., Friday, G.A., Gira, C., Vierthaler, W.A., & Michaels, L. Teaching self-management skills to asthmatic children and their parents in an ambulatory care setting. *Pediatrics*, 1981, **68**, 341–348.

Fischl, M.A., Pitchenik, A., & Gardner, L.B. An index predicting relapse and need for hospitalization in patients with actue bronchial asthma. *New England Journal of Medicine*, 1981, **305**, 783–789.

Fleegler, F.M., Rogers, K.D., Drash, A., Rosenbloom, A.C., Travis, L.B., & Court, J.M. Age, sex, and season of onset of juvenile diabetes in different geographic areas. *Pediatrics*, 1979, **63**, 374–379.

Fowler, J.E., Budzynski, & VandenBergh, R.L. Effects of an EMG biofeedback relaxation program on the control of diabetes. *Biofeedback and Self-Regulation*, 1976, **1**, 105–112.

Gilbert, B.O., Johnson, S.B., Spillar, R., McCallum, M., Silverstein, J.H., & Rosenbloom, A. The effects of a peer-modeling film on children learning to self-inject insulin. *Behavior Therapy*, 1982, **13**, 186–193.

Greydanus, D.E., & Hofmann, A.D. Psychological factors in diabetes mellitus: A review of the literature with emphasis on adolescence. *American Journal of Diseases of Children*, 1979, **133**, 1061–1066.

Gutman, R.A., Stead, W.W., & Robinson, R.R. Physical activity and employment status of patients on maintenance dialysis. *New England Journal of Medicine*, 1981, **304**, 309–313.

Hart, R.R. Utilization of token economy within a chronic dialysis unit. *Journal of Consulting and Clinical Psychology*, 1979, **47**, 646–648.

Hartman, P.E., & Becker, M.H. Noncompliance with prescribed regimen among chronic hemodialysis patients: A method of prediction and educational diagnosis. *Dialysis and Transplantation*, 1978, **7**, 978–989.

Hauser, S.T., & Pollets, D. Psychological aspects of diabetes mellitus: A critical review. *Diabetes Care*, 1979, **2**, 277–282.

Hochstadt, N.J., Shepard, J., & Lulla, S.H. Reducing hospitalizations of children with asthma. *Journal of Pediatrics*, 1980, **97**, 1012–1015.

Johnson, S.B. Psychosocial factors in juvenile diabetes: A review. *Journal of Behavioral Medicine*, 1980, **3**, 95–116.

Kannel, W.B., & McGee, D.L. Diabetes and cardiovascular risk factors: The Framingham study. *Circulation*, 1979, **59**, 8–13.

King, N.J. The behavioral management of asthma and asthma-related problems in children: A critical review of the literature. *Journal of Behavioral Medicine*, 1980, **3**, 169–189.

Kolata, G.B. Blood sugar and the complications of diabetes. *Science*, 1979, **203**, 1098–1099.

Korsch, B.M., Fine, R.N., & Negrete, V.F. Noncompliance in children with renal transplants. *Pediatrics*, 1978, **61**, 872–876.

Kutner, N.G., & Cardenas, D.D. Rehabilitation status of chronic renal disease patients undergoing dialysis: Variations by age category. *Archives of Physical Medicine and Rehabilitation*, 1981, **62**, 626–631.

Lane, D.S., & Evans, D. Measures and methods in evaluating patient education programs for chronic illness. *Medical Care*, 1979, **17**, 30–42.

Langdon, D.R., James, F.D., & Sperling, M.A. Comparison of single- and split-dose insulin regimens with 24-hour monitoring. *Journal of Pediatrics*, 1981, **99**, 854–861.

Lira, F.T., & Mlott, S.R. A behavioral approach to hemodialysis training. *Journal of American Association of Nephrology Nurses and Technicians*, 1976, **3**, 180–188.

Lowe, K., & Lutzker, J.R. Increasing compliance to a medical regimen with a juvenile diabetic. *Behavior Therapy*, 1979, **10**, 57–64.

Magrab, P.R., & Papadopoulou, Z.L. The effect of a token economy on dietary compliance for children on hemodialysis. *Journal of Applied Behavior Analysis*, 1977, **10**, 573–578.

Malone, J.I., & Root, A.W. Plasma free insulin concentrates: Keystone to effective management of diabetes mellitus in children. *Journal of Pediatrics*, 1981, **99**, 862–867.

Martin, A.J., McLennan, L.A., Landau, L.I., & Phelan, P.D. The natural history of childhood asthma to adult life. *British Medical Journal*, 1980, **280**, 1397–1400.

Martin, D.C. Renal transplantation. In J.H. Harrison, R.F. Gittes, A.D. Perlmutter, T.A. Stamey, & P.C. Walsh (Eds.), *Campbell's Urology*. Vol. 3. Philadelphia: W.B. Saunders, 1979.

Merrill, J.P. Normal and abnormal renal function. In J.H. Harrison, R.F. Gittes, A.D. Perlmutter, T.A. Stamey, & P.C. Walsh (Eds.), *Campbell's Urology*. Vol. 1. Philadelphia: W.B. Saunders, 1978.

Merrill, J.P. The management of renal failure. In J.H. Harrison, R.F. Gittes, A.D. Perlmutter, T.A. Stamey, & P.C. Walsh (Eds.), *Campbell's Urology*. Vol. 3. Philadelphia: W.B. Saunders, 1979.

Miklich, D.R., Renne, C.M., Creer, T.L., Alexander, A.B., Chai, H., Davis, M.H., Hoffman, A., & Danker-Brown, P. The clinical utility of behavior therapy as an adjunctive treatment for asthma. *Journal of Allergy and Clinical Immunology*, 1977, **60**, 285–294.

Neisworth, J.T., & Moore, F. Operant treatment of asthmatic responding with the parent as therapist. *Behavior Therapy*, 1972, **3**, 95–99.

Reimold, E.W. Chronic progressive renal failure: Rate of progression monitored by change of serum creatinine concentrate. *American Journal of Diseases of Children*, 1981, **135**, 1039–1043.

Renne, C.M., & Creer, T.L. Training children with asthma to use inhalation therapy equipment. *Journal of Applied Behavior Analysis*, 1976, **9**, 1–11.

Richter, E.A., Ruderman, N.B., & Schneider, S.H. Diabetes and exercise. *American Journal of Medicine*, 1981, **70**, 201–209.

Russo, D.C., Bennett, A.K., Harmon, W.E., & Brown, D. Behavioral medicine issues in the management of children with end-stage renal disease. *Behavioral Medicine Update*, 1981, **3**, 15–19.

Salvatierra, O., & Feduska, N.J. Renal transplantation. In D.R. Smith (Ed.), *General Urology*. Los Altos, CA: Lange, 1978.

Schafer, L.C., Glasgow, R.E., & McCaul, K.D. Increasing the adherence of diabetic adolescents. *Journal of Behavioral Medicine*, 1982, **5**, 353–362.

Seeburg, K.N., & DeBoer, K.F. Effects of EMG biofeedback on diabetes. *Biofeedback and Self-Regulation*, 1980, **5**, 289–293.

Simonds, J.F. Emotions and compliance in diabetic children. *Psychosomatics*, 1979, **20**, 544–551.

Soman, V.R., Koivisto, V.A., Deibert, D., Felig, P., & DeFronzo, R.A. Increased insulin sensitivity and insulin binding to monocytes after physical training. *New England Journal of Medicine*, 1979, **301**, 1200–1204.

Steidl, J.H., Finkelstein, F.O., Wexler, J.P., Feigenbaum, H., Kitsen, J., Kliger, A.S., & Quinlan, D.M. Medical condition, adherence to treatment regimens, and family functioning: Their interactions in patients receiving long-term dialysis treatment. *Archives of General Psychiatry*, 1980, **37**, 1025–1027.

Sublett, J.L., Pollard, S.J., Kadlec, G.J., & Karibo, J.M. Noncompliance in asthmatic children: A study of theophylline levels in a pediatric emergency room population. *Annals of Allergy*, 1979, **43**, 95–97.

Sullivan, B.J. Adjustment in diabetic adolescent girls: I. Development of the diabetic adjustment scale. *Psychosomatic Medicine*, 1979, **41**, 119–126. (a)

Sullivan, B.J. Adjustment in diabetic adolescent girls: II. Adjustment, self-esteem, and depression in diabetic adolescent girls. *Psychosomatic Medicine*, 1979, **41**, 127–138. (b)

Taplin, P.S., & Creer, T.L. A procedure for using peak expiratory flow rate data to increase the predictability of asthma episodes. *Journal of Asthma Research*, 1978, **16**, 15–19.

Tarnow, J.D., & Silverman, S.W. The psychophysiologic aspects of stress in juvenile diabetes mellitus. *International Journal of Psychiatry in Medicine*, 1981, **11**, 25–44.

Tattersall, R., & Gale, E. Patient self-monitoring of blood glucose and refinements of conventional insulin treatment. *American Journal of Medicine*, 1981, **70**, 177–182.

White, N.H., Waltman, S.R., Krapin, T., & Santiago, J.V. Reversal of neuropathic and gastrointestinal complications related to diabetes mellitus in adolescents with improved metabolic control. *Journal of Pediatrics*, 1981, **99**, 41–45.

Wishner, W.J., & O'Brien, M.S. Diabetes and the family. *Medical Clinics of North America*, 1978, **62**, 849–856.

Wolpe, J. *The Practice of Behavior Therapy.* New York: Pergamon Press, 1973.

# Part V

## Behavioral and Psychosocial Problems

# Behavioral and Psychosocial Problems: Behavior Problems, Biobehavioral Disorders, Social Skills Deficits

## BEHAVIOR PROBLEMS

Common behavior problems include noncompliance, temper tantrums, aggression, hyperactivity, mealtime problems, and bedtime problems (see Christophersen & Abernathy, 1982, for review). Behavioral parent training is an essential component in the treatment of most behavior problems in the childhood population (see Christophersen, 1982, for review).

### Noncompliance

Forehand and McMahon (1981) in their text *Helping The Noncompliant Child* provide an excellently detailed description of an empirically derived set of practical guidelines for assessing and treating noncompliant children within a behavioral parent training model.

Varni (1980a) employed a behavioral parent training approach to the management of home and school behavior problems with a 4½-year-old hemophilic child. In discussion with the child's mother, two classes of behavior were identified for home intervention: appropriate and inappropriate. The inappropriate behaviors category included noncompliance, temper tantrums, threatening language, answering back, and hitting peers. Appropriate behaviors included two household chores: making his bed in the morning and putting his clothes away. The mother also reported that the child's schoolteacher had been complaining of a high rate of misbehavior. Ten appropriate classroom behaviors were identified for intervention, including following directions, not physically disturbing others, staying in seat, not talking inappropriately, paying attention, and similar classroom-related behaviors (see Schumaker, Hovell, & Sherman, 1977).

For the home intervention, the target behaviors were written on a home contingency program chart (Table 12.1). The chart was placed on a wall and provided for the daily monitoring of appropriate and inappropriate behaviors. The occurrence of one of the appropriate behaviors resulted in a + 1 being placed on the chart, which could be exchanged within the developed point system for a preferred activity from a list of previously agreed upon reinforcers (e.g., special television program, time with particular toys, trip to the movies). Inappropriate behaviors resulted in a − 1 being placed on the chart, which was

Table 12.1.    Home Contingency Program Chart.

| Name: | | | Week of: | | | | |
|---|---|---|---|---|---|---|---|
| Target Behavior | Sun | Mon | Tue | Wed | Thurs | Fri | Sat |
| | | | | | | | |
| | | | | | | | |
| | | | | | | | |
| | | | | | | | |
| | | | | | | | |
| | | | | | | | |
| | | | | | | | |
| | | | | | | | |
| | | | | | | | |

Daily Total =

Total for Week:

consequated with a 10-minute time-out (chair facing the corner) (see Drabman & Jarvie, 1977; Leitenberg, 1965 for reviews) or a response cost contingency (the loss of a daily preferred activity, such as a preferred television program or to bed earlier than usual, separate from the items on the reinforcement list). Additionally, the mother was instructed to read Patterson's parent manual, *Families: Applications of Social Learning to Family Life,* for further instructions on behavioral parenting techniques.

For the school intervention, the ten classroom behaviors were written on a behavior checklist within an occurred/did not occur format (see Schumaker et al., 1977 for the teacher checklist). The checklist was completed daily by the teacher, signed, and then returned by the child to his mother (returning the signed checklist was also consequated). A home-based contingencies program was developed (see Schumaker et al., 1977) whereby a previously agreed upon daily occurrence of six appropriate behaviors on the checklist resulted in a + 1 being placed on the home contingency chart, with less than that number resulting in a − 1. The criterion number of appropriate behaviors for a + 1 was gradually increased to nine of ten appropriate classroom behaviors as the child succeeded at each lower criterion (shaping). These points were then consequated in the same manner as the home behaviors.

As shown in Figure 12.1, following the 3-week baseline assessment in the home, the intervention resulted in a gradual and steady increase in appropriate behaviors accompanied by a similar decrease in inappropriate behaviors. Follow-up over a 12-month period showed the maintenance of the treatment gains. The intervention demonstrated a similar positive effect in the school setting, with treatment gains maintained over a 7-month period after the initial baseline and treatment phases, with the follow-up at 6 and 7 months conducted during the first 2 months of first grade, after a 2½-month vacation.

## Hyperactivity

The constellation of behaviors associated with the term *hyperactivity* typically includes impulsivity, overactivity, short-attention span, and aggression (O'Leary & Steen, 1982). In the home setting, behavioral parent training is the modal intervention approach (e.g., Firestone & Witt, 1982). Interventions in the school setting have involved a teacher-controlled contingency program (Ayllon, Layman, & Kandel, 1975) and more recently, a self-regulation approach (Barkley, Copeland, & Sivage, 1980; Varni & Henker, 1979). Additionally, interpersonal aggression has been treated using a social skills training approach (Bornstein, Bellack, & Hersen, 1980). The primary theme of many of these interventions is the provision of a structured environment whereby the hyperactive child can clearly recognize the consequences for his behavior through reinforcement for appropriate behavior and aversive contingencies (e.g., time-out, response cost) for inappropriate behaviors.

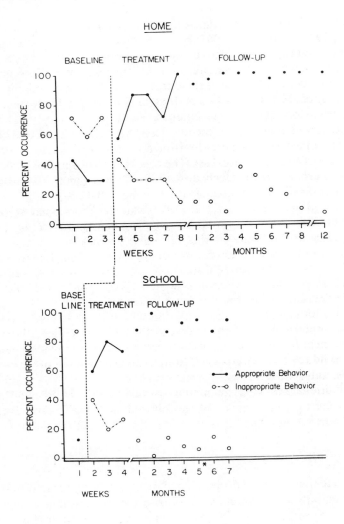

Fig. 12.1.   Percent occurrences of appropriate and inappropriate behaviors across baseline, treatment, and follow-up in the home and school. The asterisk on the school graph represents a 2½-month summer vacation and the beginning of first grade (6- and 7-month follow-up assessments).

Source: Reprinted with permission from J.W. Varni. Behavior therapy in the management of home and school behavior problems with a 4½-year-old hemophilic child. *Journal of Pediatric Psychology,* 1980, 5, 17–23.

## Mealtime Behavior Problems

Bernal (1972) taught behavioral techniques to the mother of a 4-year-old child who refused to feed herself or eat table foods. The child would eat only strained foods which consisted exclusively of oatmeal, cottage cheese and occasionally some types of fruit; however, she refused to eat other fruits, strained vegetables, or meats as well as any regular adult table foods. Because of her restricted food intake, her pediatrician had found it necessary to prescribe multivitamins to maintain the child's physical health.

The goal of the treatment program was for the child to eat a variety of basic table food groups, including meats, cereals, dairy products, fruits and vegetables by self-feeding. To accomplish the goal of eating table foods, a shaping program was initiated to teach the parents to gradually exert increasing control over the child's eating habits rather than to require an abrupt shift from her initial eating pattern to the final goal.

Baseline observations showed that the child received social attention for such behaviors as playing with the baby food, chatting, and messiness, all of which interfered with eating. Consequently, the first step of the program involved training the mother to withhold her social attention (smiling, chatting pleasantly, looking at the child) until the child had put the food in her mouth and had swallowed it. At this first step, the child received contingent social reinforcement for self-feeding preferred foods. The next step involved allowing the child to eat a preferred food only if she first ate nonpreferred strained vegetables and fruits. The third step consisted of using television viewing time as an additional reinforcer for eating new table foods. This shaping program resulted in the child subsequently eating the table foods served to the rest of her family, with her self-feeding of the family meal being consequated with dessert.

Hatcher (1979) worked with a 2-year-old child who refused to accept solid foods, subsisting on milk, juices, and a few strained foods, resulting in a gradual weight loss. The treatment consisted of making a preferred food (liquids) contingent on the eating of a nonpreferred food (solid foods). Mealtimes were timed for 30 minutes, following which all food and drink was removed. Social reinforcement was contingent on appropriate eating, with food refusal consequated by withdrawal of social attention and the preferred food. The intervention resulted in a return to normal weight gain. Additional studies have reported success using similar procedures, including social reinforcement and preferred foods contingent on the ingestion of nonpreferred foods (Palmer, Thompson, & Linscheid, 1975), social reinforcement and manual guidance (Reidy, 1979), social reinforcement and a token reinforcement program (Fox & Roseen, 1977) and a treatment package consisting of social reinforcement, a token reinforcement program, and gradually requiring the attainment of eating a meal within 20 minutes (Sanok & Ascione, 1978).

McMahon and Forehand (1978) assessed the effectiveness of a brochure in teaching mothers to modify their preschool children's inappropriate mealtime behaviors. A mealtime behavior checklist was developed, which was divided into two general categories: (1) inappropriate eating behaviors, e.g., spilling food onto the table and/or floor on purpose, playing with food, eating food with fingers, spitting out food; (2) misconduct, e.g., not coming to the table when called, leaving table before end of meal, stealing food, throwing food, banging utensils, hitting others at table, whining or crying, screaming or yelling. The intervention consisted of the use of differential attention and time-out to reduce the children's inappropriate mealtime behaviors. Appropriate mealtime behaviors resulted in social reinforcement (praise, attention). When inappropriate mealtime behavior occurred, the parent was instructed to issue a command to stop the behavior. If compliance to the command did not occur, the parent was instructed to place the child in a 2-minute time-out. The behavioral parent training intervention resulted in substantial decreases in inappropriate mealtime behaviors for all the children.

## Bedtime Behavior Problems

The two most common bedtime behavior problems are crying and getting out of bed at night (Christophersen, 1982). Rapoff, Christophersen, and Rapoff (1982) studied six children (mean, 36 months of age, range 24 to 54 months) whose parents reported that the children cried, called out to them frequently, and got out of bed. Two child and one parent verbal behaviors were defined and recorded on a cassette tape recorder placed in the child's bedroom at bedtime. The two child verbal behaviors recorded were: (1) Cry/whine, operationally defined as when the child complained, demanded something, or called out to the parent in a whining tone of voice; and (2) child vocalization, defined as when the child was talking (without crying or whining), singing, humming, or laughing. Parent verbal behavior was scored when the parents said anything to the child.

Two separate written guidelines on how to manage crying at bedtime and getting out of bed were given to the parents so they could refer to them after the clinic visit (see Christophersen, 1982). The management procedures combined extinction and mild punishment:

1. A reasonable time for bedtime was established and the child was put to bed at that time on a consistent basis.
2. Approximately 30 minutes prior to the child's bedtime the parents were instructed to have their children engage in quiet activities (e.g., reading) rather than active (roughhousing) play.
3. Following the normal bedtime routine (e.g., bedtime story, kisses, bathroom), the parents were instructed to say goodnight to their child, turn off the lights, and leave the child's room.

4. If the child cried, called out to them, or vocalized in any way, the parents were asked to ignore this behavior (extinction).
5. If the child left her room the parents were instructed to administer one swat and without talking, return their child to bed. For the parents who objected to the swat, they were asked to return their child to bed without talking.

The parents were warned that their child would be very disruptive for the first few nights that the procedures were in effect, but that they were to consistently employ the recommended procedures. The intervention resulted in three of the six children exhibiting low levels of crying or whining at a stable rate following treatment. The three children whose bedtime problem behavior did not decrease appeared to continue to receive intermittent reinforcement (attention) from their parents, suggesting that parental noncompliance to the treatment instructions was instrumental in maintaining their children's bedtime behavior problems.

## BIOBEHAVIORAL DISORDERS

Biobehavioral disorders not specifically covered in previous chapters include sleep disorders, some forms of habit disorders, and chronic rumination and vomiting.

## Sleep Disorders

The prevalence of pediatric sleep disturbance has been found to be as high as 50 percent in one study (Price, Coates, Thoresen, & Grinstead, 1978). In preschool and school-age children, the most common disorders of sleep include nightmares, night terrors, sleepwalking, sleeptalking, and certain patterns of enuresis (Anders, Carskadon, & Dement, 1980). In adolescents, additional sleep disorders exhibited include disorders of initiating and maintaining sleep (the insomnias), disorders of excessive somnolence (hypersomnias), and dyssomnias associated with disruptions of the 24-hour sleep-wake cycle (Anders et al., 1980).

### Nightmares and Night Terrors

Nightmares are nocturnal episodes of intense anxiety and fear associated with vivid mental recollections. They occur during REM sleep, typically late in the night (Anders et al., 1980). Nightmares are common in children and may persist into adulthood (Kales, Soldatos, Caldwell, Charney, Kales, Markel, & Cadieux, 1980).

Cellucci and Lawrence (1978) worked with college undergraduate students who reported an average of 3.2 nightmares per week during baseline. The major themes of the nightmares consisted of threat of physical harm to self, injury and death of others, interpersonal conflicts, fear of harm from animals, and other anxiety-related themes. As a guideline, nightmares were operationally defined as subjectively disturbing or anxiety-provoking dreams from which a person usually awakens. The intervention consisted of a systematic desensitization procedure, whereby a hierarchy for each subject was individualized in terms of the disturbing themes and images in that subject's nightmares. The themes and images on the hierarchy were then systematically paired with relaxation training, resulting in a significant decrease in the frequency of nightmares, averaging 0.6 nightmares per week during the seventh week of treatment.

Framer and Sanders (1980) treated a 13-year-old with a history of sleeptalking, sleepwalking, and nightmares dating back to early childhood, averaging four episodes of sleep disturbance per week according to parental report. The treatment did not specifically target the patient's disturbed sleep *per se,* but rather attempted to reduce daytime stress that was occurring because of conflict between the patient and his parents over parental rules, his rights, and what constituted reasonable behavior for a child of his age. The intervention consisted of developing a contingency contract to increase the patient's compliance with parental requests in exchange for an increase in the number and type of activities and privileges granted to the patient by his parents. A 1-year follow-up evaluation evidenced only one incident of sleep disturbance during a 3-week assessment. This approach of reducing daytime stress is consistent with the findings by Kales et al. (1980) that 90 percent of their adult subjects reported that daytime stress increased the frequency of their nightmares.

Night terrors (*pavor nocturnus*) are found with greatest frequency in preschool-age children (Anders et al., 1980). Night terrors are not associated with dream recall; instead, the child suddenly sits upright in bed, screams, and has no recollection of the experience in the morning (Anders et al., 1980). Night terrors typically occur early in the night during slow wave sleep.

Kellerman (1979) reported on a 3-year-old child with acute lymphocytic leukemia in remission who presented with a 1-month history of persistent, recurring night terrors, occurring from one to six times nightly. The mother's description of the sleep disturbance conformed to the pattern of night terror, in that the child sat up, screamed "Terry scared," or "Terry doesn't want to," appeared extremely anxious, and then went back to sleep. The parents had been previously advised to take the child into their bed contingent upon the occurrence of the night terror; however, this was discontinued when it appeared to be ineffective in reducing the night terrors.

Kellerman (1979) hypothesized that the night terrors represented an anxiety reaction. Trauma in the child's life included the diagnosis of leukemia and the multiple medical procedures (e.g., bone marrow aspirations) related to its treatment. The mother reported that on nights following BMAs the patient's sleep appeared to be more disturbed than usual. The intervention consisted of decreasing the child's anxiety during BMAs through preparatory play with syringes, swabs, and other medical apparatus, simulated medical procedures with a variety of dolls, and ameliorating separation anxiety by teaching the mother progressive muscle relaxation techniques so that she could be present during her child's BMAs. Additionally, when the child first began to experience one restful night of sleep without night terrors, a positive reinforcement system was set up in which the child was able to earn a specified treat each morning following a restful night. When the child did experience a night terror, the parents were instructed to offer minimal reassurance using the phrases "Mommy's here" or "Daddy's here" and to refrain from hovering over the child for prolonged periods or removing her from her bed. This was done to reduce any reinforcing qualities the night terrors may have assumed in terms of eliciting parental attention. The intervention resulted in a steady decline in the weekly incidence of night terrors, with the child experiencing her first completely restful night on the 24th day following the initiation of treatment.

Roberts and Gordon (1979) treated the night terrors of a 5-year-old girl subsequent to being severely burned over 20 percent of her body on her chest, arms, neck, and ears. The burn accident occurred 8 weeks prior to behavioral treatment, when the child and her younger brother were playing with matches in their bedroom after having been put to bed for the night. While she was striking a match, her nightgown caught on fire. She was hospitalized the night of the accident for a period of 6 weeks and had two skin graft operations prior to behavioral treatment. According to parental report, the child began exhibiting night terrors from the first night in the hospital. The parents reported that the night terrors followed a specific sequence from the beginning, suggestive that the child was dreaming of the fire itself. The sequence would frequently begin with the child clutching her nightgown and moving her hands toward her upper body until they were on her neck where the most severe burns had occurred. At this point, the child would begin to scream and kick her bed with her feet until awakened by the nurses in the hospital. At no time was she able to remember the content of her dreams. Typically, the nurses would quiet the child with some juice or ice cream and offer her reassurance. The hospital records from the nurses' notes indicated that the child's night terrors occurred 8 to 15 times a night during her hospitalization.

Once the child returned home, the night terrors continued at a rate of 10 to 20 times per night, almost every night. The parents would verbally comfort the child and frequently gave her something to drink. Additionally, the child would frequently go into her parents' bedroom sometime during the night and either climb into bed with them or fall asleep at the foot of their bed on the floor. However, night terrors occurred even in the parents' bedroom. Even placing the child in another bedroom other than the one in which the fire occurred had no effect on the frequency or intensity of the night terrors.

Roberts and Gordon (1979) suggested that the consequences for the night terrors prior to treatment consisted of a number of potentially reinforcing events, including ice cream and juice, physical comfort, and adult attention. Consequently, the initial step was to remove these potentially reinforcing consequences of the night terrors. Additionally, since the night terrors followed a specific sequence ending in wild thrashing, it was decided to awaken the child early in the chain of behaviors (i.e., clutching her nightgown) in an attempt to interrupt the sequence at an early stage. The parents' instructions were to arouse their daughter as soon as she clutched her nightgown and to allow her to go back to sleep immediately. Additionally, the child was to remain in her room all night.

Since the parents also reported that the child was increasingly fearful of fire during the daytime hours, including the gas stove in the kitchen, lit cigarettes, and fires that she saw on television, the second phase of treatment included systematic desensitization. The desensitization hierarchy consisted of ten magazine pictures of fires selected to represent fire in a wide variety of settings and uses. The child rated each picture on a 5-point scale, from 1 (not scary at all) to 5 (very scary). After each exposure trial, the child was allowed to play with her favorite toys for several minutes as a component of the counterconditioning procedure. The combination of nonreinforcement (extinction) of night terrors and desensitization of the fire anxious reaction during the daytime hours resulted in a complete cessation of night terrors over a 6-month follow-up period.

*Insomnia*

Disorders of initiating and maintaining sleep that originally develop during childhood may persist into adulthood if untreated (Hauri & Olmstead, 1980). The Institute of Medicine has delineated the many contraindications of sleep-inducing medications for chronic insomnia, while emphasizing the development and evaluation of psychosocial and behavioral interventions (Solomon, White, Parron, & Mendelson, 1979).

Anderson (1979) treated a 13-year-old with a 4-month history of insomnia. The parents reported that the patient would become tense and agitated after dinner, pacing the floor, and occasionally crying. The patient would lie awake for 2 to 3 hours before falling asleep, with his mother sitting up with him throughout. If the patient awakened during the night, he would go to his parents' bedroom and complain of vague somatic symptoms. Once again, his mother would sit up with him until he fell asleep. A 3-week baseline indicated an average of 6.3 nights per week of disturbed sleep. In order to deal with the patient's agitation and general level of tension, he was taught progressive muscle relaxation techniques. The patient was instructed to practice the techniques once each day, to engage in the techniques just prior to bedtime, and to employ the techniques should he awaken during the night. Additionally, his parents were instructed to gradually reduce their social reinforcement of sleep-incompatible behaviors, eventually simply instructing their son to return to his room and employ the relaxation techniques. The combination of patient utilization of relaxation techniques and parental nonreinforcement of sleep-incompatible behaviors resulted in an almost complete cessation of insomnia over an 8-month follow-up.

Varni (1980b) designed a treatment package consisting of progressive muscle relaxation, meditative breathing, cognitive refocusing, and stimulus control procedures. The patient had severe, classical hemophilia. Because of the development of an anticoagulant inhibitor (high titer Factor VIII antibody), treatment of bleeding episodes with Factor VIII replacement was not possible, further complicating his medical care with increased severity and duration of each bleeding episode. The patient had a history of chronic insomnia, which was further aggravated 1 year prior to the investigation when his older hemophilic brother died as a result of a severe internal hemorrhage. At that time the patient's antibody titer was also found to be higher than previously noted, resulting in even greater feelings of his own vulnerability. At the time of referral, he reported that these factors resulted in his constant worrying at bedtime about the potential consequences of a severe hemorrhage.

Four dependent measures were delineated for assessment: (1) total number of hours of uninterrupted sleep per night averaged to the half hour; (2) daily tension rating on a scale from 1 (relaxed) to 10 (most tense); (3) number of days per week in which bleeding was evident; and (4) bleeding pain intensity on a scale from 1 (mild) to 10 (most severe). A daily questionnaire checklist was developed for the self-recording of these parameters. Sleep duration in hours was recorded in the morning, bleeding episodes were recorded when they occurred, and the pain and tension ratings averaged for the whole day were recorded at night.

During the initial evaluation, the patient was instructed in the self-monitoring techniques. After an analysis of the information provided from the initial evaluation and a 3-week self-recording baseline, three areas were targeted for intervention: (1) presleep and daily tension, (2) presleep intrusive cognitions, and (3) sleep incompatible activities while in bed. Training in the self-management of insomnia and chronic tension consisted of a 4-component treatment package: (1) A 25-step progressive muscle relaxation sequence involving the alternative tensing and relaxing of major muscle groups. (2) Meditative breathing consisting of medium deep breaths inhaled through the nose and slowly exhaled through the mouth. While exhaling, the patient was instructed to say the word *relax* silently to himself and to visualize the word *relax* in colors, as if written in color chalk on a blackboard. (3) Cognitive refocusing techniques involving a detailed multisensory image of a previously experienced pleasant scene. (4) Stimulus control techniques, including delaying bedtime until very sleepy, using the bed only for sleep-compatible behaviors (no television viewing or reading), getting out of bed within 15 minutes if unable to sleep and engaging in an activity such as reading with a return to bed only when very sleepy, and no daytime naps.

After the 3-week baseline, the patient was instructed in the various techniques during the first treatment session, with the recommendation to practice the progressive muscle relaxation exercises three times daily and the meditative

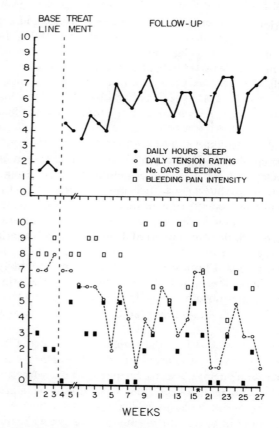

Fig. 12.2. Daily number of hours spent in uninterrupted sleep, daily tension ratings, bleeding frequency per week, and bleeding pain intensity across baseline, treatment, and follow-up. The asterisk represents a 4-week hospitalization.

Source: Reprinted with permission from J.W. Varni. Behavioral treatment of disease-related chronic insomnia in a hemophiliac. *Journal of Behavior Therapy and Experimental Psychiatry,* 1980, **11**, 143–145.

breathing techniques once an hour during the 2-week treatment phase. The protocol during the follow-up period specified the gradual reduction of the meditative breathing exercises to stress-related times or on an as needed basis, with the progressive muscle relaxation sequence practiced once daily just before bedtime. The other aspects of the treatment program were maintained unchanged across treatment and follow-up periods. As indicated by Figure 12.2, the implementation of the treatment package significantly increased the daily number of hours spent in uninterrupted sleep, as well as decreased the daily tension ratings, even during very painful bleeding episodes.

## Habit Disorders

Three habit disorders will be discussed that have not been described in previous chapters (e.g., tics in Chapter 8): chronic destructive scratching associated with neurodermatitis and exfoliative dermatitis, trichotillomania, and pica.

*Chronic Destructive Scratching: Neurodermatitis and Exfoliative Dermatitis*

Chronic destructive scratching is typically associated with neurodermatitis and exfoliative dermatitis. The common sequence in these disorders involves the itch-scratch cycle, whereby excessive scratching exacerbates the skin disorder. The skin condition usually begins with a minor trauma, infection or skin lesion that produces itching and subsequent scratching. The scratching relieves the itching, however, chronic scratching may result in cutaneous inflammation, lichenification, exfoliation (scaling off of dead tissue), and excoriations or deep lesions on the skin.

Carr and McDowell (1980) treated the self-injurious scratching behavior of a 10-year-old child using a combination of time-out for scratching plus reinforcement for reductions in the number of body sores. The child's scratching had begun 3 years prior to the behavioral intervention as a result of contact dermatitis caused by poison oak. The chronic scratching was evidenced by the numerous scars and lesions over the child's skin, even though the contact dermatitis had been successfully treated with medication 3 years earlier. Virtually all of the scratching occurred at home. A functional analysis of the scratching behavior suggested that it was maintained by social attention. The treatment package of time-out contingent on scratching occurrence and positive reinforcement (e.g., trip to the science museum, roller skating) contingent on the weekly reduction of at least two sores on his body (compared to the sore count at the start of the week) resulted in near zero rates of scratching and skin sores.

Latimer (1979) treated a 12-year-old girl with numerous scabs and scars covering her face, arms and legs. An allergic skin reaction and a dog bite lesion were suspected to be the initial etiologies of the itch-scratch cycle. The treatment package consisted of differential parental attention (e.g., ignoring scratching and attending to the child when she was not scratching), an incompatible behavior to scratching (pressing her finger and thumb together for 60 seconds), and a point system for reinforcing nonscratching behaviors and scratching-free periods of time. A 3-year follow-up subsequent to the treatment evidenced a complete cessation of the scratching behavior.

Rosenbaum and Ayllon (1981a) worked with a 16-year-old patient referred for treatment of neurodermatitis on the shins of both legs. The patient had a 1-year history of scratching her shins in response to their itching. The patient reported that her scratching was most severe when she worked on her homework or studied for a test. The principal treatment technique was the competing response practice procedure, whereby the patient was taught an isometric exercise characterized by being incompatible with the scratching behavior (e.g., placing her hands in her lap or by her side and clenching her fists when the urge to scratch occurred). At the 6-month follow-up subsequent to treatment, scratching behavior had decreased substantially, and the patient's shins had begun to heal.

Cataldo, Varni, Russo, and Estes (1980) treated a patient with exfoliative dermatitis whose condition was so severe that he had to be hospitalized. Six years prior to the behavioral intervention, a localized dermatitis had developed subsequent to an insect bite on one arm. Over 3 months, the eruption had become generalized despite vigorous medical treatment. Skin biopsy specimens over the next several years always demonstrated a subacute and chronic dermatitis. On the patient's sixth admission to the hospital 6 years after the precipitating insect bite, skin examination demonstrated almost total-body lichenification with scaling and areas of hypopigmentation and hyperpigmentation. Numerous areas showed underlying erythema and scattered linear excoriations with deep ulcers, especially on the patient's extremities. Alopecia of the scalp, axillae, and pubic hair was noted. Additionally, a chronic tachycardia was present. After cardiac consultation, it was believed that his tachycardia resulted from a high output state because of increased cutaneous blood flow caused by his generalized dermatitis. In spite of a vigorous medical regimen, daily examination by the dermatologist indicated numerous fresh excoriations. The patient's continuous scratching behavior was also observed on the hospital ward. In conjunction with the continuation of the same medical regimen, a behavioral treatment program was begun to control the scratching. All treatment and evaluation were conducted in the patient's hospital room.

Two sets of behavior were measured: the scratching of hands and arms and the scratching of other parts of the body. A measure of the patient's scratching behavior was obtained via an interval recording procedure in which scratching was recorded for the duration of a session during a series of observation and recording sequences. After the behavioral treatment for scratching had been

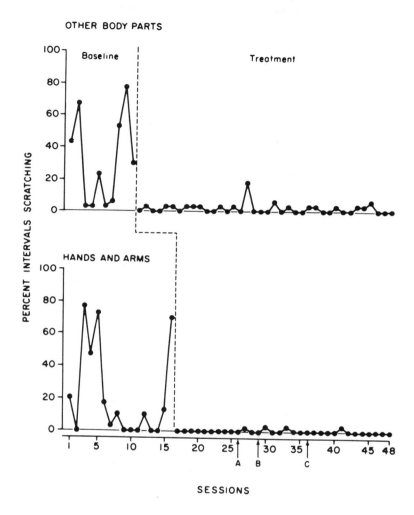

Fig. 12.3.    Data on scratching of hands and arms and other body parts during both baseline and treatment periods in the multiple-baseline design. Letter "A" on the abscissa at session 26 indicates a change in session length from 10 to 20 minutes. Letter "B" at session 29 indicates a session length of 30 minutes for the remainder of the study. Letter "C" at session 36 indicates the start of the excoriation counts.

Source: Reprinted with permission from M.F. Cataldo, J.W. Varni, D.C. Russo, & S.A. Estes. Behavior therapy techniques in treatment of exfoliative dermatitis. *Archives of Dermatology,* 1980, **116**, 919–922.

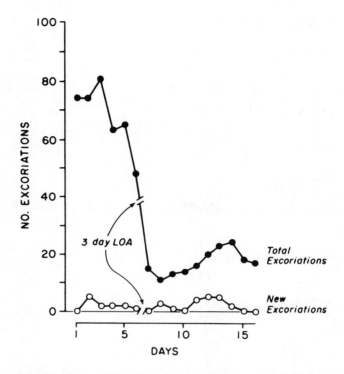

Fig. 12.4.    Total number and number of new excoriations from session 36 of treat-ment to the time of discharge from the hospital. Excoriation counts were made daily at morning rounds by the dermatologist. The arrow indicates a 3-day leave of absence from the hospital.

Source: Reprinted with permission from M.F. Cataldo, J.W. Varni, D.C. Russo, & S.A. Estes. Behavior therapy techniques in treatment of exfoliative dermatitis. *Archives of Dermatology,* 1980, **116**, 919–922.

started, an additional measure was initiated—i.e., the number of new and total excoriations was measured daily by the dermatologist beginning with session 36. An excoriation was operationally defined as any full-thickness erosion of the epidermis produced by scratching.

A multiple-baseline design across other-parts-of-the-body-scratching be-havior and hands-and-arm-scratching behavior was implemented. During the baseline sessions, the therapist simply interacted with the patient in a pleasant manner, discussing any issues or topics initiated by the patient (all sessions were conducted while the patient was in his bed). After baseline, the therapist described to the patient the ramifications of his scratching behavior (e.g., increased itching or tachycardia) and obtained the patient's agreement to work on decreasing his scratching. The treatment procedures consisted of the therapist ceasing his social interaction with the patient for 1 minute when the patient began to scratch (a form of time-out). Just prior to time-out and as soon as the patient scratched himself, the therapist also called the patient by name and said, "You're scratching," and then asked the patient to fold his hands (a competing or incompatible response to scratching) and to think of some pleasant scene (distraction or refocusing of attention away from the itch sensation). These reminders (prompts) that the patient was scratching were gradually discontinued (fading procedure) as the patient began spontaneously folding his hands. The combination of the incompatible response and the distraction technique were designed to interrupt the itch-scratch cycle. The use of differential social attention provided the social reinforcement for non-scratching periods. As shown in Figure 12.3, the treatment package resulted in almost complete cessation of scratching behavior. Figure 12.4 demonstrates that the reduction in scratching behavior resulted in a low level of new excoriations and a steady decrease in the number of new excoriations.

### Trichotillomania

Trichotillomania (chronic hairpulling) is a habit disorder that may result in tissue irritation and alopecia, often in such areas as the scalp, eyebrows, and eyelashes.

Gray (1979) reported on a 5-year-old child who had been pulling out her scalp hair since age one and had been almost totally bald since that time. The treatment program consisted of a variety of positive reinforcement and punishment procedures delivered by the child's parents. For every waking hour in which there had been no hairpulling, a marble (token) was dropped into a transparent jar, and the child was often socially reinforced. When the jar was filled with marbles, the child received a toy previously selected by her and purchased by her parents. This procedure usually resulted in receiving a toy approximately once a week. Since progress was slow (probably somewhat due to the lack of consistent immediate reinforcement), a punishment contingency (four slaps on the hand) was also initiated for each instance of hairpulling, resulting in a steady reduction of hairpulling to a zero rate by the 53rd day. Follow-up at 16 months by photograph showed thick, shoulder length hair.

Sanchez (1979) described a 27-month-old child who had been pulling out his scalp hair for approximately 6 months. A sequence or chain of behaviors was observed, with hairpulling preceded and followed by finger sucking. The treatment consisted of time-out for each instance of hairpulling, reinforcement for behavior that was judged incompatible with hairpulling (e.g., playing with toys and siblings), and finally, punishment for prehairpulling finger sucking (taping his fingers together). The intervention resulted in zero rates of hairpulling and finger sucking and complete regrowth of scalp hair.

Azrin, Nunn, and Frantz (1980) worked with 34 patients who evidenced trichotillomania, four of whom were children 13 or 14 years old. The habit reversal training package consisted of the following components:

1. *Competing response training,* consisting of the inconspicuous competing response of grasping or clenching the hands for 3 minutes whenever hair-pulling occurred or was likely to occur;
2. *Awareness training,* involving teaching the patients to become acutely aware of the specific movements involved in the hairpulling, especially by observing themselves in a mirror;
3. *Identifying response precursors,* involving identifying a common response that was a precursor to hairpulling such as face-touching or hair-straightening;
4. *Identifying habit prone situations,* such as watching television, reading, studying, and driving;
5. *Relaxation training,* through deep regular breathing and postural adjustment;
6. *Self-recording* of each instance of hairpulling to further increase the patient's awareness of the habit;
7. *Social reinforcement.*

The four adolescents treated with this comprehensive program evidenced no incidents of hairpulling (scalp, eyebrows, eyelashes) at a 4-week follow-up. Rosenbaum and Ayllon (1981b) also found this habit reversal program to be successful with a 10-year-old child, who at a 12-month posttreatment follow-up demonstrated no instances of hairpulling.

*Pica*

Pica is the habit behavior of ingesting inedible material, such as paint, clay, plaster, and ashes. Although infants exhibit mouthing of inedible objects during the first year of life, they gradually discriminate inedible from edible objects. Pica becomes a clinical problem for the ambulatory child who actively seeks out inedible substances and swallows them. This can be a particularly serious problem when the child ingests inedible substances that contain lead, particularly bits of plaster and lead-based paint available on the walls of older houses; dust containing lead may be ingested when the child puts toys or body parts exposed to the dust in her mouth. Such ingestion of lead containing inedible material can lead to lead poisoning, which may result in permanent neurological impairment, mental retardation, or even death.

Madden, Russo, and Cataldo (1980a) studied three young children who were hospitalized for asymptomatic lead intoxication diagnosed by high lead levels during routine lead screening. In a simulated environment in the hospital,

Madden et al. (1980a) found that the mouthing behavior of these children occurred to differing degrees in different environmental settings. A major determinant of the observed mouthing behavior was the relative enrichment of the environment in terms of activities, toys, and adult and child contact. In impoverished environments in which a minimum of activities were available, mouthing behavior of inedible objects was significantly higher for each of the children, while little or no mouthing behavior was observed in the stimulating environment. This finding suggests that the environmental deprivation involved in the natural environment (home setting) of these children may be a factor that in itself increases the likelihood of lead ingestion through pica.

In a subsequent study, Madden, Russo, and Cataldo (1980b) utilized behavioral procedures to eliminate pica in three young children with lead poisoning. Observations of pica were conducted in a simulated impoverished environment, containing few toys and activities. Additionally, a board coated with a nontoxic material resembling flaking lead paint (made from flour paste) was placed against one wall of the room, with some of these simulated paint chips also placed on a table, a windowsill, and on the floor near the board. The treatment program involved three components implemented sequentially:

1. *Discrimination training,* in which the child was taught to recognize that paint and several other objects were not edible;
2. *Correspondence training and reinforcement* for nonpica, during which the child was taught to report accurately whether or not she had put anything in her mouth and was reinforced for accurate reporting of no pica behavior;
3. *Differential reinforcement of other behavior (DRO) and overcorrection,* which consisted of reinforcing the child for nonpica behavior and the absence of pica behavior (DRO) and brushing the child's mouth and teeth for 1 minute with a child's soft-bristle toothbrush that had been dipped in Listerine for each instance of pica (overcorrection procedure).

Pica was eliminated in all three children treated by one, two, or all three components of the above treatment package when applied sequentially. A subsequent study by Finney, Russo, and Cataldo (1982) replicated and extended the above treatment package to four additional children, once again substantially reducing pica behavior in these children.

## Chronic Rumination and Vomiting

In this section, chronic rumination and vomiting are defined as the regurgitation of food and liquid *not* secondary to chemotherapy, radiation therapy, or disease (as discussed in Chapter 9), nor associated with anorexia nervosa and bulimia (see Chapter 7). Chronic rumination and vomiting may lead to serious health problems, with the regular loss of large amounts of ingested food and liquids causing malnutrition, dehydration, acute gastrointestinal distress, lowered resistance to disease, and even death in some cases (see Davis & Cuvo, 1980, for review). In reviewing the behavioral treatment literature, Davis and Cuvo (1980) found that in most cases, chronic rumination and vomiting appeared to be behaviors maintained by positive and negative reinforcement contingencies, such as: adult social and physical attention, reconsumption of the food and liquid, and avoidance of an undesired activity. The behavioral studies reviewed have attempted to rearrange these contingencies so as to decrease chronic rumination and vomiting through aversive contingencies, extinction, and/or positive reinforcement for their nonoccurrence.

When rumination and vomiting have become life-threatening in infants and young children, aversive contingencies have been most commonly utilized to decrease these maladaptive behaviors rather quickly. Distasteful liquids placed directly in the child's mouth contingent on rumination and vomiting are commonly utilized aversive stimuli.

Sajwaj, Libet, and Agras (1974) treated the chronic, life-threatening rumination of a 6-month-old infant by squirting a small amount of unsweetened lemon juice into her mouth when rumination or its precursors were detected. Prior to treatment, the patient was emaciated and rapidly losing weight secondary to chronic rumination. Malnutrition and dehydration were pressing problems, and death, resulting from possible complications, was a distinct possibility. Immediately after each feeding, ruminative behavior would begin. The infant would open her mouth, elevate and fold her tongue, and then vigorously thrust her tongue forward and backward. Within a few minutes milk would appear at the back of her mouth and then slowly flow out. This behavior would continue for about 20 to 40 minutes until she apparently lost all of the milk she had previously consumed. Rumination could be interrupted by touches, pokes, or mild slaps, but would resume immediately. Lemon-juice therapy consisted of squirting about 5 to 10 cc of unsweetened lemon juice into the infant's mouth with a 30-cc medical syringe as soon as vigorous tongue movements were detected. If ruminative tongue movements persisted after 60 seconds, lemon juice was reapplied. This intervention decreased rumination to essentially a zero rate of occurrence and resulted in a normal weight gain curve. Similar positive findings were observed using lemon-juice therapy with a 3-year-old profoundly retarded child (Becker, Turner, & Sajwaj, 1978).

Murray, Keele, and McCarver (1977) employed a behavioral program including stimulus control, an aversive, distasteful liquid (Tabasco sauce), and continuous massive social and physical attention for a 6-month-old emaciated, dehydrated, malnourished child who vomited after every feeding. Following each feeding, the infant voluntarily began to protrude his tongue repeatedly and make chewing motions with his jaws. This was followed in approximately 30 seconds by regurgitation of food into his mouth, which subsequently rolled out onto the front of his shirt. He would continue this activity until the entire gastric contents were emptied. The multicomponent treatment program consisted of: (1) Decreasing the child's rumination through intervening at the initial phase of the sequence of the emetic behaviors, i.e., the tongue rolling; (2) Continuing to thicken the child's formula with cereal to make the initiation of rumination more difficult; (3) Holding the child during the actual feeding; (4) When the child began the emetic behavior by tongue manipulation, placing him in his crib (time-out). Also, two drops of Tabasco sauce were placed on his tongue; (5) If the tongue rolling began again, the Tabasco sauce was reapplied; (6) When tongue manipulation ceased, the child was immediately picked up and held and rocked for 20 minutes. The treatment program was effective in bringing the rumination under control within a few days, resulting in a return to normal developmental weight gain. This combination of an aversive liquid, time-out, differential reinforcement of nonemetic behavior, plus a mild physical punishment (a rap on the knuckles with a plastic comb), was also successfully utilized with a 26-month-old developmentally delayed child (O'Neil, White, King, & Carek, 1979).

Munford and Pally (1979) described the elimination of an 8-year intermittent chronic vomiting pattern in an 11-year-old child that occurred daily during the 6 months prior to behavioral treatment. During a 1-week baseline, the patient vomited 29 times, often consequated by family members with sympathy and assistance in cleaning up any soiling. The intervention consisted of shifting attention away from vomiting-related behaviors to adaptive, age-appropriate behaviors (e.g., daily bedmaking, trash removal, and completion of homework assignments). This combination of extinction for vomiting and positive reinforcement for appropriate behaviors (DRO schedule) resulted in a total cessation of vomiting by the third week of treatment, maintained over a 1-year follow-up. A similar differential attention procedure combining time-out for vomiting and social and physical attention for nonvomiting behaviors was also utilized to reduce ruminating in a 9-month-old infant (Wright, Brown, & Andrews, 1978).

Ingersoll and Curry (1977) worked with a 14-year-old patient whose onset of chronic vomiting occurred after a 24-hour episode of nausea and malaise. Twenty-seven days after its onset, vomiting continued to occur during or immediately following a meal. A shaping procedure was designed to gradually return to normal food and beverage intake along the dimensions of: (1) the time food was retained; (2) the type of food or drink; and (3) the amount eaten and retained. The patient was fed specified amounts of food within designated intervals. These intervals were gradually lengthened from 5 minutes to the time required for a full meal; the type of food was gradually changed from a liquid to a solid diet; and the amount ingested at each feeding was gradually increased from 2 ounces to a full meal portion. A timer was activated to record the time of food retention. Reinforcement (attention, praise, trips, games) was contingent upon eating and retaining the specific food amounts. In addition, for each minute of food retention the patient earned a token that could be exchanged for money or television viewing time. Finally, a 15-minute time-out was contingent immediately upon each incident of vomiting behavior, with the patient removed from the feeding area and placed in a chair in a corner. At the end of the time-out, the patient returned to the feeding area, and food of the same type and amount previous to time-out was offered in addition to the contingent reinforcers. Within 5 days, vomiting had completely stopped, maintained without reoccurrence over a 1-year follow-up.

## SOCIAL SKILLS DEFICITS

Children with chronic physical disorders often experience a disruption in their social relations with peers, siblings, and parents secondary to illness-imposed limitations, outpatient treatment, and hospitalization (Zeltzer, Kellerman, Ellenberg, Dash, & Rigler, 1980). The potential of social skills training in overcoming these disruptions in normal social development may result not only in improved relationships in the present, but may also prevent later psychosocial problems. Handicapped children may not only be taught the requisite social skills for effective social interaction and peer acceptance (Gresham, 1982), but social skills training may even aid the targeted child to excel in interpersonal skills beyond the level of nonhandicapped children (e.g., Matson, Kazdin, & Esveldt-Dawson, 1980).

### Social Skills Assessment

Green and Forehand (1980) identified four methods primarily utilized in the assessment of children's social skills: sociometric instruments, behavioral observations, teacher reports, and child self-report. Sociometric assessment typically involves obtaining a measure of peer acceptance by the peer nomination technique, that is, the number of nominations a child receives from her classmates on their desire to play or work with her or have her as a friend.

Behavioral measures of social skills in the natural environment have included rate, frequency, or percentage of interactions between a target child and his peers in a play or classroom situation (see Van Hasselt, Hersen, Whitehill, & Bellack, 1979, for review). In the clinic setting, the specific behavioral components of social skills have been identified, including the ratio of eye contact to duration of response, smiles, duration of reply, number of words, affect, ratio of speech disturbances to duration of speech, appreciation, spontaneous positive behavior, and regard (Reardon, Hersen, Bellack, & Foley, 1979).

Teachers scoring of children's social skills typically involves either ranking the children in their classroom or rating targeted children on a 100-point scale along the dimensions of withdrawn, prosocial, aggressive, and passive behavior. Self-report measures by children involve having the children check their responses to described social situations (Reardon et al., 1979) or checking off characteristics descriptive of themselves, for example, "I don't have any friends" (Weissman, Orvaschel, & Padian, 1980).

Three major problems in the validity of the current assessment methodology for children's social skills include: (1) whether the measures in the clinic are reflective of social skills in the natural environment (Van Hasselt, Hersen, & Bellack, 1981); (2) whether the target social behaviors observed in the natural environment are critical to adaptive social functioning (Forster & Ritchey, 1979); and (3) the lack of correlation between behavioral, sociometric, teacher, and clinic measures of social skills (Green & Forehand, 1980; Reardon et al., 1979; Van Hasselt et al., 1979). In view of these assessment issues, the following intervention studies should be considered as initial findings until assessment methodology is improved.

## Social Skills Training

Teaching social skills to children typically involves some form of modeling, behavioral rehearsal, corrective feedback, and reinforcement of selected pro-social behaviors (see Cartledge & Milburn, 1980). Social skills selected for intervention include improving conversational skills and increasing cooperative play, positive peer interactions, peer acceptance, and friendship making (Ladd, 1981; La Greca & Mesibov, 1979; Oden & Asher, 1977; Whitehill, Hersen, & Bellack, 1980).

In young children, increasing prosocial behaviors, such as sharing, helping, defending, sympathy, rescuing, and cooperation (Yarrow & Waxler, 1976), has typically involved film modeling, based on the concept of observational learning. O'Connor (1969, 1972) studied socially withdrawn preschool children using film modeling as the intervention. The children observed a sound film depicting peers engaged in progressively more active social interaction. The prosocial behavior of the children in the film was reinforced by peer approval, either verbal or expressional (smiling, nodding) and peer acceptance of the model into a game or conversation. The intervention resulted in the target children increasing their level of social interaction to that of the other children in the nursery school classroom. Strain, Shores, and Kerr (1976), also working with preschool children, used a combination of verbal and physical prompts, plus verbal praise contingent on appropriate social behaviors, implemented by the classroom teacher, resulting in an increase in positive social behaviors and a decrease in negative social behaviors.

Increasing the social skills of school-age children has typically involved direct training in the components of appropriate social interaction, with or without some form of modeling. Gottman, Gonso, and Schuler (1976) described a three-step treatment package:

1. The first step attempted to teach the child how to initiate interaction by having the child view a videotape with vignettes showing children contemplating cooperative play and subsequently receiving peer positive consequences for joining in cooperative play.
2. During the second step an attempt was made to teach the child how to make friends using a friend-making sequence (i.e., name greeting, asking for information, giving information, extending an offer of inclusion, and effective leave taking). In this stage, the child role-played (behavioral rehearsal) with an adult coach who played the part of another child.
3. In the third step, the child practiced communication skills and active listening.

The two target children who received social skills training improved significantly in sociometric ratings in comparison to two control children. Cooke and Appolloni (1976) taught four children four positive social-emotional behaviors: smiling, sharing, positive physical contacting, and verbal complimenting, using instructions, modeling, and praise, resulting in an increase in all these behaviors.

Bornstein, Bellack, and Hersen (1977) operationally defined three specific components of assertiveness: (1) ratio of eye contact to speech duration, (2) loudness of speech, and (3) requests for new behavior. Nine role-played scenes, consisting of situations that the children were likely to engage in daily with other children, served as the training and generalization context for the intervention package of instructions, performance, feedback, modeling, behavioral rehearsal, and social reinforcement for four unassertive children. All four children demonstrated an increase in the target behaviors and received a higher rating on an overall assertiveness scale subsequent to training. Whitehill, Hersen and Bellack (1980) used a similar method to increase the overall conversational ability of four socially isolated children, operationally defining three specific components of conversational skills: (1) informative statements, (2) open-ended questions, and (3) requests for shared activity. Matson, Esveldt-Dawson, Andrasik, Ollendick, Petti, and Hersen (1980) again used similar methodology to treat the social skills deficits of four children between 9 and 11 years of age in a social skills training group format. The component skills identified were: (1) appropriate verbal content, including giving compliments, giving help, and making appropriate requests (e.g., "Will you play with me?"); (2) appropriate affect, including voice pitch and volume and facial mannerisms (e.g., smiles when complimented); (3) appropriate eye contact; and (4) appropriate body posture. Initially, two children received social skills training while the other two observed this training. This procedure was used to evaluate the effects of observational learning. The observational learning alone condition was of minimal benefit. The effects of direct social skills training, however, were immediate and positive, maintained over a 15-week follow-up.

La Greca and Santogrossi (1980) identified eight skill areas for training 30 children, grades 3 to 5, who were selected on the basis of low peer acceptance ratings. The eight social skill areas included smiling/laughing, greeting others, joining ongoing activities, extending invitations, conversational skills, sharing and cooperation, verbal complimenting, and physical appearance/grooming. The main treatment procedures were modeling, coaching, and behavioral rehearsal and videotaped feedback within a group format. During the initial meeting, the children were informed that the purpose of the group was to learn better ways of playing and working with others. During treatment, for each of the eight target skill areas, the children viewed videotapes of peer models demonstrating the skill and then discussed the videotape and how they might use the skill in their daily activities with peers. The next step involved coaching the children in their use of the skills and providing opportunities to rehearse the skills in role-playing situations within the group. Role-playing situations were based on the real-life experiences the children reported encountering (e.g., joining games at recess, cooperating during gym activities, complimenting others on their work). This role-playing was videotaped, and the children were given immediate feedback on their performance, with suggestions for improvement. Finally, to encourage the children to use the skills with their peers, the children were given homework assignments that focused on practicing the social skills with peers outside the group sessions (e.g., greeting a classmate at least once a day for the next week).

The treatment outcome measures included: (1) A skills knowledge measure to assess whether the children learned the skills that were trained, involving verbally describing what a film model should do in a variety of play and work situations, and what the child herself would do in a similar situation (the situations included all eight skill areas covered in the training program); (2) A role-playing situation that assessed the children's observable skill in a structured social situation by an individual role-play of making friends with a new child in school; (3) Naturalistic situations where the children were observed during a variety of situations conducive to peer interactions (e.g., recess, gym period, and club meetings); and (4) Sociometric measures that required children in the classroom to rate each child on how much they would like to play with and work with the child on a 5-point scale (1 = very much, to 5 = not at all). In comparison to an attention-placebo group and a waiting-list control group, the social skills training group demonstrated increased skill in the role-play situation, a greater verbal knowledge of how to interact with peers, and more initiation of peer interactions in the school setting.

Future research on social skills training for children would benefit from greater attention to the following three issues: (1) the role of social perception in determining the appropriate context and timing for emitting specific social behaviors (Morrison & Bellack, 1981); (2) the role that social anxiety may play in inhibiting the emission of appropriate social behavior (Alden & Cappe,

1981); and (3) the systematic programming of generalization through some form of *in vivo* social skills training in the natural environment (Linden & Wright, 1980).

# REFERENCES

Alden, L., & Cappe, R. Nonassertiveness: Skill deficit or selective self-evaluation? *Behavior Therapy,* 1981, **12**, 107–114.

Anders, T.F., Carskadon, M.A., & Dement, W.C. Sleep and sleepiness in children and adolescents. *Pediatric Clinics of North America,* 1980, **27**, 29–43.

Anderson, D.R. Treatment of insomnia in a 13-year-old boy by relaxation training and reduction of parental attention. *Journal of Behavior Therapy and Experimental Psychiatry,* 1979, **10**, 263–265.

Ayllon, T., Layman, D., & Kandel, H.J. A behavioral-educational alternative to drug control of hyperactive children. *Journal of Applied Behavior Analysis,* 1975, **8**, 137–146.

Azrin, N.H., Nunn, R.G., & Frantz, S.E. Treatment of hairpulling (trichotillomania): A comparative study of habit reversal and negative practice training. *Journal of Behavior Therapy and Experimental Psychiatry,* 1980, **11**, 13–20.

Barkley, R.A., Copeland, A.P., & Sivage, C. A self-control classroom for hyperactive children. *Journal of Autism and Developmental Disorders,* 1980, **10**, 75–89.

Becker, J.V., Turner, S.M., & Sajwaj, T.E. Multiple behavioral effects of the use of lemon juice with a ruminating toddler-age child. *Behavior Modification,* 1978, **2**, 267–278.

Bernal, M.E. Behavioral treatment of a child's eating problem. *Journal of Behavior Therapy and Experimental Psychiatry,* 1972, **3**, 43–50.

Bornstein, M.R., Bellack, A.S., & Hersen, M. Social skills training for highly aggressive children: Treatment in an inpatient psychiatric setting. *Behavior Modification,* 1980, **4**, 173–186.

Bornstein, M.R., Bellack, A.S., & Hersen, M. Social-skills training for unassertive children: A multiple-baseline analysis. *Journal of Applied Behavior Analysis,* 1977, **10**, 183–195.

Carr, E.G., & McDowell, J.J. Social control of self-injurious behavior of organic etiology. *Behavior Therapy,* 1980, **11**, 402–409.

Cartledge, G., & Milburn, J.F. (Eds.). *Teaching Social Skills to Children: Innovative Approaches.* New York: Pergamon Press, 1980.

Cataldo, M.F., Varni, J.W., Russo, D.C., & Estes, S.A. Behavior therapy techniques in treatment of exfoliative dermatitis. *Archives of Dermatology,* 1980, **116**, 919–922.

Cellucci, A.J., & Lawrence, P.S. The efficacy of systematic desensitization in reducing nightmares. *Journal of Behavior Therapy and Experimental Psychiatry,* 1978, **9**, 109–114.

Christophersen, E.R. Incorporating behavioral pediatrics into primary care. *Pediatric Clinics of North America,* 1982, **19**, 261–296.

Christophersen, E.R., & Abernathy, J.E. Research in ambulatory pediatrics. In D.C. Russo & J.W. Varni (Eds.), *Behavioral Pediatrics: Research and Practice.* New York: Plenum Press, 1982.

Cooke, T.P., & Apolloni, T. Developing positive social-emotional behaviors: A study of training and generalization effects. *Journal of Applied Behavior Analysis,* 1976, **9**, 65–78.

Davis, P.K., & Curo, A.J. Chronic vomiting and rumination in intellectually normal and retarded individuals: Review and evaluation of behavioral research. *Behavior Research of Severe Developmental Disabilities,* 1980, **1**, 31–59.

Drabman, R.S., & Jarvie G. Counseling parents of children with behavior problems: The use of extinction and time-out techniques. *Pediatrics,* 1977, **59**, 78–85.

Finney, J.W., Russo, D.C., & Cataldo, M.F. Reduction of pica in young children with lead poisoning. *Journal of Pediatric Psychology,* 1982, **7**, 197–207.

Firestone, P., & Witt, J.E. Characteristics of families completing and prematurely discontinuing a behavioral parent-training program. *Journal of Pediatric Psychology,* 1982, **7**, 209–222.

Forehand, R.L., & McMahon, R.J. *Helping the Noncompliant Child: A Clinician's Guide to Parent Training.* New York: Guilford Press, 1981.

Forster, S.L., & Ritchey, W.L. Issues in the assessment of social competence in children. *Journal of Applied Behavior Analysis,* 1979, **12**, 625–638.

Fox, R.A., & Roseen, D.L. A parent administered token program for dietary regulation of phenylketonuria. *Journal of Behavior Therapy and Experimental Psychiatry,* 1977, **8**, 441–443.

Framer, E.M., & Sanders, S.H. The effects of family contingency contracting on disturbed sleeping behaviors in a male adolescent. *Journal of Behavior Therapy and Experimental Psychiatry,* 1980, **11**, 235–237.

Gottman, J., Gonso, J., & Schuler, P. Teaching social skills to isolated children. *Journal of Abnormal Child Psychology,* 1976, **4**, 179–197.

Gray, J.J. Positive reinforcement and punishment in the treatment of childhood trichotillomania. *Journal of Behavior Therapy and Experimental Psychiatry,* 1979, **10**, 125–129.

Green, K.K., & Forehand, R. Assessment of children's social skills: A review of methods. *Journal of Behavioral Assessment,* 1980, **2**, 143–159.

Gresham, F.M. Misguided mainstreaming: The case for social skills training with handicapped children. *Exceptional Children,* 1982, **48**, 422–433.

Hatcher, R.P. Treatment of food refusal in a two-year-old child. *Journal of Behavior Therapy and Experimental Psychiatry,* 1979, **10**, 363–367.

Hauri, P., & Olmstead, E. Childhood-onset insomnia. *Sleep,* 1980, **3**, 59–65.

Ingersoll, B., & Curry, F. Rapid treatment of persistent vomiting in a 14-year-old female by shaping and time-out. *Journal of Behavior Therapy and Experimental Psychiatry,* 1977, **8**, 305–307.

Kales, A., Soldatos, C.R., Caldwell, A.B., Charney, D.S., Kales, J.D., Markel, D., & Cadieux, R. Nightmares: Clinical characteristics and personality patterns. *American Journal of Psychiatry,* 1980, **137**, 1197–1201.

Kellerman, J. Behavioral treatment of night terrors in a child with acute leukemia. *Journal of Nervous and Mental Disease,* 1979, **167**, 182–185.

Ladd, G.W. Effectiveness of a social learning method for enhancing children's social interaction and peer acceptance. *Child Development,* 1981, **52**, 171–178.

La Greca, A.M., & Mesibov, G.B. Social skills intervention with learning disabled children: Selecting skills and implementing training. *Journal of Clinical Child Psychology,* 1979, **8**, 234–241.

La Greca, A.M., & Santogrossi, D.A. Social skills training with elementary school students: A behavioral group approach. *Journal of Consulting and Clinical Psychology,* 1980, **48**, 220–227.

Latimer, P.R. The behavioral treatment of self-excoriation in a twelve-year-old girl. *Journal of Behavior Therapy and Experimental Psychiatry,* 1979, **10**, 349–352.

Leitenberg, H. Is time-out from positive reinforcement an aversive event? A review of the experimental evidence. *Psychological Bulletin,* 1965, **64**, 428–441.

Linden, W., & Wright, J. Programming generalization through social skills training in the natural environment. *Behavioural Analysis and Modification,* 1980, **4**, 239–251.

Madden, N.A., Russo, D.C., & Cataldo, M.F. Environmental influences on mouthing in children with lead intoxication. *Journal of Pediatric Psychology,* 1980, **5**, 207–216. (a)

Madden, N.A., Russo, D.C., & Cataldo, M.F. Behavioral treatment of pica in children with lead poisoning. *Child Behavior Therapy,* 1980, **2**, 67–81. (b)

Matson, J.L., Esveldt-Dawson, K., Andrasik, F., Ollendick, T.H., Petti, T., & Hersen, M. Direct, observational, and generalization effects of social skills training with emotionally disturbed children. *Behavior Therapy,* 1980, **11**, 522–531.

Matson, J.L., Kazdin, A.E., & Esveldt-Dawson, K. Training interpersonal skills among mentally retarded and socially dysfunctional children. *Behaviour Research and Therapy,* 1980, **18**, 419–427.

McMahon, R.J., & Forehand, R. Nonprescription behavior therapy: Effectiveness of a brochure in teaching mothers to correct their children's inappropriate mealtime behaviors. *Behavior Therapy,* 1978, **9**, 814–820.

Morrison, R.L., & Bellack, A.S. The role of social perception in social skill. *Behavior Therapy,* 1981, **12**, 69–79.

Munford, P.R., & Pally, R. Outpatient contingency management of operant vomiting. *Journal of Behavior Therapy and Experimental Psychiatry,* 1979, **10**, 135–137.

Murray, M.E., Keele, D.K., & McCarver, J.W. Treatment of ruminations with behavioral techniques: A case report. *Behavior Therapy,* 1977, **8**, 999–1003.

O'Connor, R.D. Relative efficacy of modeling, shaping, and the combined procedures for modification of social withdrawal. *Journal of Abnormal Psychology,* 1972, **79**, 327–334.

O'Connor, R.D. Modification of social withdrawal through symbolic modeling. *Journal of Applied Behavior Analysis,* 1969, **2**, 15–22.

Oden, S., & Asher, S.R. Coaching children in social skills for friendship making. *Child Development,* 1977, **48**, 495–506.

O'Leary, S.G., & Steen, P.L. Subcategorizing hyperactivity: The Stony Brook Scale. *Journal of Consulting and Clinical Psychology,* 1982, **50**, 426–432.

O'Neil, P.M., White, J.L., King, C.R., & Carek, D.J. Controlling childhood rumination through differential reinforcement of other behavior. *Behavior Modification,* 1979, **3**, 355–372.

Palmer, S., Thompson, R.J., & Linscheid, T.R. Applied behavior analysis in the treatment of childhood feeding problems. *Developmental Medicine and Child Neurology,* 1975, **17**, 333–339.

Patterson, G.R. *Families: Applications of Social Learning to Family Life.* Champaign, Illinois: Research Press, 1975.

Price, V.A., Coates, T.J., Thoresen, C.E., & Grinstead, O.A. Prevalence and correlates of poor sleep among adolescents. *American Journal of Diseases of Children,* 1978, **132**, 583–586.

Rapoff, M.A., Christophersen, E.R., & Rapoff, K.E. The management of common childhood bedtime problems by pediatric nurse practitioners. *Journal of Pediatric Psychology,* 1982, **7**, 179–196.

Reardon, R.C., Hersen, M., Bellack, A.S., & Foley, J.M. Measuring social skill in grade school boys. *Journal of Behavioral Assessment,* 1979, **1**, 87–105.

Reidy, T.J. Training appropriate eating behavior in a pediatric rehabilitation setting: Case study. *Archives of Physical Medicine and Rehabilitation,* 1979, **60**, 226–230.

Roberts, R.N., & Gordon, S.B. Reducing childhood nightmares subsequent to a burn trauma. *Child Behavior Therapy,* 1979, **1**, 373–381.

Rosenbaum, M.S., & Ayllon, T. The behavioral treatment of neurodermatitis through habit-reversal. *Behaviour Research and Therapy,* 1981, **19**, 313–318. (a)

Rosenbaum, M.S., & Ayllon, T. The habit-reversal technique in treating trichotillomania. *Behavior Therapy,* 1981, **12**, 473–481. (b)

Sajwaj, T., Libet, J., & Agras, S. Lemon-juice therapy: The control of life-threatening rumination in a six-month-old infant. *Journal of Applied Behavior Analysis,* 1974, **7**, 557–563.

Sanchez, V. Behavioral treatment of chronic hair pulling in a two year old. *Journal of Behavior Therapy and Experimental Psychiatry,* 1979, **10**, 241–245.

Sanok, R.L., & Ascione, F.R. The effects of reduced time limits on prolonged eating behavior. *Journal of Behavior Therapy and Experimental Psychiatry,* 1978, **9**, 177–179.

Schumaker, J.B., Hovell, M.F., & Sherman, J.A. An analysis of daily report cards and parent-managed privileges in the improvement of adolescents' classroom performance. *Journal of Applied Behavior Analysis,* 1977, **10**, 449–464.

Solomon, F., White, C.C., Parron, D.L., & Mendelson, W.B. Sleeping pills, insomnia, and medical practice. *New England Journal of Medicine,* 1979, **300**, 803–808.

Strain, P.S., Shores, R.E., & Kerr, M.M. An experimental analysis of "spillover" effects on the social interaction of behaviorally handicapped preschool children. *Journal of Applied Behavior Analysis,* 1976, **9**, 31–40.

Van Hasselt, V.B., Hersen, M., & Bellack, A.S. The validity of role play tests for assessing social skills in children. *Behavior Therapy,* 1981, **12**, 202–216.

Van Hasselt, V.B., Hersen, J., Whitehill, M.B., & Bellack, A.S. Social skill assessment and training for children: An evaluative review. *Behaviour Research and Therapy,* 1979, **17**, 413–437.

Varni, J.W. Behavior therapy in the management of home and school behavior problems with a 4½-year-old hemophilic child. *Journal of Pediatric Psychology,* 1980, **5**, 17–23. (a)

Varni, J.W. Behavioral treatment of disease-related chronic insomnia in a hemophiliac. *Journal of Behavior Therapy and Experimental Psychiatry,* 1980, **11**, 143–145. (b)

Varni, J.W., & Henker, B. A self-regulation approach to the treatment of three hyperactive boys. *Child Behavior Therapy,* 1979, **1**, 171–192.

Weissman, M.M., Orvaschel, H., & Padian, N. Children's symptom and social functioning self-report scales: Comparison of mothers' and children's reports. *Journal of Nervous and Mental Disease,* 1980, **168**, 736–740.

Whitehill, M.B., Hersen, M., & Bellack, A.S. Conversational skills training for socially isolated children. *Behaviour Research and Therapy,* 1980, **18**, 217–225.

Wright, D.F., Brown, R.A., & Andrews, M.E. Remission of chronic ruminative vomiting through a reversal of social contingencies. *Behaviour Research and Therapy,* 1978, **16**, 134–136.

Yarrow, M.R., & Waxler, C.Z. Dimensions and correlates of prosocial behavior in young children. *Child Development,* 1976, **47**, 118–125.

Zeltzer, L., Kellerman, J., Ellenberg, L., Dash, J., & Rigler, D. Psychological effects of illness in adolescence. II. Impact of illness in adolescents—crucial issues and coping styles. *Journal of Pediatrics,* 1980, **97**, 132–138.

# Afterword

The application of biobehavioral techniques to pediatrics represents an endeavor of unlimited possibilities. The potentially greatest long-term influence of behavioral pediatrics on the general population of children and adolescents may be ultimately most evident in the prevention of serious health problems and the promotion and maintenance of healthy lifestyles. Biobehavioral interventions targeting eating, exercise, diet, smoking, and alcohol patterns in children and adolescents may have a profound influence on the primary prevention of such highly prevalent chronic disorders as cardiovascular disease and cancer. Additionally, improvements in health-related behaviors may significantly enhance the prognosis of children with chronic disorders. For example, the synergistic effect of excessive weight, lack of exercise, and disease activity in juvenile rheumatoid arthritis may result in greater disability. The promotion of a regimen combining appropriate eating, exercise, diet, and medication adherence might result in the secondary prevention of further morbidity, leading to an improved prognosis for the most optimal quality of life for the growing child into adulthood.

A common and potentially serious problem evident in essentially all pediatric health care is the varying degrees of adherence to therapeutic regimens and to a healthy lifestyle. Assessment and management of therapeutic adherence and noncompliance will increasingly be a prominent component of behavioral pediatrics research as the field grows and has wider application. Three areas of investigation, *behavioral health care professional training, behavioral parent training,* and *child self-regulation training,* hold the promise for enhancing parent and child therapeutic adherence. Essentially, there is an unlimited number of potential contributions of behavioral pediatrics to pediatric comprehensive care where health-related behaviors and therapeutic adherence may influence the etiology and course of the disease or disability. With careful and systematic biobehavioral clinical research, clinical behavioral pediatrics may make a major contribution to the quality of life for children and adolescents and help to establish a healthy lifestyle as a habit pattern that will be maintained into adulthood. This is a promise as yet unfulfilled, but it may now be within our grasp.

# Author Index

# Subject Index

# About the Author

James W. Varni received his Ph.D. from the Department of Psychology, University of California, Los Angeles, and was a Postdoctoral Fellow in Pediatric Psychology, Department of Pediatrics, Johns Hopkins University School of Medicine and John F. Kennedy Institute, Johns Hopkins Medical Center. Dr. Varni is currently Co-Director, Behavioral Pediatrics Program, Orthopaedic Hospital, Los Angeles, Associate Clinical Professor of Pediatrics and Psychiatry, University of Southern California School of Medicine, and Clinical Associate Professor of Psychology, University of Southern California, Los Angeles.